A Clinical Approach to Fractures

A Clinical Approach to Fractures

Editor: Brandon Gomez

AMERICAN
MEDICAL PUBLISHERS
www.americanmedicalpublishers.com

AMERICAN
MEDICAL PUBLISHERS
www.americanmedicalpublishers.com

Cataloging-in-Publication Data

A clinical approach to fractures / edited by Brandon Gomez.
p. cm.
Includes bibliographical references and index.
ISBN 978-1-63927-388-1
1. Fractures. 2. Bones--Wounds and injuries. I. Gomez, Brandon.
RD771.B217 H36 2022
617.15--dc23

American Medical Publishers,
41 Flatbush Avenue,
1st Floor, New York,
NY 11217, USA

ISBN 978-1-63927-388-1 (Hardback)

Contents

Preface

This book was inspired by the evolution of our times; to answer the curiosity of inquisitive minds. Many developments have occurred across the globe in the recent past which has transformed the progress in the field.

A fracture is a clinical condition in which there is a complete or partial break in the continuity of a bone. In severe cases of bone fracture, bone continuity can be broken at several sites. It can arise as a result of a high force stress or impact or a minimal trauma injury occurring due to conditions that weaken the bones such as osteopenia, bone cancer, osteoporosis or osteogenesis imperfecta. The most common sign of bone fracture is pain. If there is damage incurred in adjacent structures such as muscles, blood vessels, nerves, spinal cord, etc. other signs and symptoms may appear. If such fractures are not assessed and treated, they may lead to complications such as non-union and mal-union of the fractured bone compartment syndrome that may require amputation of the affected limb. The objective of this book is to give a general view of the different types of bone fractures and their clinical presentations. It attempts to understand the various interventions used for the management and correction of bone fractures. For all readers who are interested in orthopedics, the case studies included in this book will serve as an excellent guide to develop a comprehensive understanding.

This book was developed from a mere concept to drafts to chapters and finally compiled together as a complete text to benefit the readers across all nations. To ensure the quality of the content we instilled two significant steps in our procedure. The first was to appoint an editorial team that would verify the data and statistics provided in the book and also select the most appropriate and valuable contributions from the plentiful contributions we received from authors worldwide. The next step was to appoint an expert of the topic as the Editor-in-Chief, who would head the project and finally make the necessary amendments and modifications to make the text reader-friendly. I was then commissioned to examine all the material to present the topics in the most comprehensible and productive format.

I would like to take this opportunity to thank all the contributing authors who were supportive enough to contribute their time and knowledge to this project. I also wish to convey my regards to my family who have been extremely supportive during the entire project.

Editor

1

Effect of a resistance and balance exercise programme for women with osteoporosis and vertebral fracture

Brita Stanghelle[1*], Hege Bentzen[2], Lora Giangregorio[3], Are Hugo Pripp[4] and Astrid Bergland[5]

Abstract

Background: Osteoporotic vertebral fractures are common, and are associated with reduced functioning and health related quality of life. The primary aims of this randomized controlled trial are to examine the immediate and long-term effects of a 12-weeks supervised group exercise programme on habitual walking speed in older women with osteoporosis and a history of vertebral fracture. The secondary aims are to examine the immediate and long-term effects of the exercise program on physical fitness, fear of falling and quality of life.

Methods: The study is a single-blinded randomized controlled trial. Women aged 65 years or older with osteoporosis and a history of vertebral fracture are included. The intervention group receives a 12-week multicomponent exercise programme, including resistance training combined with balance training. The control group receives usual care. Adherence to the programme will be of importance for the internal validity of the study. Participants in the exercise group who don't attend will be followed up with motivational phone calls. The primary outcome is habitual walking speed over 10 m. Secondary outcomes are health related quality of life (Qualeffo-41, SF-36), physical activity (I-PAQ), Patient Specific Functional Scale, Fear of falling (FES-1) and physical fitness (Senior Fitness test, Functional reach test, 4 square step test, grip strength). Sample size, based on the primary outcome, is 150 participants randomized into the two arms on a 1:1 allocation, including an estimated 20% drop out. Descriptive data will be reported as mean (standard deviation), median (range) or count (percent) as appropriate. The data will be analysed following the intention-to-treat principle. Between group differences in primary and secondary outcomes at 3 months follow-up will be assessed using linear regression models with respective outcome at baseline as covariate and the randomised group as factor.

Discussion: This trial will generate new knowledge on the effects of a multicomponent exercise programme among women over 65 years with osteoporosis and a history of vertebral fracture, knowledge that is of importance for clinicians, health managers and policy makers.

Keywords: Osteoporosis, Vertebral fracture, Exercise, Physical function, Health related quality of life

* Correspondence: brita.stanghelle@hioa.no
[1]Faculty of Health Sciences, Department of Physiotherapy, Oslo and Akershus University College of Applied Sciences, PO box 4, St. Olavs plass, 0130 Oslo, Norway
Full list of author information is available at the end of the article

Background

Osteoporosis is a worldwide health problem. Approximately 30% of all postmenopausal women in Europe and the United States have osteoporosis. More than 40% of these women will sustain one or more fragility fractures in their remaining course of life [1] Osteoporosis is usually defined as an overall bone mineral density (BMD) that is less than or equal to 2.5 standard deviations below the mean BMD for young, female adults [2]. The prevalence of osteoporosis is more frequent among women than men [2]. Osteoporosis is a systemic skeletal disease characterised by low bone mass and deterioration of bone tissue leading to bone fragility and an increased risk of fractures [2].

An osteoporotic fracture, also called a fragility fracture, is a fracture that occurs with minimal trauma [3]. Vertebral fractures, the most common type of osteoporotic fractures, are associated with height loss, kyphosis, back pain and reduced balance, mobility and activity of daily life (ADL), as well as reduced physical activity [4, 5]. Women with osteoporotic vertebral fractures have an increased risk of subsequent vertebral fractures [6] and experience reduced health related quality of life (HRQOL) compared to those who have not experienced fractures [2, 7, 8]. Several studies have shown that people with vertebral fractures experience reduced HRQOL, both in short and long term perspective [9–11]. Further, women with fragility fractures are more likely to experience fear of falling, anxiety, depression and loss of social roles [12–15].

Good physical fitness can contribute to maintenance of functional independence in older people [16]. According to Rikli and Jones [17] physical fitness is defined as the capacity to perform activities of daily living safely and independently without fatigue. The concept is multidimensional and includes muscle strength, aerobic endurance, flexibility, body composition, dynamic balance and agility/mobility [17]. Recent recommendations specify that older adults with osteoporosis or osteoporotic vertebral fractures should engage in a multicomponent exercise programme that includes resistance training combined with balance training [18, 19]. The mode of exercise, dosage and effects on different outcomes for this group has not yet been well established by research [3, 20]. Safety considerations are necessary when it comes to exercise for individuals with vertebral fractures since adverse events have happened in previous randomized trials [3, 18, 19]. Examples include modifying or avoiding rapid, repetitive, weighted and sustained or end-range flexion or twisting of the spine [18, 21]. Although individual trials of exercise in individuals with vertebral fractures did report benefits for some pain, physical function and quality of life outcomes, the quality of evidence is low. A recent Cochrane review concluded that there is insufficient evidence to determine whether exercise interventions reduce fear of falling beyond the end of the intervention, and their effect on other outcomes from designed randomised trials is required [22]. However, Olsen and Bergland [23] concluded that a group-based exercise programme and an educational session had a positive and durable effect on fear of falling in community-dwelling elderly women with osteoporosis and a history of vertebral fracture.

The main focus of this project is to develop evidence-based knowledge regarding exercise as an intervention for improving physical fitness and HRQOL in older women with osteoporosis and a history of vertebral fracture. Finding safe and feasible interventions to improve physical fitness and increase HRQOL in this group will have great potential benefits. This study builds on a previous study conducted by Bergland et al. [24]. However, the intervention in this study will to a greater degree conform to recent exercise recommendations regarding dosage and difficulty level [18]. In this trial we have left out the education component to be able to explore solely the effect of exercise, and we aim to include a larger sample.

Aims

Primary aim

To assess the effects of a 12-weeks supervised strengthening and balance programme on habitual walking speed among older women with osteoporosis and a history of vertebral fracture.

Secondary aims

To assess the effects of the same programme on physical fitness, fear of falling and health related quality of life among women with osteoporosis and a history of vertebral fracture.

Hypotheses

An intervention consisting of a 12- weeks supervised group exercise programme will improve habitual walking speed as well as physical fitness, fear of falling and quality of life among older women with osteoporosis and a history of vertebral fracture.

Methods/design

Study design

This is a parallel-group, single blinded randomized controlled trial. The participants will be randomly assigned in a 1:1 ratio to the intervention group and the control group after baseline assessment. A computer-generated, permuted block randomization scheme is used to allocate the participant, block sizes varying from 4 to 8. The allocation of the participants is administered by an individual not involved in any testing or contact with the participants, and the allocation sequence is kept on that individual's computer. Following randomisation, the participant receives information by telephone on which group they are allocated to. See flow chart in Fig. 1.

Study setting

The present study will be undertaken at facilities in Oslo and Akershus University College of Applied Sciences, and at two different community based facilities in the area around Oslo, Norway.

Recruitment and study population

Participants will be recruited from a specialty outpatient clinic for osteoporosis in Oslo, and from two outpatient clinics at hospitals in and around Oslo.

Exclusion/inclusion

We will include women at the age of 65 or over, living at home and able to walk independently with or without walking aid. Further, to be found eligible, the women must have a t-score − 2.5 SD or less verified by Dual X-ray Absorptometry (DXA) scan and at least one vertebral fracture classified grade 1, 2 or 3 [6] verified by DXA or X-ray. Patients will be excluded if they are not able to speak and understand Norwegian. Individuals who have self-reported severe diseases or other health conditions like severe lung- or heart diseases that make it unsafe to exercise will be excluded. In cases of uncertainty the participants will be asked to consult their physician to make sure that it is safe for them to exercise.

Intervention group

The intervention will be informed by recent exercise recommendations for people with osteoporosis and vertebral fracture [18], which recommend progressive resistance training for all major muscle groups in combination with balance training. The expert panel recommends that older people with osteoporosis and vertebral fracture do not engage in aerobic exercise to the exclusion of resistance and balance training [18]. The recommendations for exercise prescription for people with osteoporosis and vertebral fracture are based on the GRADE process [3] to evaluate the quality of existing evidence and generate recommendations for exercise prescription [18]. The programme should be performed at a minimum of twice a week. Alongside with the mentioned recommendations [18], the exercise program of this study is also based on the guidelines from the position stand on Exercise and Physical Activity for Older Adults from the American College of Sports Medicine [25], recommendations for fall prevention exercises [26]

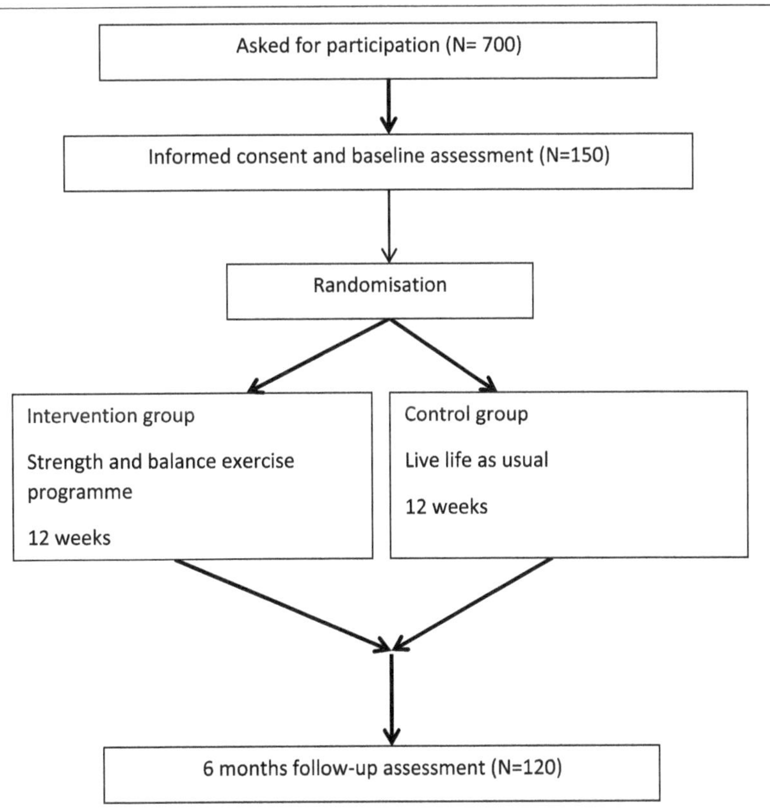

Fig. 1 Flow of participants in the study

and guidelines for treatment in postmenopausal and senile osteoporosis [27].

The intervention is designed as a group-based circuit exercise programme of eight different exercises. Emphasis is put on resistance and balance exercises with some aerobic components as well. The majority of the exercises will be carried out in a weight bearing position, with or without support. Besides different exercises to improve leg strength and balance, exercises for upper limb strength, upper and lower back strength and posture are also integrated in the programme. The intervention will be led by an experienced physiotherapist. The participants with increased risk of falls, restrictions in movement or weight-bearing during training and activity will be focused upon to avoid injuries. The physiotherapists will be trained in instructing the resistance and balance exercise programme and to make sure the participants have support objects nearby when necessary.

The programme will last for 1 h and will be carried out twice a week for 12 weeks. The physiotherapist supervising the exercise session, will also be responsible for individual tailoring and suitable dosage and progression of the exercises. The exercise session starts with 10 min warm up consisting of stretching, breathing exercises, flexibility and dynamic balance carried out with background music. The warm up is followed by two rounds of stationary circuit sessions with strength- and balance exercises. The participants will work 1.5 min at each station, with a short break of 30 s to rest and move to the next station. The exercise session ends with 10 min cool down and stretching. The participants are encouraged to report any serious adverse events caused by the exercise like muscle soreness, joint tenderness and increased level of pain.

When designing the exercise programme all the chosen exercises were evaluated according to safety cautions for people with osteoporosis and vertebral fractures [3, 18, 21]. Exercises that includes flexion and rotation of the spine are not considered safe and therefore not included in the programme. We also had in mind that the participants should be able to support themselves on a chair or a bar when performing exercises that challenged the balance if needed. Correct techniques in the different exercises is also a priority in the programme, and for the two first weeks of the programme this is emphasized for the participants by thoroughly instructions of the physiotherapists. The exercise group will have no more than 8–10 participants at the time, making sure that the physiotherapist can supervise and instruct the participants in a safe way. After a few weeks of adaption, the participants are encouraged to intensify their exercise and work until volitional fatigue without jeopardizing safety so that they perceive it as somewhat hard. This corresponds with an intensity level of 13–14 on the Borg Rating of Perceived Exertion Scale [28]. Weight belts, elastic bands, manual weights and frequency will be used for the progression of the strength exercises. Advancing to more challenging positions will be used to progress in balance exercises [29]. See Table 1 for a detailed description of the exercises.

Control group

Participants allocated to the control group receive treatment as usual. They are asked to maintain their current physical activity level and continue life as usual. They will be contacted for their follow up tests at 3 months and 6 months. After the 6-months test, participants in the control group are offered to participate in the same strength and balance exercise programme as the participants of the intervention group.

Time plan of the study

Recruitment started January 2016 and is expected to be completed by spring 2018. The intervention will continue 12 weeks after the last inclusion. Data collection will last for 6 months after recruitment is completed. Thereafter, we will write up and publish peer-reviewed articles.

Outcome measures

Assessments will be performed at baseline, and at 3 and 6 months. The participants are randomised after the baseline assessment by a person not involved in the recruitment, assessment or intervention of the study. Assessors (certified physiotherapists) are blinded to participants' group allocation for all outcomes and the participants are instructed not to reveal group allocation to the assessors during the study period. The assessors are taking part in a training programme to ensure consistency in how the tests are performed and to ensure that the protocol is standardized. The time window between baseline assessment and start of intervention is aimed to be within two week(s) and the same time window for assessment due at 3 and 6 months.

Adverse events

Adverse events such as falls, pain, fracture, and joint pain will be recorded by the instructor of the group during the exercise sessions. The participants will be instructed to report any adverse events outside the exercise session to the instructor of the group.

Demographic variables and descriptive

We will record the following variables: age, living alone (yes/no), BMI, smoking (yes/no), are you afraid of falling (yes/no), have you fallen the last year (yes/no), injuries caused by falls the last year, number and name of medications, taking analgesics (yes/no), pain level last week

Table 1 Resistance and balance programme, description of exercises

Exercise	Therapeutic goal	Level	Description	Progression or modify
Squats	Leg strength	1	Raise from a chair (sit to stand)	Tempo, weightbelt
		2	Deep squats (lower than 90 degrees kneeflexion)	Weightbelt, Degrees of kneeflexion
		3	Lounges	Weightbelt
Step up	Leg strength, dynamic balance	1	Go up and down from a step, change legs	Height of steps, tempo, Weightbelt. support
		2	Step up and one leg stance, go down	Tempo, height of steps
Sideways step up	Hip stability, dynamic balance, leg strength	1	Step up sideways on a step	Height of the step, tempo, weightbelt
Upright row	Posture, upper back strengthening	1	Row exercise with elastic bands	Three different resistance levels on the elastic bands
Balance pad	Balance, static and dynamic	1	Standing on balance pad, semitandem	Open/closed eyes, turning head from one side to the other
		2	Standing on balance pad, tandem	
		3	One leg standing	
Chest press	Chest and arm strengthening	1	Chest press against the wall	
		2	Chest press against a bench	
		3	Chest press resting on the knees on the floor	
Hip raise	Lower back strengthening	1	Lying on back with knees bent, raise hip	
		2	One leg hip raise	
Diagonal lift		1	Standing on all four, lift left arm and right leg, alternate	Choose either hip raise or diagonal lift
Biceps curl	Upper arm strengthening	1	Seated armcurls with dumbbells	Increase load of dumbbells (1, 2, 3, 4 or 5 kg)

by score from 0 to 10 on a Numeric Rating Scale [30, 31] and comorbidities.

Primary outcome

Physical function, measured by 10 m habitual walking speed, is the primary outcome of this study. Walking speed is considered as a robust measure and is a valid, reliable and sensitive measure for assessing functional status and overall health in a wide range of populations [32, 33]. Walking speed is indicative of an individual's functional capacity and general health status, but also predictive of a range of outcomes including rehabilitation response, frailty and mobility disability. There is also an observed association between slow selected walking speed and lower quality of life [32, 34].

There is no standardized protocol available for measuring walking speed, and a variety of procedures exist that differ in regards to distance [32, 35]. In this study habitual walking speed of a straight path of 10 m will be measured from a static position, using a stopwatch as timing instrument. No acceleration or deceleration phase will be used. The stopwatch is started as the participant crosses the start line with her first foot, and stopped when crossing the finishing line with the first foot [35]. The participant will be instructed to walk at a comfortable pace, in the speed she normally chooses when walking from one point to another. A walking aid can be used when necessary, and the test will be performed with the same walking aid at the post tests if needed.

Secondary outcomes

Secondary outcomes are physical fitness, HRQOL, Falls-efficacy Scale International (FES-1) and International Physical Activity Questionnaire short form (IPAQ –SF).

Physical fitness

Alongside habitual walking speed as a measure of physical fitness, we apply tests like functional reach (FR), the four square step test (FSST), grip strength and Senior Fitness Test (SFT).

FR is a reliable and valid measure of proactive balance [36], and is a sensitive measure strongly connected to physical frailty [37]. FR is a measure of the maximal distance one can reach forward from a standing static position. The test will be performed three times, after one test trial to make sure that the participant understands the instructions. A mean of three recorded attempts will be reported.

FSST is a balance test for dynamic standing balance [38]. Four sticks or canes are resting on the floor forming four squares. The participant is instructed to step as fast as she can from square to square, with both feet resting in one square before she can move to the next. The FSST will be performed starting in square 1 then moving to 2,3,4,1,4,3,2,1. This test requires that the participant steps forward, backward and sideways, both to the left and right. A stopwatch is used to measure time it takes to complete, starting when the first foot touches square 2 and stops when the last foot has landed in square 1. The participant will first be shown the test, before one trial attempt is performed. The best of two successful attempts will be recorded as the score. Tested on a group of community dwelling elderly adults, the FSST is shown to be valid and reliable test, with a sensitivity of 85% and a specificity of 88–100% [38].

Grip strength is measured with a hydraulic handheld dynamometer, using the second position of the handle position for all participants. The handgrip test is a simple and reliable [39] method of measuring muscle strength [40]. Grip strength measurement has shown to have predictive validity, and falls, disability, low health related quality of life have been associated with low values of grip strength [40]. The test will be performed with the subject sitting at a chair, holding the instrument with the shoulder in a neutral position, elbow flexed to 90 degrees. The participant will perform one submaximal test of each hand, before performing three maximal tests of each side. The dominant hand will be tested first. The highest score of each hand is recorded.

SFT is a valid and reliable test for physical fitness [41] designed to assess underlying physical components associated with mobility in older people, such as muscle strength, aerobic endurance, flexibility, body composition (assessed as BMI in kg/m2) and agility/dynamic balance [42]. The test consists of: number of Chair Stands in 30 s, number of Arm Curls in 30 s, Chair-Sit-and-Reach-Test (CSRT) (cm), Back Scratch Test (cm), 2.45 m Up-and-Go test (seconds) and 6 min walk test (6 MWT) and BMI (weight/height^2). All of the tests have high reliability and validity and the procedures for administering SFT are standardized and described in detail [41, 42]. The CSRT was excluded due to safety reasons for our study population, as it requires flexion of the back. The 6 MWT will of practical reasons be performed walking around a 40 m course. In a study from Sciurba et al. [43] there was reported no significant difference between walking courses of 15 to 50 m.

Health-related quality of life

HRQOL will be measured by the Quality of Life Questionnaire of the European Foundation for Osteoporosis (QUALEFFO-41) which is a disease-specific self-reported quality of life questionnaire containing 41 questions or items in five sections; pain, physical function, social function, perception of general health and mental function. These five sections can be evaluated separately or represented in a total score of all the 41 items [7]. Futhermore HR-QoL will also be measured by the Short Form 36 (SF-36). The SF-36 is divided into eight sub-scales (physical function, role limitations-physical, bodily pain, general health, vitality, social function, role limitations-emotional and mental health). The instrument is scored to a 0–100 scale for each sub-scale, the higher the score, the better the health status [44]. The SF-36 is shown to have high reliability and validity among older people [45].

Fear of falling

The Norwegian version of the Falls-Efficacy Scale international (FES-I) [46, 47] will be used to examine fear of falling. The FES-I assesses level of concern about falling on a 4 point scale during 16 activities of daily living. Scores range from 16 to 64 with higher scores indicating greater concern about falling.

Physical activity

To measure level of physical activity we will use the International Physical Activity Questionnaire Short Form (IPAQ –SF). IPAQ-SF measures self reported physical activity over the previous 7 days. It records 4 levels of physical activity; vigorous- intensity, moderate intensity, walking and sitting. The IPAQ-SF is frequently used as a measure of physical activity and is reported to have high reliability [48], its validity against objective measures of physical activity is questioned by Lee et al. [49].

Adherence

Adherence will be calculated as the percentage completed of the total intervention days prescribed (24 sessions = 100%).

Sample size estimation

The sample size is based on a substantial meaningful change in 10 m habitual walking speed [50]. Perera [50] defined the minimal detectable change as 0.05 m/s. A substantial meaningful change is defined as 0.10 m/s and the expected standard deviation in habitual walking speed is assumed to be 0.2 m/s based on findings by Perera [50]. This estimate requires 128 patients, 64 in each group, to obtain 80% statistical power with 5% significance level for an independent samples t-test. We will aim to include 150 in order to compensate for an estimate of 20% drop outs.

Statistical procedure

The results of the study will be reported in accordance with CONSORT [51]. Statistical analysis is performed using statistical software as e.g. SPSS, Stata or R. The level of significance is 5%. Descriptive data will be reported as mean (standard deviation), median (range) or count (percent) as appropriate. The data will be analysed following the intention-to-treat principle. Between group differences in primary and secondary outcomes at 3 months follow-up will be assessed using linear regression models with respective outcome at baseline as covariate and the randomised group as factor (dummy variable), i.e. an ANCOVA analysis [52]. In addition, we will perform linear mixed model analysis for repeated measurements. We expect few or none missing data in baseline characteristics. However, due to possible drop-outs or participants unable to complete the outcome measurements, there might be missing data for both primary and secondary outcomes during follow-up. Linear mixed model for repeated measurement is able to statistically adjust for missing data associated with variables in the model, i.e. missing at random (MAR) structure. Further, we will also assess multiple imputation methods and sensitivity analysis for missing data in longitudinal studies. All tests will be two-sided. A statistical analysis plan will be performed in advance of each paper from the study.

Discussion

The main purpose of the study is to evaluate the impact of a resistance and balance programme informed by expert panel recommendations for older women with osteoporosis and a history of vertebral fracture. We anticipate that the intervention described will have a positive impact on the primary outcome, 10 m habitual walking speed, as well as secondary outcomes such as HRQOL [3, 18, 23, 24]. Our study has a range of secondary outcomes which can give a broad picture of the women's health and life situation. The presence of one or more osteoporotic vertebral fractures has a large impact on HRQOL [10], and findings from a 7 year follow up study shows that lowered scores on pain and disability does not fade away unless effective treatment is given [9]. QUALEFFO-41 and SF-36 are outcome measures applied to examine HRQOL and can add valuable knowledge whether exercise can improve HRQOL.

We rely on a systematic approach which corresponds with the guidance on developing and evaluating complex interventions [53]. Several issues related to the quality of the study have to be discussed, such as internal and external validity. Examples of methodological issues that may influence internal validity in a RCT include random allocation, blinding, outcome measures, sample size, drop-outs, statistical methods, and the participants' adherence to the intervention. In the present study we are particularly concerned with the outcome measures and the participants' adherence to the programme. Adherence to the programme will be of importance for the internal validity of the study. For some women it can be a challenge to be able to attend to the course twice a week for 12 weeks. In particular this can be challenging for the frailest of the participants. Motivational factors can also affect the adherence. Participants who don't attend will be followed up with phone calls to motivate and find solutions so they can complete the programme as intended.

Implementation of research into clinical practice is of importance for the overall quality in health research [53]. If the intervention of this present study appears effective, one of its advantages is its applicability in the health care system. The programme requires little equipment, has low material costs and can easily be implemented in community based facilities. The women can perform many of the exercises at home without too much space and equipment to maintain strength and balance after the completion of the programme. The exercise programme can be performed in groups and is therefore more cost effective than one-on-one supervision. The design of group-based stationary circuit session allows the maintenance of the need for individual tailoring. Furthermore, the programme can also be used as a home-based exercise programme under supervision of health care professionals for those who are too fragile to attend to a community based group. Last but not least the exercise programme can also be used as home based"self-training" exercise based on welfare technology/telerehabilitation. The intervention will have potential to promote evidence-based decision-making and empower women with osteoporosis and vertebral fracture to remain in charge of their own lives.

Limitations

Some limitations of this study should be noted. First, this study evaluates the programme in an urban area, which may limit its generalizability to rural parts and other states with varying demographic characteristics of older adult populations. Second, in this study we don't recruit people with low walking speed in particular, and it therefore be less likely that we see an effect on the primary outcome. Furthermore, the Hawthorne effect should be considered [54]. Exercise intervention studies appeal to healthier and better-motivated individuals [55]. In this study the intervention is based on an exercise intervention of 12 weeks, twice a week. Frail women with osteoporosis and a history of vertebral fracture in particular may not be able to attend community-based classes twice a week, even though they might benefit even more than healthy women from an exercise intervention. Another limitation is the inclusion criteria, which restrict our findings to individuals living on their own and being free from severe cognitive symptoms. Again the frailest may not be included. General conclusions can only be drawn with caution and no conclusions about training results should be drawn beyond the female osteoporosis population with a history of vertebral fracture living at home. It is a risk of drop-outs and thereby missing data during follow-up. Impact of missing data will be assess with appropriate statistical methods as e.g. linear mixed models, multiple imputations and sensitivity analysis.

Conclusion

There are a limited number of studies examining the effects of practical exercise programmes on health and quality of life in individuals with osteoporotic vertebral fractures. The proposed study will assess whether an evidence-based multicomponent exercise programme can enhance physical function as well as quality of life for women with osteoporosis and at least one vertebral fracture, as compared to no intervention. Further, the study will assess the effects of the exercise programme immediately post-exercise, and whether they are maintained after cessation. Findings from this study will contribute to the body of evidence available to clinicians to inform the management of people with osteoporotic vertebral fractures.

Abbreviations

6MWT: 6 Minutes walk test; ADL: Activity of daily life; BMD: Bone mineral density; BMI: Body mass index; DXA: Dual X-ray absorptometry; FES-1: Falls-efficacy scale international; FR: Functional reach; FSST: Four square step test; HRQOL: Health related quality of life; IPAQ-SF: International Physical Activity Questionnaire Short Form; QUALEFFO-41: Quality of life questionnaire of the european foundation for osteoporosis; SF-36: Short form 36; SFT: Senior fitness test

Acknowledgements

We are greatly thankful to the participants for their participation. We also want to thank the dedicated physiotherapists who contributes in the intervention and assessment of the participants this study.

Funding

The project receives internal funding from Oslo and Akershus University College of Applied Sciences. The funding body has no role in the design of the study, in writing the manuscript and in collecting, analysis and interpretation of data. The study has no external funding. LG has received salary support from the Canadian Institutes of Health Research, and is a Schlegel Research Chair in Mobility and Aging.

Authors' contributions

BS was involved in designing the exercise program as well as outcome measures, and will administer the intervention programme. AB was responsible for the internal grant application for this trial. BS, AB and HB contributed to the design of the study. BS has made contributions to conception and design of the project protocol as well as being the main responsible in drafting the initial manuscript and revising it critically for important intellectual content. HB has contributed with drafting the manuscript and revising it critically for important intellectual content. AHP has contributed with the statistical plan for this study. GL has contributed with drafting the manuscript and revising it critically for important intellectual content. AB has made contributions to conception and design of the project protocol as well as being the main responsible in drafting the initial manuscript and revising it critically for important intellectual content. All authors read, critically revised, and approved the final version of this manuscript.

Consent for publication

Not applicable

Competing interests

The authors declare that they have no competing interests.

Author details

[1]Faculty of Health Sciences, Department of Physiotherapy, Oslo and Akershus University College of Applied Sciences, PO box 4, St. Olavs plass, 0130 Oslo, Norway. [2]Department of Physiotherapy, Oslo and Akershus University College of Applied Sciences, Oslo, Norway. [3]Department of Kinesiology, University of Waterloo, Waterloo, Canada. [4]Faculty of Health Sciences, Oslo and Akershus University College of Applied Sciences, Oslo, Norway. [5]Faculty of Health Sciences, Leader of the research group Age, Health and Welfare and the PhD- program in Health Sciences, Oslo and Akershus University College of Applied Sciences, Oslo, Norway.

References

1. Melton LJ 3rd, Chrischilles EA, Cooper C, Lane AW, Riggs BL. Perspective. How many women have osteoporosis? J Bone Miner Res. 1992;7(9):1005–10.
2. Kanis JA, McCloskey EV, Johansson H, Cooper C, Rizzoli R, Reginster JY. European guidance for the diagnosis and management of osteoporosis in postmenopausal women. Osteoporos Int. 2013;24(1):23–57.
3. Giangregorio LM, Macintyre NJ, Thabane L, Skidmore CJ, Papaioannou A. Exercise for improving outcomes after osteoporotic vertebral fracture. Cochrane Database Syst Rev. 2013;1:Cd008618.
4. Cummings SR, Melton LJ. Epidemiology and outcomes of osteoporotic fractures. Lancet (London, England). 2002;359(9319):1761–7.
5. Sinaki M, Brey RH, Hughes CA, Larson DR, Kaufman KR. Balance disorder and increased risk of falls in osteoporosis and kyphosis: significance of kyphotic posture and muscle strength. Osteoporos Int. 2005;16(8):1004–10.
6. Kendler DL, Bauer DC, Davison KS, Dian L, Hanley DA, Harris ST, McClung MR, Miller PD, Schousboe JT, Yuen CK, et al. Vertebral fractures: clinical importance and management. Am J Med. 2016;129(2):221.e221–10.
7. Lips P, Cooper C, Agnusdei D, Caulin F, Egger P, Johnell O, Kanis JA, Kellingray S, Leplege A, Liberman UA, et al. Quality of life in patients with vertebral fractures: validation of the quality of life questionnaire of the European Foundation for Osteoporosis (QUALEFFO). Working Party for Quality of life of the European Foundation for Osteoporosis. Osteoporos Int. 1999;10(2):150–60.
8. Felsenberg D, Silman AJ, Lunt M, Armbrecht G, Ismail AA, Finn JD, Cockerill WC, Banzer D, Benevolenskaya LI, Bhalla A, et al. Incidence of vertebral fracture in europe: results from the European prospective osteoporosis study (EPOS). J Bone Miner Res. 2002;17(4):716–24.
9. Hallberg I, Bachrach-Lindstrom M, Hammerby S, Toss G, Ek AC. Health-related quality of life after vertebral or hip fracture: a seven-year follow-up study. BMC Musculoskelet Disord. 2009;10:135.
10. Hallberg I, Rosenqvist AM, Kartous L, Lofman O, Wahlstrom O, Toss G. Health-related quality of life after osteoporotic fractures. Osteoporos Int. 2004;15(10):834–41.
11. Lips P, van Schoor NM. Quality of life in patients with osteoporosis. Osteoporos Int. 2005;16(5):447–55.
12. Adachi JD, Adami S, Gehlbach S, Anderson FA Jr, Boonen S, Chapurlat RD, Compston JE, Cooper C, Delmas P, Diez-Perez A, et al. Impact of prevalent fractures on quality of life: baseline results from the global longitudinal study of osteoporosis in women. Mayo Clin Proc. 2010;85(9):806–13.

13. Gold DT. The nonskeletal consequences of osteoporotic fractures. Psychologic and social outcomes. Rheum Dis Clin N Am. 2001;27(1):255–62.
14. Salkeld G, Cameron ID, Cumming RG, Easter S, Seymour J, Kurrle SE, Quine S. Quality of life related to fear of falling and hip fracture in older women: a time trade off study. BMJ. 2000;320(7231):341–6.
15. Papaioannou A, Adachi JD, Winegard K, Ferko N, Parkinson W, Cook RJ, Webber C, McCartney N. Efficacy of home-based exercise for improving quality of life among elderly women with symptomatic osteoporosis-related vertebral fractures. Osteoporos Int. 2003;14(8):677–82.
16. World report on ageing and health. http://www.who.int/ageing/events/world-report-2015-launch/en/. Accessed 9 Apr 2017.
17. Rikli RE, Jones CJ, Hanson T. Senior fitness test : fysisk formåen hos ældre : manual og referenceværdier. København: FADL's Forlag; 2004.
18. Giangregorio LM, Papaioannou A, Macintyre NJ, Ashe MC, Heinonen A, Shipp K, Wark J, McGill S, Keller H, Jain R, et al. Too fit to fracture: exercise recommendations for individuals with osteoporosis or osteoporotic vertebral fracture. Osteoporos Int. 2014;25(3):821–35.
19. Giangregorio L, El-Kotob R. Exercise, muscle, and the applied load-bone strength balance. Osteoporos Int. 2017;28(1):21–33.
20. Cheung AM, Detsky AS. Osteoporosis and fractures: missing the bridge? JAMA. 2008;299(12):1468–70.
21. Sinaki M. Exercise for patients with osteoporosis: management of vertebral compression fractures and trunk strengthening for fall prevention. PM R. 2012;4(11):882–8.
22. Kendrick D, Kumar A, Carpenter H, Zijlstra GA, Skelton DA, Cook JR, Stevens Z, Belcher CM, Haworth D, Gawler SJ, et al. Exercise for reducing fear of falling in older people living in the community. Cochrane Database Syst Rev. 2014;11:Cd009848.
23. Olsen CF, Bergland A. The effect of exercise and education on fear of falling in elderly women with osteoporosis and a history of vertebral fracture: results of a randomized controlled trial. Osteoporos Int. 2014;25(8):2017–25.
24. Bergland A, Thorsen H, Karesen R. Effect of exercise on mobility, balance, and health-related quality of life in osteoporotic women with a history of vertebral fracture: a randomized, controlled trial. Osteoporos Int. 2011;22(6): 1863–71.
25. Chodzko-Zajko WJ, Proctor DN, Fiatarone Singh MA, Minson CT, Nigg CR, Salem GJ, Skinner JS. American College of Sports Medicine position stand. Exercise and physical activity for older adults. Med Sci Sports Exerc. 2009;41(7):1510–30.
26. Vieira ER, Palmer RC, Chaves PH. Prevention of falls in older people living in the community. BMJ. 2016;353:i1419.
27. Bonaiuti D, Arioli G, Diana G, Franchignoni F, Giustini A, Monticone M, Negrini S, Maini M. SIMFER rehabilitation treatment guidelines in postmenopausal and senile osteoporosis. EuraMedicophys. 2005;41(4):315–37.
28. Borg GA. Psychophysical bases of perceived exertion. Med Sci Sports Exerc. 1982;14(5):377–81.
29. Howe TE, Rochester L, Neil F, Skelton DA, Ballinger C. Exercise for improving balance in older people. Cochrane Database Syst Rev. 2011;11:Cd004963.
30. Farrar JT, Young JP Jr, LaMoreaux L, Werth JL, Poole RM. Clinical importance of changes in chronic pain intensity measured on an 11-point numerical pain rating scale. Pain. 2001;94(2):149–58.
31. Von Korff M, Jensen MP, Karoly P. Assessing global pain severity by self-report in clinical and health services research. Spine. 2000;25(24):3140–51.
32. Middleton A, Fritz SL, Lusardi M. Walking speed: the functional vital sign. J Aging Phys Act. 2015;23(2):314–22.
33. Rydwik E, Bergland A, Forsen L, Frandin K. Investigation into the reliability and validity of the measurement of elderly people's clinical walking speed: a systematic review. Physiother Theory Pract. 2012;28(3):238–56.
34. Middleton A, Fulk GD, Beets MW, Herter TM, Fritz SL. Self-selected walking speed is predictive of daily ambulatory activity in older adults. J Aging Phys Act. 2016;24(2):214–22.
35. Graham JE, Ostir GV, Fisher SR, Ottenbacher KJ. Assessing walking speed in clinical research: a systematic review. J Eval Clin Pract. 2008;14(4):552–62.
36. Duncan PW, Weiner DK, Chandler J, Studenski S. Functional reach: a new clinical measure of balance. J Gerontol. 1990;45(6):M192–7.
37. Weiner DK, Duncan PW, Chandler J, Studenski SA. Functional reach: a marker of physical frailty. J Am Geriatr Soc. 1992;40(3):203–7.
38. Dite W, Temple VA. A clinical test of stepping and change of direction to identify multiple falling older adults. Arch Phys Med Rehabil. 2002;83(11):1566–71.
39. Peolsson A, Hedlund R, Oberg B. Intra- and inter-tester reliability and reference values for hand strength. J Rehabil Med. 2001;33(1):36–41.
40. Roberts HC, Denison HJ, Martin HJ, Patel HP, Syddall H, Cooper C, Sayer AA. A review of the measurement of grip strength in clinical and epidemiological studies: towards a standardised approach. Age Ageing. 2011;40(4):423–9.
41. Rikli J. Functional fitness normative scores for community-residing older adults, ages 60-94. / Normes pour l ' evaluation de la condition physique fonctionnelle pour des personnes agees de 60 a 94 ans, residant en maison de retraite. J Aging Phys Act. 1999;7(2):162–81.
42. Rikli J. Development and validation of criterion-referenced clinically relevant fitness standards for maintaining physical independence in later years. Gerontologist. 2013;53(2):255–67.
43. Sciurba F, Criner GJ, Lee SM, Mohsenifar Z, Shade D, Slivka W, Wise RA. Six-minute walk distance in chronic obstructive pulmonary disease: reproducibility and effect of walking course layout and length. Am J Respir Crit Care Med. 2003;167(11):1522–7.
44. Ware JE Jr. SF-36 health survey update. Spine. 2000;25(24):3130–9.
45. Haywood KL, Garratt AM, Fitzpatrick R. Quality of life in older people: a structured review of generic self-assessed health instruments. Qual Life Res. 2005;14(7):1651–68.
46. Helbostad JL, Taraldsen K, Granbo R, Yardley L, Todd CJ, Sletvold O. Validation of the falls efficacy scale-international in fall-prone older persons. Age Ageing. 2010;39(2):259.
47. Yardley L, Beyer N, Hauer K, Kempen G, Piot-Ziegler C, Todd C. Development and initial validation of the falls efficacy scale-international (FES-I). Age Ageing. 2005;34(6):614–9.
48. Craig CL, Marshall AL, Sjostrom M, Bauman AE, Booth ML, Ainsworth BE, Pratt M, Ekelund U, Yngve A, Sallis JF, et al. International physical activity questionnaire: 12-country reliability and validity. Med Sci Sports Exerc. 2003;35(8):1381–95.
49. Lee PH, Macfarlane DJ, Lam TH, Stewart SM. Validity of the international physical activity questionnaire short form (IPAQ-SF): a systematic review. Int J Beha Nutr Phys Act. 2011;8:115.
50. Perera S, Mody SH, Woodman RC, Studenski SA. Meaningful change and responsiveness in common physical performance measures in older adults. J Am Geriatr Soc. 2006;54(5):743–9.
51. CONSORT statement. http://consort-statement.org. Accessed 11 Sept 2017.
52. Altman DG. Practical statistics for medical research. 2nd ed. London; New York: Chapman and Hall; 2016.
53. Craig P, Dieppe P, Macintyre S, Michie S, Nazareth I, Petticrew M. Developing and evaluating complex interventions: the new Medical Research Council guidance. Int J Nurs Stud. 2013;50(5):587–92.
54. De Amici D, Klersy C, Ramajoli F, Brustia L. More about the Hawthorne effect. Anesth Analg. 2000;91(4):1043.
55. Pacala JT, Judge JO, Boult C. Factors affecting sample selection in a randomized trial of balance enhancement: the FICSIT study. J Am Geriatr Soc. 1996;44(4):377–82.

2

Comparison and analysis of reoperations in two different treatment protocols for trochanteric hip fractures – postoperative technical complications with dynamic hip screw, intramedullary nail and Medoff sliding plate

Johnny Paulsson, Josefine Corin Stig and Ola Olsson*

Abstract

Background: In treatment of unstable trochanteric fractures dynamic hip screw and Medoff sliding plate devices are designed to allow secondary fracture impaction, whereas intramedullary nails aim to maintain fracture alignment. Different treatment protocols are used by two similar Swedish regional emergency care hospitals. Dynamic hip screw is used for fractures considered as stable within the respective treatment protocol, whereas one treatment protocol (Medoff sliding plate/dynamic hip screw) uses biaxial Medoff sliding plate for unstable pertrochanteric fractures and uniaxial Medoff sliding plate for subtrochanteric fractures, the second (intramedullary nail/dynamic hip screw) uses intramedullary nail for subtrochanteric fractures and for pertrochanteric fractures with intertrochanteric comminution or subtrochanteric extension. All orthopedic surgeries are registered in a regional database.

Methods: All consecutive trochanteric fracture operations during 2011–2012 (n = 856) and subsequent technical reoperations (n = 40) were derived from the database. Reoperations were analysed and classified into the categories adjustment (percutaneous removal of the locking screw of the Medoff sliding plate or the intramedullary nail, followed by fracture healing) or minor, intermediate (reosteosynthesis) or major (hip joint replacement, Girdlestone or persistent nonunion) technical complications.

Results: The relative risk of intermediate or major technical complications was 4.2 (1.2–14) times higher in unstable pertrochanteric fractures and 4.6 (1.1–19) times higher in subtrochanteric fractures with treatment protocol: intramedullary nail/dynamic hip screw, compared to treatment protocol: Medoff sliding plate/dynamic hip screw. Overall rates of intermediate and major technical complications in unstable pertrochanteric and subtrochanteric fractures were with biaxial Medoff sliding plate 0.68%, with uniaxial Medoff sliding plate 1.4%, with dynamic hip screw 3.4% and with intramedullary nail 7.2%.

Conclusions: The treatment protocol based on use of biaxial Medoff sliding plate for unstable pertrochanteric and uniaxial Medoff sliding plate for subtrochanteric fractures reduced the risk of severe technical complications compared to using the treatment protocol based on dynamic hip screw and intramedullary nail.

Keywords: Pertrochanteric, Subtrochanteric, Fracture, Reoperation, Intramedullary nail, Medoff sliding plate, Dynamic hip screw

* Correspondence: ola.a.olsson@skane.se
Department of Orthopedics, Helsingborg Hospital, S-251 87 Helsingborg, Sweden

Background

Stable two-fragment pertrochanteric fractures are treated with good result with dynamic hip screw (DHS) devices [1, 2], but controversy remains regarding treatment of unstable pertrochanteric and subtrochanteric fractures. Dynamic fixation methods are designed to allow secondary fracture impaction to improve interfragmentary stress transfer, thereby facilitating fracture healing and unloading the implant. DHS allows dynamic compression along the axis of the femoral neck, which, depending on fracture geometry, may be more or less appropriate or effective [3, 4].

The Medoff sliding plate [5] (MSP) adds compression along the axis of the femoral shaft, thus allowing biaxial dynamisation. Lag screw sliding is optional and may be blocked by a locking screw to prevent medialisation of the femoral shaft, thereby creating uniaxial dynamisation.

Intramedullary nail (IMN) fixation is most commonly used worldwide for unstable pertrochanteric and subtrochanteric fractures and provides a strong and rigid fixation [6]. However, poor load transfer may subject the implant to high loads with increased risk of non-union, implant failure or fracture due to stress concentration [2, 7].

In Skåne, Sweden, two similar regional emergency care hospitals use different treatment protocols for trochanteric fractures. For pertrochanteric fractures considered as stable both hospitals use DHS, whereas for fractures considered as unstable within the respective treatment protocol, Helsingborg Hospital uses MSP, and Kristianstad Hospital uses IMN. All orthopedic operations performed are consecutively registered in a mutual regional database and both hospitals cover similar population based catchment areas.

The aim of this consecutive retrospective study was to analyse and compare all performed reoperations and related technical complications in all pertrochanteric and subtrochanteric fractures, treated during two years according to two different treatment protocols in two parallel consecutive case series.

Methods

The two treatment protocols for choice of fixation methods (MSP/DHS or IMN/DHS) are described in Table 1. In short, DHS was used in fractures considered as stable, whereas treatment protocol: MSP/DHS aimed to use MSP in all pertrochanteric fractures with 3 or more fragments and treatment protocol: IMN/DHS aimed to use IMN in fractures with intertrochanteric comminution or fracture extension below the trochanters. In subtrochanteric fractures treatment protocol: MSP/DHS used locked MSP and treatment protocol: IMN/DHS used IMN. The implants used were the Medoff sliding plate (MSP) or Hansson plate (DHS) (Swemac Orthopaedics, Linköping, Sweden), or IM nails (Gamma Nail (Stryker, Kalamazoo, MI, USA), Intertan and Trochanteric Anterior Nail (Smith&Nephew, Memphis, TN, USA). The DHS and MSP were combined with either a Twin hook [8] (n = 697) (Swemac, Orthopaedics, Linköping, Sweden) or a lag screw (n = 5). The Twin hook wings may be retracted, which allowed percutaneous technique with the plate left in situ when adjustment, replacement or removal of the Twin hook was needed. The MSP was used in biaxial or uniaxial mode (locking screw for the Twin hook/ lag screw). In treatment protocol: MSP/DHS repeat radiographs were obtained 10 days postoperatively when MSP was used in uniaxial mode. If axial sliding capacity of the plate was consumed (25 mm), or migration of the Twin

Table 1 Treatment protocols for pertrochanteric and subtrochanteric fractures in the two treatment groups

Fracture type	Fixation method	
	Treatment protocol: MSP/DHS[a]	Treatment protocol: IMN/DHS[b]
Pertrochanteric		
Stable - 2 fragments[c]	DHS	
Unstable - 3 or more fragments[c]	MSP biaxial	
Unstable - no lateral and/or no posterior support[c]	MSP uniaxial (locked)	
Stable[d]		DHS
Intertrochanteric comminution and/or subtrochanteric extension[d]		IMN
Subtrochanteric	MSP uniaxial (locked)	IMN
Fracture extension below >2 of	IMN or	
MSP plate screws[e]	long DHS	

[a]Medoff sliding plate (MSP) / dynamic hip screw (DHS)
[b]Intramedullary nail (IMN) / dynamic hip screw (DHS)
[c]Choice of treatment based on Jensen Michaelsen and Seinsheimer classifications including analysis of lateral and posterior support
[d]Choice of treatment based on intertrochanteric fracture comminution or subtrochanteric fracture extension
[e]Approximately 10 cm below the lesser trochanter

hook/lag screw was observed, the locking screw was routinely removed to allow biaxial dynamisation.

From the mutual regional orthopedic surgery database all orthopedic operations performed in the two Skåne regional hospitals during 2011 and 2012 were assessed. Data on all operations with a surgical procedure code for plate or intramedullary nail, and any of the International Code of Disease (ICD-10) codes S7200/01 (femoral neck fracture), S7210/11 (pertrochanteric fracture) or S7220/21 (subtrochanteric fracture), were retrieved (n = 892). The total number of previously performed trochanteric hip fracture surgeries was also derived from the database for each individual non-specialist surgeon.

All fractures were classified by evaluation of available pre-, intra- and postoperative radiographs. Following exclusion of femoral neck and basicervical fractures, a final study group of 856 patients was set (Fig. 1).

Pertrochanteric fractures were classified according to Jensen Michaelsen (JM) [9], and subtrochanteric fractures according to Seinsheimer (SH) [10]. In the study analysis JM types 1–2 (2 fragments) were considered as stable and JM types 3–4-5 (3 or more fragments) and all subtrochanteric fractures as unstable.

Fractures were also classified regarding lateral and/or posterior support, defined as the presence of intact cortical bone of the femoral shaft at the level of or above the center of the lag screw entry hole.

Fracture classification was performed by a single examiner. To assess interobserver variability 75 randomly selected fractures were also classified by a second independent observer.

To find relevant reoperations all additional orthopedic operations performed in any Skåne regional hospital after the index operation on the 856 study patients between

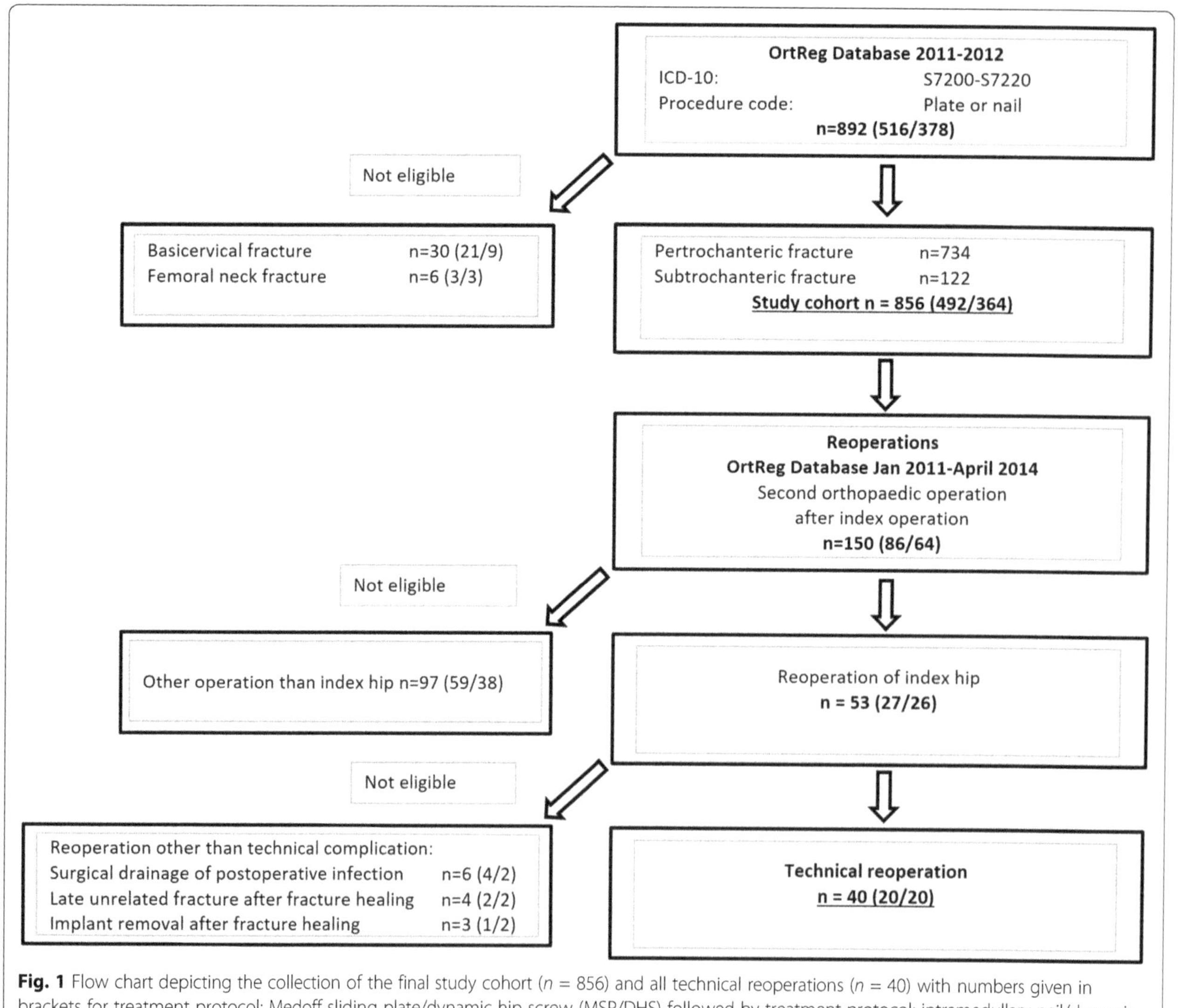

Fig. 1 Flow chart depicting the collection of the final study cohort (n = 856) and all technical reoperations (n = 40) with numbers given in brackets for treatment protocol: Medoff sliding plate/dynamic hip screw (MSP/DHS) followed by treatment protocol: intramedullary nail/dynamic hip screw (IMN/DHS)

January 2011 and April 2014, thus with a follow-up time span from 16 to 40 months, were derived from the regional database. After exclusion of other orthopedic surgical procedures and of reoperations other than technical, a final total of 40 technical reoperations was set (Fig. 1). For these cases, technical reoperations and the postoperative course of events were analysed in detail using all available postoperative radiographs and medical charts. Quality of fracture reduction and implant positioning was classified as good, acceptable or poor [11–13] and definitions were set to analyse reoperations, final outcome and related technical complications in the four categories adjustment (removal of locking screw, no technical complication) or minor (percutaneous withdrawal, replacement or removal of Twin Hook/lag screw due to penetration, followed by fracture healing), intermediate (reosteosynthesis due to non-union, femoral shaft stress fracture or varisation/cut-out) or major (loss of hip joint integrity with Girdlestone procedure or hip joint replacement, or persistent nonunion).

Statistical analysis

Statistical analyses were made using Analyse-it Standard Edition 3.20 (Analyse-it Software, Ltd. Leeds, UK). Median was given with 25th and 75th percentiles. Comparisons between groups were made using the chi-squared test or by calculation of relative risk (RR) with 95% C.I. Results with a $p < 0.05$ were considered as significant.

Results

Study group

The treatment protocol: MSP/DHS (n = 492) and treatment protocol: IMN/DHS (n = 364) groups were similar regarding age, gender, distribution of different fracture subtypes, number of surgeons and surgeons experience. Median age was 85 (79–89) years and two thirds of the patients were female. The operations were made by a surgeon having performed 25 or more previous trochanteric hip fracture surgeries in 68% of the patients in treatment protocol MSP/DHS and in 87% in treatment protocol IMN/DHS, respectively. 16% of all fractures were classified as stable pertrochanteric, 70% unstable pertrochanteric and 14% subtrochanteric. Lack of lateral support was noted in 19% and of posterior support in 48% of all fractures.

In assessment of interobserver variability, classification agreement was 75% (56/75) for specific JM/SH fracture subtypes, whereas 97% (73/75) were uniformly classified as stable or unstable.

Fixation methods

A vast majority of stable pertrochanteric fractures were treated using DHS in both treatment groups. Unstable pertrochanteric fractures, according to study fracture classification, were operated with MSP in biaxial mode (82%) or in uniaxial mode (9%) in treatment protocol: MSP/DHS. In 9% DHS was used, not compliant with the treatment protocol. In treatment protocol: IMN/DHS 35% were operated with IMN and 65% with DHS, but of all fractures JM types 3–4-5 only 2% (6/251) had lack of lateral support and were treated with DHS, contradicting the treatment protocol. Subtrochanteric fractures were treated using IMN (92%) or DHS (8%) in treatment protocol: IMN/DHS, and with MSP in uniaxial (61%) or biaxial mode (7%), with IMN (23%) or with DHS (9%) in treatment protocol: MSP/DHS (Table 2).

Treatment groups and reoperations

There was a total of 40 technical reoperations in 856 patients, 20 in treatment protocol: MSP/DHS (4.1%, Table 3) and 20 (5.5%) in treatment protocol: IMN/DHS (p = 0.33, Table 4). Quality of fracture reduction and of implant positioning in the 40 reoperated patients appeared to be similar in the 2 treatment groups (Tables 3 and 4). 13 technical complications (2.6%) occurred in treatment protocol: MSP/DHS and 19 (5.2%) in treatment protocol: IMN/DHS (p = 0.049). The rate of intermediate and major complications was more than 3 times higher (RR 3.6, 1.5–8.9) in treatment protocol: IMN/DHS (16/364, 4.4%) than in treatment protocol: MSP/DHS (6/492, 1.2%) (p = 0.0037). Documented absence of fracture healing (joint replacement, Girdlestone procedure or persisting nonunion) occurred in 10 cases in treatment protocol: IMN/DHS (2.7%) and in 3 cases (0.61%) in treatment protocol: MSP/DHS (p = 0.011, RR = 4.5, 1.3–15) (Fig. 2).

Stable pertrochanteric fractures had a total reoperation rate of 0.75%, unstable pertrochanteric 3.2% and subtrochanteric 16%. Intermediate and major technical complications were more than 4 times more frequent in treatment protocol: IMN/DHS than in treatment protocol: MSP/DHS in both unstable pertrochanteric fractures (p = 0.018) and in subtrochanteric fractures (p = 0.031, Table 5).

Implants and reoperations

Total reoperation rate with biaxial MSP was 1.3%, with DHS 3.1% and with IMN 8.4% (Fig. 3). With MSP in uniaxial mode 13 of 74 (18%) were reoperated, 92% of these were adjustments (n = 7) or minor technical complications (n = 5). Overall rate of intermediate and major technical complications in all unstable pertrochanteric and subtrochanteric fractures was with uniaxial MSP 1.4% and was lower with biaxial MSP (0.68%) than with IMN (7.2%, p = 0.0001) and with DHS (3.4%, p = 0.023). For unstable pertrochanteric fractures separately rate of intermediate and major technical complications was lower with biaxial MSP (0.69%) than with IMN (4.5%, p = 0.011), and was

Table 2 Number of fractures, and fraction within fracture type group, treated with each fixation method for different fracture subtypes in the 2 treatment groups

Fracture type[c]	Treatment protocol: MSP/DHS[a]				Treatment protocol: IMN/DHS[b]	
	DHS	MSP biaxial	MSP locked uniaxial	IMN	DHS	IMN
Stable pertrochanteric	56 (77%)	17 (23%)	0	0	59 (98%)	1 (2%)
JM1	28 (88%)	4 (12%)			39 (98%)	1 (2%)
JM2	28 (68%)	13 (32%)			20 (100%)	0
Unstable pertrochanteric	30 (9%)	288 (82%)	32 (9%)	0	163 (65%)	88 (35%)
JM3	13 (16%)	60 (74%)	8 (10%)		67 (89%)	8 (11%)
JM4	12 (20%)	43 (73%)	4 (7%)		13 (59%)	9 (41%)
JM5	5 (2%)	185 (88%)	20 (10%)		83 (54%)	71 (46%)
Subtrochanteric	6 (9%)	5 (7%)	42 (61%)	16 (23%)	4 (8%)	49 (92%)
Divergence from treatment protocol[d]						
JM1-JM2 with no lateral or no posterior support or JM3-JM4-JM5	31 (1[e])					
JM 3–4-5 with no lateral support					6 (2[e])	
JM3-JM4-JM5 with no lateral or no posterior support or subtrochanteric		8 (0[e])				

[a]Treatment protocol: Medoff sliding plate (MSP)/dynamic hip screw (DHS)
[b]Treatment protocol: Intramedullary nail (IMN)/dynamic hip screw (DHS)
[c]*JM* Jensen Michaelsen fracture classification
[d]The number of operations among the above with fixation methods with main divergence from the respective treatment protocol for grouped fracture subtypes
[e]Among these, number of reoperations with technical complication

with DHS 3.1% and with uniaxial MSP none (Table 5). In 42 subtrochanteric fractures operated with uniaxial MSP one intermediate technical complication (2.4%) occurred and in 65 operated with IMN 7 intermediate or major technical complications occurred (11%, p = 0.11).

Lateral/posterior support

In total, 5 reoperations (1.6%) were performed in 308 unstable pertrochanteric fractures with intact lateral and posterior support. Of the 4 technical complications 3 were minor and only one (0.32%) was major. In the 293 unstable pertrochanteric fractures with lack of lateral or posterior support 14 (4.8%) reoperations and technical complications occurred, 11 (3.8%) of these intermediate (n = 3) or major (n = 8, 2.7%). Lack of posterior support was more frequent than lack of lateral support, but only one of the 14 reoperations had intact posterior support compared to 10 with intact lateral support.

Implants and lateral/posterior support

In unstable pertrochanteric fractures with intact lateral and posterior support, reoperation rates were with DHS 2/136 (1.5%), with biaxial MSP 1/143 (0.70%) and none of the 24 fractures operated with IM. If either lateral or posterior support also was lacking, 6 (11%) technical complications occurred with DHS, 5 of these intermediate (n = 1) or major (n = 4, 7.0%) and with biaxial MSP 2.1% (3/145, p = 0.0063), one intermediate and one (0.70%) major. All reoperations with IMN in unstable pertrochanteric fractures (4/88, 4.5%) lacked lateral or posterior support.

Discussion

The major finding in this study was the more than 4 times higher rate of technical complications with loss of hip integrity, persistent non-union or need for revision osteosynthesis, following treatment of both unstable pertrochanteric and subtrochanteric fractures according to treatment protocol: IMN/DHS compared to treatment protocol: MSP/DHS. The low technical complication rate with MSP in both unstable pertrochanteric and subtrochanteric fractures is in line with results reported in previous studies [4, 12, 14–16]. The main mechanisms behind major technical complications were malalignment with varus dislocation and cut-out due to anteromedialisation of the femoral shaft in fractures without lateral or posterior support operated with DHS or biaxial MSP, varus dislocation and cut-out in fractures treated with DHS or IMN due to insufficient load-sharing, or bone or implant stress fracture or nonunion due to load-bearing in fractures treated with IMN.

The retrospective study design was observational using post-hoc analysis of existing data, which usually provides less solid information due to limited control of systematic and consecutive study inclusion and incomplete outcome data. However, the regional orthopedic surgery database structure warranted complete consecutive inclusion of all operated patients as well as complete registration of the

Table 3 Details of all reoperations (n = 20) and analysis of mechanisms of technical complications in treatment protocol: Medoff sliding plate/dynamic hip screw

Fracture type	Fixation	Analysis of mechanism	Reflection on mechanism of complication	Reoperation	Technical complication category	Surgeon's experience[a]	Fracture reduction	Twin hook/lag screw position	Outcome[b]
JM5	MSP uniaxial	Sliding plate consumed	In line with treatment protocol	Locking screw removed	No; adjustment	2	Acceptable	Good	Fracture healing
SH2C						3			
SH3A						4	Good		
SH5						1			
SH5						2	Acceptable		
SH5						3			
SH5						2	Poor		
JM5	MSP biaxial	Intraoperative error -TH wing in hip joint	Avoidable	TH replaced	Minor	3	Poor	To distal	Fracture healing
JM5	MSP uniaxial	TH penetration – sliding plate consumed, but locking screw not removed	Locking screw should have been removed postoperatively, since plate sliding capacity was consumed	TH replaced locking screw removed	Minor	2	Poor	Good	Fracture healing
JM5						4	Good		
SH2C						2			
SH5						3			
SH3A						3	Acceptable		
SH3A						4			
JM3	DHS	Medialisation and varus dislocation	DHS allowed anteromedialisation due to lack of lateral/posterior support	Hip joint replacement	Major	1	Good	Good	Hip joint replacement
JM5	MSP biaxial	TH penetration –medialisation	MSP should have been locked. Biaxial MSP allowed anteromedialisation due to lack of lateral/posterior support	MSP biaxial replaced with MSP uniaxial	Intermediate	3	Acceptable	Good	Fracture healing
JM5		Medialisation and varus dislocation		Hip joint replacement	Major	4	Good		Hip joint replacement
JM2	DHS	Varus dislocation and cut-out	Fracture impaction occured - DHS load-sharing was insufficient with unloading of fracture site	Hip joint replacement	Major	2	Good	Posterior	Hip joint replacement
SH5	IMN	Nonunion with broken IMN	IMN was load-bearing with unloading of fracture site and with stress concentration	IMN replaced with uniaxial MSP	Intermediate	4	Acceptable	Good	Fracture healing

JM Jensen Michaelsen fracture classification, *SH* Seinsheimer fracture classification
TH Twin hook, *DHS* dynamic hip screw, *MSP* Medoff sliding plate, *IMN* intramedullary nail
[a]Documented number of previous trochanteric hip fracture surgeries performed by index operation surgeon: Less than 10[1], 10 to 24[2], 25 or more[3], or specialist orthopaedic surgeon[4]
[b]Fracture considered as healing if no documentation of diversion from fracture healing at final follow-up

Table 4 Details of all reoperations (n = 20) and analysis of mechanisms of technical complications in treatment protocol: intramedullary nail / dynamic hip screw

Fracture type	Fixation	Analysis of mechanism	Reflection on mechanism of complication	Reoperation	Technical complication category	Surgeon's experience[a]	Fracture reduction	Twin hook/lag screw position	Outcome[b]
SH2A	IMN	No fracture impaction	IMN was load-bearing with unloading of fracture site	Locking screw removed	No; adjustment	4	Acceptable	Good	Fracture healing
JM5	DHS	Intraoperative error -TH wing in hip joint	Avoidable	TH replaced	Minor	3	Acceptable	Posterior	Fracture healing
JM3	DHS	TH penetration –anteriorisation	DHS allowed anteromedialisation due to lack of lateral/posterior support	TH replaced	Minor	4	Acceptable	Posterior	Fracture healing[c]
JM5		TH penetration – medialisation		DHS/TH replaced with new DHS	Intermediate	4	Good	Good	Fracture healing
SH2C		Medialisation		DHS replaced with IMN		4	Acceptable		
JM3		Nonunion – anteromedialisation		Girdlestone	Major	4	Good		Girdlestone
JM5						3			
JM3	DHS	Varus dislocation and nonunion	Fracture impaction occured - DHS load-sharing was insufficient with unloading of fracture site	Hip joint replacement	Major	4	Good	Good	Hip joint replacement
JM5		Varus dislocation and cut-out				2			
JM4	IMN	Varus dislocation and cut-out	Fracture impaction occured -IMN was loadbearing with unloading of fracture site	Hip joint replacement	Major	4	Acceptable	Posterior	Hip joint replacement
SH5						3		Good	
SH2C	IMN	Nonunion	IMN was load-bearing with unloading of fracture site	IMN replaced with long DHS	Intermediate	4	Acceptable	Good	Fracture healing
JM5			Removal of IMN and lag screw	Major		4	Good	Posterior	Nonunion
JM5			Hip joint replacement	Major		4		Good	Hip joint replacement
SH3A						4			
SH3A						4	Poor	Proximal	
SH3A	IMN	Broken locking screw	IMN was load-bearing with unloading of fracture site and with stress concentration	IMN locking screw removed	Minor	4	Good	Good	Fracture healing
JM5		Broken IMN		IMN replaced with long IMN	Intermediate	3			
SH5		Femoral shaft stress fracture				4	Poor		
SH4		Nonunion with femoral shaft stress fracture		IMN replaced with long DHS		4			

JM Jensen Michaelsen fracture classification, *SH* Seinsheimer fracture classification
TH Twin hook, *DHS* dynamic hip screw, *MSP* Medoff sliding plate, *IMN* intramedullary nail
[a]Documented number of previous trochanteric hip fracture surgeries performed by index operation surgeon: Less than 10[1], 10 to 24[2], 25 or more[3], or specialist orthopaedic surgeon[4]
[b]Fracture considered as healing if no documentation of diversion from fracture healing at final follow-up
[c]Recurrence of Twin Hook penetration left in situ

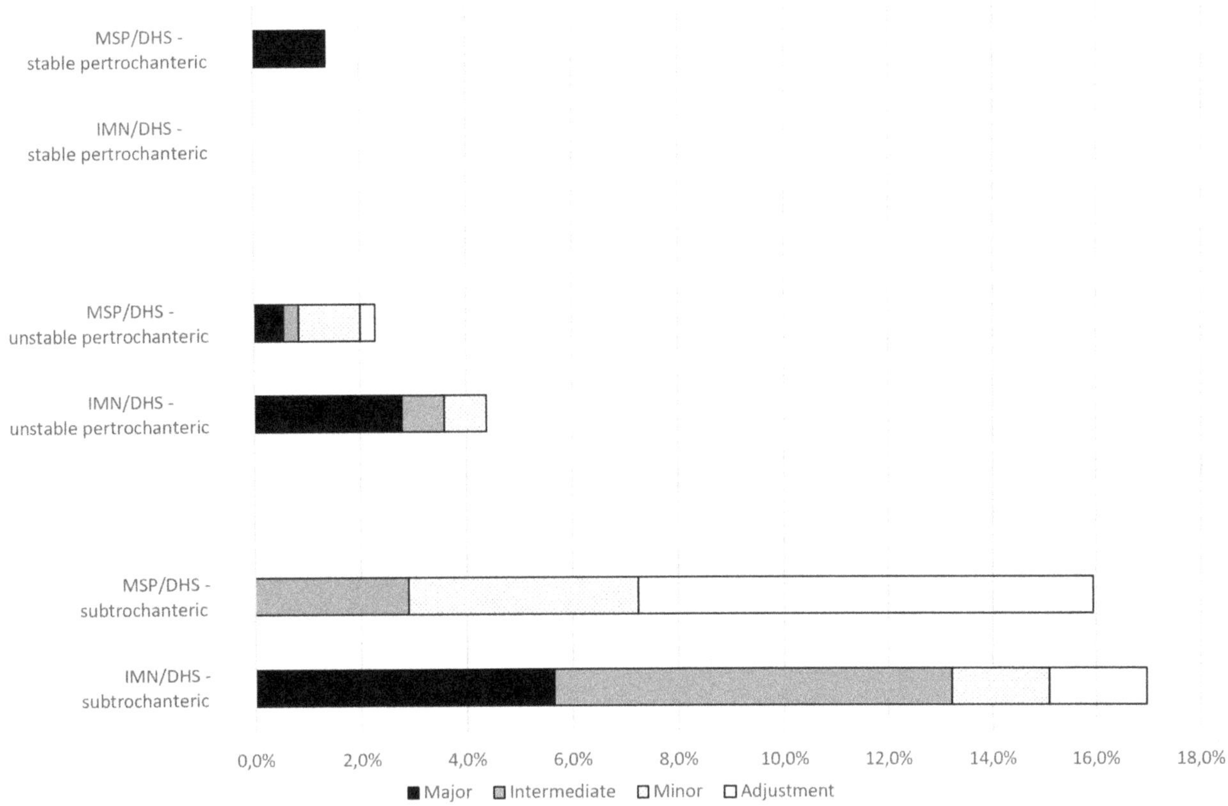

Fig. 2 Rates of adjustment reoperations and the different categories of reoperations with technical complications for stable pertrochanteric, unstable pertrochanteric and subtrochanteric fractures in treatment protocol: Medoff sliding plate/dynamic hip screw (MSP/DHS) and in treatment protocol: intramedullary nail/dynamic hip screw (IMN/DHS)

sole outcome parameter reoperation. Therefore, the study design may actually be considered a strength, since the objective of studying treatment protocol performance in regular daily care was not biased by study design, or by awareness among involved surgeons of an ongoing study. Systematic repeat radiographs after the postoperative examination were obtained only when uniaxial MSP was used. Reported rates of technical complications for the treatment protocols should therefore be considered as lower limits of true rates.

Assumed treatment group similarity to allow group comparisons appeared justified, since all fractures were consecutively included and no relevant group differences were observed regarding patient baseline data, fracture type distribution or surgical performance. Still, in addition to implants, existence of other group differing factors with possible impact on outcome, such as fracture pattern distribution or hospital specific performance, cannot be completely ruled out. Classification reliability was assessed by interobserver comparison and agreement was high, in particular in the important distinction between stable and unstable fractures.

Similar to other reports [2, 4, 14], the main technical complications with DHS in unstable pertrochanteric fractures were varus dislocation with lag screw cut-out or nonunion, frequently related to femoral shaft medialisation. With MSP in biaxial mode, lower rate of fixation failure in unstable pertrochanteric fractures was reproduced in this study. The sliding mechanism of both the DHS and the MSP lag screw barrel is aligned parallel to the femoral neck. Hence, compression along this axis will induce anteromedial translation of the femoral shaft relative to the head and neck fragment, which may compromise stable contact and load transfer between the main proximal and distal fracture fragments. A sevenfold increase of technical fixation failures with DHS has been reported with a medialisation of 30% or more [17]. As with DHS, the main mechanism behind major complications with biaxial MSP is femoral shaft anteromedialisation, which however appeared to be less frequent and less pronounced than with DHS in this study as well as in others [4, 16], probably due to facilitated axial fracture impaction and interdigitation of fracture fragments. Still, as with DHS, biaxial MSP may be inappropriate if the fracture extends below the level of the lag screw entry hole with subsequent loss of lateral and or posterior support. Fracture malalignment has severe consequences and the vast majority of reoperations related to femoral

Table 5 Number of technical complications in unstable pertrochanteric and in subtrochanteric fractures in the 2 treatment groups

Fracture type	Implant	Treatment protocol		Relative risk[c]
		MSP/DHS[a]	IMN/DHS[b]	
Unstable pertrochanteric		All technical complications		
		7/350 (2,0%)	11/251 (4,4%)	2.9 (0.89–5.4)
	DHS	1/30	7/163	
	MSP biaxial	4/288	-	
	MSP uniaxial	2/32	-	
	IMN	-	4/88	
		Intermediate and major technical complications		
		3/350 (0,86%)	9/251 (3,6%)	4.2 (1.2–14)
	DHS	1/30	5/163	
	MSP biaxial	2/288	-	
	MSP uniaxial	0/32	-	
	IMN	-	4/88	
		Major technical complications		
		2/350 (0,57%)	7/251 (2,8%)	4.9 (1.2–21)
	DHS	1/30	4/163	
	MSP biaxial	1/288	-	
	MSP uniaxial	0/32	-	
	IMN	-	3/88	
Subtrochanteric		All technical complications		
		5/69 (7,2%)	8/53 (15%)	2.1 (0.78–5.8)
	DHS	0/6	1/4	
	MSP biaxial	0/5	-	
	MSP uniaxial	4/42	-	
	IMN	1/16	7/49	
		Intermediate and major technical complications		
		2/69 (2,9%)	7/53 (13%)	4.6 (1.1–19)
	DHS	0/6	1/4	
	MSP biaxial	0/5	-	
	MSP uniaxial	1/42	-	
	IMN	1/16	6/49	
		Major technical complications		
		0/69	3/53 (5,7%)	8.6 (0.45–163)
	DHS	0/6	0/4	
	MSP biaxial	0/5	0	
	MSP uniaxial	0/42	0	
	IMN	0/16	3/49	

DHS dynamic hip screw, *MSP* Medoff sliding plate, *IMN* intramedullary nail
[a]Treatment protocol: Medoff sliding plate (MSP)/dynamic hip screw (DHS)
[b]Treatment protocol: intramedullary nail (IMN)/dynamic hip screw (DHS)
[c]95% CI

shaft anteromedialisation in this study were associated with major complications. According to treatment protocol: MSP/DHS MSP should be used in uniaxial mode in the absence of lateral or posterior support. This strategy prompted some adjustment procedures to allow secondary dynamisation, or minor reoperations due to Twin hook/lag screw penetration, but no major complications occurred.

The IMN maintains alignment and prevents femoral shaft anteromedialisation. Still, due to poor load transfer from implant to fracture site, varus dislocation and

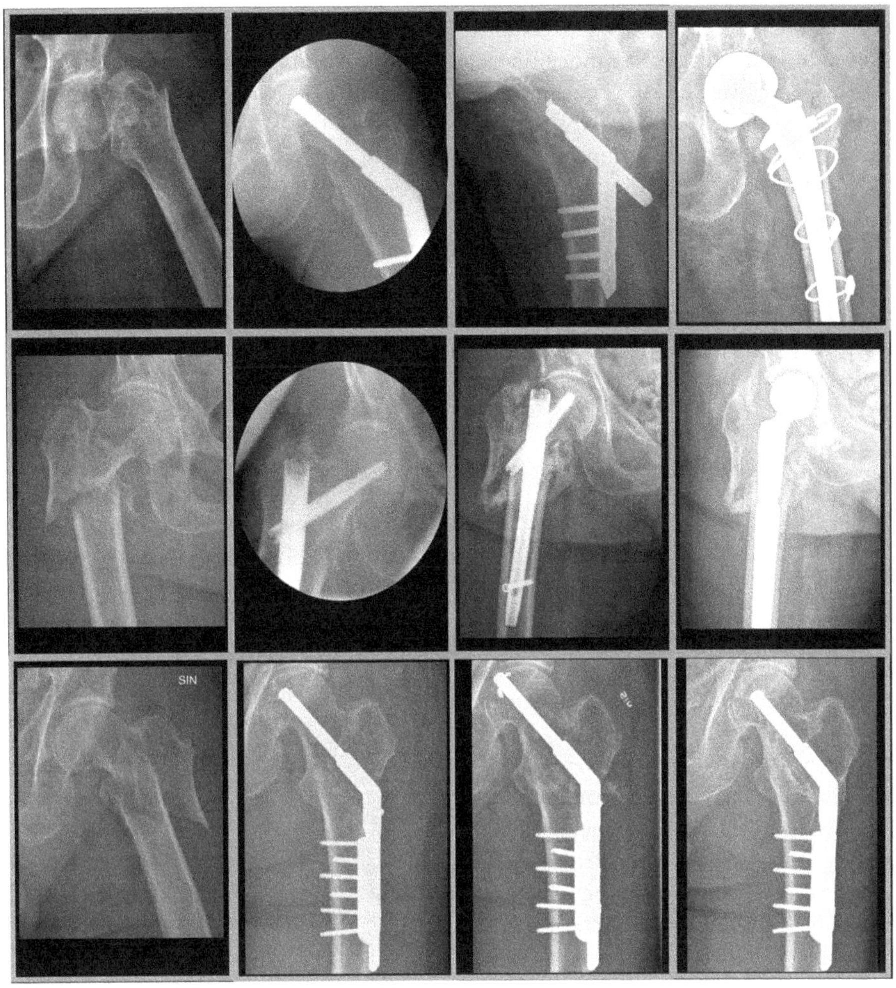

Fig. 3 From left to right preoperative, intra/postoperative, post technical complication and final radiographs of the typical and most frequent type of technical complication that occurred with dynamic hip screw (medialisation and nonunion followed by hip joint replacement, upper panels), intramedullary nail (nonunion followed by hip joint replacement, middle panels) and uniaxial Medoff sliding plate (Twin hook penetration followed by Twin hook replacement and fracture healing, lower panels)

cut-out may occur following loss of fixation purchase in the femoral head and neck fragment [13, 18]. If purchase is maintained, nonunion, implant breakage or femoral shaft stress fracture may occur due to persistent unloading of the fracture surfaces [19–22], typical complications that were all observed in the present study.

In subtrochanteric fractures lateral and/or posterior support is by definition always absent. Miedel [23] reported reoperations in subtrochanteric fractures operated with MSP due to medialisation. However, in this study the MSP was used in biaxial mode. In subtrochanteric fractures MSP should always be used in uniaxial mode [24, 25] to achieve efficient load-sharing and prevent malalignment, at the expense of need for secondary dynamisation in a minority of patients to avoid risk of Twin hook/lag screw penetration. Nevertheless, as noted in this and in other studies [26, 27], with MSP in uniaxial mode Twin hook/lag screw penetration should not be expected to be completely avoided. With maintained axial and varus/valgus alignment this complication is however less demanding and may be resolved with a minor procedure, particularly with the Twin hook allowing percutaneous adjustments. Compared to the MSP, the IMN had a higher rate of intermediate and major technical complications, all related to load-bearing, when used in subtrochanteric fractures.

In treatment protocol: MSP/DHS the aim was to use MSP in all cases with identification of one or more separate trochanteric fragment, that is all fractures types JM 3-4-5. In treatment protocol: IMN/DHS on the other hand, most of the intermediate unstable pertrochanteric fractures, retrospectively classified as JM3–4-5, but with intact lateral and posterior support were, in accordance with the treatment protocol, treated with DHS. Thus, as opposed to in treatment protocol: MSP/DHS, almost two thirds of pertrochanteric fractures with more than 2 main fragments were operated with DHS. The remaining third operated with IMN therefore most likely represents more complex fractures within these subgroups and implant specific complication rates cannot be directly compared in fractures with the same postoperative classification in the two treatment groups. Accordingly, group comparisons in this study refer to complete fracture type groups. It should also be pointed out that the treatment protocol: IMN/DHS pattern of chosen fixation methods is representative of the overall Swedish national use of fixation methods for pertrochanteric as well as subtrochanteric fractures [28].

The complication rate with DHS was almost as high as with the IMN, suggesting that treatment of mild to moderately complex unstable pertrochanteric fractures with DHS was not optimal. A more than sevenfold increase of the technical complication rate was observed in unstable pertrochanteric fractures treated with DHS, if in addition lack of lateral or posterior support was noted. Whether the intermediate unstable pertrochanteric fracture category would do better with IMN than with DHS cannot be answered by this study. Anteromedialisation due to lack of lateral/posterior support would be controlled by the IMN, but increasing issues related to load-bearing with stress concentration and non-union should be expected. Shortcomings in fracture classification firmly defining these fracture type subgroups limit the value of available studies, as does the fact that most fractures in this subgroup are probably not treated with IMN.

In treatment protocol: MSP/DHS, a vast majority of unstable pertrochanteric fractures were operated with biaxial MSP, which in terms of minimising risk of reoperation and technical complication appears superior to both alternatives for this spectrum of fracture types. Due to surgeons' assessment of lack of lateral or posterior support, 9% of unstable pertrochanteric fractures in treatment protocol: MSP/DHS were treated with MSP in uniaxial mode. Among these, 2 lag screw penetrations occurred but no major complications, again supporting priority of alignment control over biaxial dynamisation in appropriate fracture patterns. From analysis of mechanisms of technical complications in this study as well as others [29], fractures at increased risk of reoperation can often be identified if additional parameters such as lateral and posterior support are examined.

Reoperations with minor complications had no documented divergence from final fracture healing and were by definition performed percutaneously. This type of technical complication per se should have minor consequences for most patients. Intermediate and major technical complications should be expected to have more profound consequences and these subgroups comprise the cases that should be considered true failures from a technical orthopedic surgical point of view.

Conclusions

In summary, in this consecutive retrospective observational study comparing two different treatment protocols, technical complications in unstable pertrochanteric and subtrochanteric fractures were less frequent and less severe with a treatment protocol based on MSP fixation, compared to a treatment protocol based on IMN fixation. In this respect, a vast majority of unstable pertrochanteric fractures are best treated with MSP in biaxial mode and stand greater risk of major complications if treated with DHS, due to loss of alignment or insufficient load-sharing, or with IMN due to load-bearing. In the most challenging unstable pertrochanteric and subtrochanteric fractures proper application of the MSP in uniaxial mode, in combining maintained alignment and effective load-sharing, will minimise the risk of major technical complications compared to DHS and IMN.

Abbreviations

DHS: Dynamic hip screw; IMN: Intramedullary nail; JM: Jensen & Michaelsen classification; MSP: Medoff sliding plate; SH: Seinsheimer classification; TH: Twin hook

Acknowledgements

Not applicable.

Funding

This study was supported by grants from Stig and Ragna Gorthon Foundation, Helsingborg, Sweden. The funding body had no role in the design or in the conduction of the study.

Authors' contributions

OO and JP designed the study. JCS and JP collected all data. Data analysis was performed by JCS and JP under supervision of OO. Classification of radiographs were performed by JCS under supervision of OO and interobserver variability was assessed for JCS and OO. All authors contributed in reviewal and interpretation of data. The manuscript was drafted by JCS, reviewed by all authors and revised with contributions from all authors under supervision and final revision of OO. OO was responsible for the integrity of the work from inception to finished article. All authors read and approved the final manuscript.

Consent for publication

Not applicable.

Competing interests
The authors declare that they have no competing interests. No benefits in any form have been received or will be received from a commercial party related directly or indirectly to the subjects of this article.

References

1. Jensen JS, Sonne-Holm S, Tondevold E. Unstable trochanteric fractures. A comparative analysis of four methods of internal fixation. Acta Orthop Scand. 1980;51:949–62.
2. Matre K, Havelin LI, Gjertsen JE, Espehaug B, Fevang JM. Intramedullary nails result in more reoperations than sliding hip screws in two-part intertrochanteric fractures. Clin Orthop Relat Res. 2013;471:1379–86.
3. Kyle RF, Wright TM, Burstein AH. Biomechanical analysis of the sliding characteristics of compression hip screws. J Bone Joint Surg Am. 1980;62:1308–14.
4. Olsson O, Ceder L, Hauggaard A. Femoral shortening in intertrochanteric fractures. A comparison between the Medoff sliding plate and the compression hip screw. J Bone Joint Surg Br. 2001;83:572–8.
5. Medoff RJ, Maes K. A new device for the fixation of unstable pertrochanteric fractures of the hip. J Bone Joint Surg Am. 1991;73:1192–9.
6. Matre K, Havelin LI, Gjertsen JE, Vinje T, Espehaug B, Fevang JM. Sliding hip screw versus IM nail in reverse oblique trochanteric and subtrochanteric fractures. A study of 2716 patients in the Norwegian hip fracture register. Injury. 2013;44:735–42.
7. Miedel R, Tornkvist H, Ponzer S, Söderqvist A, Tidermark J. Musculoskeletal function and quality of life in elderly patients after a subtrochanteric femoral fracture treated with a cephalomedullary nail. J Ortho Trauma. 2011;25:208–13.
8. Olseen P, Jonsson B, Ceder L, Besjakov J, Olsson O, Sernbo I, et al. The Hansson twin hook is adequate for fixation of trochanteric fractures: 2 fixation failures in a series of 157 prospectively followed patients. Acta Orthop. 2008;79:602–8.
9. Jensen JS, Michaelsen M. Trochanteric femoral fractures treated with McLaughlin osteosynthesis. Acta Orthop Scand. 1975;46:795–803.
10. Seinsheimer F. Subtrochanteric fractures of the femur. J Bone Joint Surg Am. 1978;60:300–6.
11. Baumgaertner MR, Curtin SL, Lindskog DM, Keggi JM. The value of the tip-apex distance in predicting failure of fixation of peritrochanteric fractures of the hip. J Bone Joint Surg Am. 1995;77:1058–64.
12. Olsson O, Ceder L, Lunsjo K, Hauggaard A. Biaxial dynamization in unstable intertrochanteric fractures. Good experience with a simplified Medoff sliding plate in 94 patients. Acta Orthop Scand. 1997;68:327–31.
13. Bojan AJ, Beimel C, Taglang G, Collin D, Ekholm C, Jonsson A. Critical factors in cut-out complication after gamma nail treatment of proximal femoral fractures. BMC Musculoskelet Disord. 2013;14:1.
14. Watson JT, Moed BR, Cramer KE, Karges DE. Comparison of the compression hip screw with the Medoff sliding plate for intertrochanteric fractures. Clin Orthop Relat Res. 1998:79–86.
15. Wächtl SW, Gautier E, Jakob RP. Low reoperation rate with the Medoff sliding plate: 1 technical failure in 63 trochanteric hip fractures. Acta Orthop Scand. 2001;72:141–5.
16. McCormack R, Panagiotopolous K, Buckley R, Penner M, Perey B, Pate G, et al. A multicentre, prospective, randomised comparison of the sliding hip screw with the Medoff sliding screw and side plate for unstable intertrochanteric hip fractures. Injury. 2013;44:1904–9.
17. Parker MJ. Trochanteric hip fractures. Fixation failure commoner with femoral medialization, a comparison of 101 cases. Acta Orthop Scand. 1996;67:329–32.
18. Miedel R, Tornkvist H, Ponzer S, Tidermark J. Musculoskeletal function and quality of life after an unstable trochanteric fracture treated with the trochanteric gamma nail. Arch Orthop Trauma Surg. 2012;132:1495–503.
19. Kummer FJ, Olsson O, Pearlman CA, Ceder L, Larsson S, Koval KJ. Intramedullary versus extramedullary fixation of subtrochanteric fractures. A biomechanical study. Acta Orthop Scand. 1998;69:580–4.
20. Mahomed N, Harrington I, Kellam J, Maistrelli G, Hearn T, Vroemen J. Biomechanical analysis of the gamma nail and sliding hip screw. Clin Orthop Relat Res. 1994:280–8.
21. Mahomed MN, Harrington IJ, Hearn TC. Biomechanical analysis of the Medoff sliding plate. J Trauma. 2000;48:93–100.
22. Kouvidis G, Sakellariou VI, Mavrogenis AF, Stavrakakis J, Kampas D, Galanakis J, et al. Dual lag screw cephalomedullary nail versus the classic sliding hip screw for the stabilization of intertrochanteric fractures. A prospective randomized study. Strateg Trauma Limb Reconstr. 2012;7:155–62.
23. Miedel R, Ponzer S, Tornkvist H, Söderqvist A, Tidermark J. The standard gamma nail or the Medoff sliding plate for unstable trochanteric and subtrochanteric fractures. A randomised, controlled trial. J Bone Joint Surg Br. 2005;87:68–75.
24. Ceder L, Lunsjo K, Olsson O, Stigsson L, Hauggaard A. Different ways to treat subtrochanteric fractures with the Medoff sliding plate. Clin Orthop Relat Res. 1998:101–6.
25. Olsson O. Alternative techniques in trochanteric hip fracture surgery. Clinical and biomechanical studies on the Medoff sliding plate and the twin hook. Acta Orthop Scand Suppl. 2000;295:1–31.
26. Lunsjo K, Ceder L, Thorngren KG, Skytting B, Tidermark J, Berntsson PO, et al. Extramedullary fixation of 569 unstable intertrochanteric fractures: a randomized multicenter trial of the Medoff sliding plate versus three other screw-plate systems. Acta Orthop Scand. 2001;72:133–40.
27. Ekstrom W, Karlsson-Thur C, Larsson S, Ragnarsson B, Alberts KA. Functional outcome in treatment of unstable trochanteric and subtrochanteric fractures with the proximal femoral nail and the Medoff sliding plate. J Ortho Trauma. 2007;21:18–25.
28. Swedish Hip Fracture Registry Annual Report 2011. Rikshöft Web Site Available at: http://rikshoft.se/wp-content/uploads/2013/07/arsrapport2011.pdf. Accessed June 2, 2016.
29. Palm H, Jacobsen S, Sonne-Holm S, Gebuhr P. Integrity of the lateral femoral wall in intertrochanteric hip fractures: an important predictor of a reoperation. J Bone Joint Surg Am. 2007;89:470–5.

3

Influence of subject discontinuation on long-term nonvertebral fracture rate in the denosumab FREEDOM Extension study

Jonathan D. Adachi[1*], Henry G. Bone[2], Nadia S. Daizadeh[3], Paula Dakin[3], Socrates Papapoulos[4], Peyman Hadji[5], Chris Recknor[6], Michael A. Bolognese[7], Andrea Wang[3], Celia J. F. Lin[3], Rachel B. Wagman[3] and Serge Ferrari[8]

Abstract

Background: Denosumab treatment for up to 8 years in the FREEDOM study and Extension was associated with low fracture incidence. It was not clear whether subjects who discontinued during the study conduct had a higher risk of fracture than those who remained enrolled, thereby underestimating the true fracture risk for the entire trial cohort. Thus, we explored the influence of early withdrawals on nonvertebral fracture incidence during the Extension study.

Methods: To understand the potential effect of depletion of susceptible subjects on fracture incidence, we first evaluated subject characteristics in patients who were enrolled in the Extension vs those who were not. We subsequently employed a Kaplan-Meier multiple imputation (KMMI) approach to consider subjects who discontinued as if they remained enrolled with a 0%, 20%, 50%, and 100% increase in fracture risk compared with participants remaining on study.

Results: Extension enrollees were generally similar to nonparticipants in median age (71.9 and 73.1 years, respectively), mean total hip bone mineral density T-score (−1.9 and −2.0, respectively), and probability of fracture risk by Fracture Risk Assessment Tool (FRAX®) at FREEDOM baseline (16.9% and 17.7% for major osteoporotic fracture and 6.7% and 7.4% for hip fracture, respectively). When we assumed a doubled fracture risk (100% increase) after discontinuation in KMMI analyses, nonvertebral fracture rate estimates were only marginally higher than the observed rates for both the crossover group (10.32% vs 9.16%, respectively) and the long-term group (7.63% vs 6.63%, respectively).

Conclusion: The observation of continued denosumab efficacy over 8 years of treatment was robust and does not seem to be explained by depletion of susceptible subjects.

Keywords: Denosumab, Osteoporosis, Selection bias, Extension study, FREEDOM

Background

Osteoporosis is a chronic disease requiring continuing treatment, and information on the long-term safety and efficacy of treatments is therefore essential. In the 3-year FREEDOM study, treatment with the receptor activator of nuclear factor kappa-B ligand inhibitor denosumab significantly reduced the incidence of vertebral, nonvertebral, and hip fractures compared with placebo [1]. To assess the safety and efficacy of denosumab for up to 10 years, the FREEDOM study was extended. FREEDOM subjects who were eligible and desired to participate in the Extension were transitioned to denosumab if they had formerly received placebo (crossover group) or continued denosumab treatment (long-term group). Denosumab treatment for up to 8 years was associated with low fracture incidence, continued bone mineral density (BMD) increases, and an adverse event profile similar to what was previously reported [2–6].

The interpretation of the continued low incidence of fractures in the Extension study is limited by the lack of a placebo control group as a reference for the incidence

* Correspondence: jd.adachi@sympatico.ca
[1]McMaster University, 501-25 Charlton Ave E., Hamilton, ON L8N 1Y2, Canada

of fracture in untreated subjects. Therefore, it is conceivable that changes in study population characteristics might affect interpretation of efficacy and safety outcomes. Subjects may discontinue participation in an osteoporosis clinical trial for a variety of reasons. The nature of long-term follow-up with prescribed visits may prove to be a hindrance in an aging population. In addition, the occurrence of fracture or adverse events may discourage participation. As in all long-term studies, subject discontinuation has the potential to bias results through the depletion of available susceptible subjects.

The primary aim of the present analyses [7, 8] was to evaluate the possible influence of early withdrawals on nonvertebral fracture incidence during the Extension study. For this evaluation, we used a Kaplan-Meier multiple imputation (KMMI) approach [9]. We created four scenarios, where we assumed different increases in fracture risk for the subjects who discontinued the Extension study early compared to the participants who remained on study. We then compared results from the KMMI scenarios to those obtained from the Extension primary analyses.

Methods

Study design

As described previously, FREEDOM was a phase 3, multicenter, randomized, double-blind, placebo-controlled study with a duration of 3 years [1]. Subjects were randomized to receive either denosumab 60 mg or placebo by subcutaneous (SC) injection every 6 months. In the Extension, all subjects were to receive denosumab 60 mg SC every 6 months for a total of 7 years (Additional file 1). Description of the Extension study has been published elsewhere [2, 3] and is summarized briefly. This manuscript includes data from the first 5 years of the Extension, representing up to 8 years of denosumab treatment for the long-term group and up to 5 years of denosumab treatment for the crossover group.

Key eligibility criteria to participate in the Extension required that the patients:

- did not discontinue investigational medicine and completed the 36-month visit in the FREEDOM study,
- did not miss more than one dose of investigational medicine during the FREEDOM study, and
- provided consent to participate in the Extension.

A full list of criteria is shown in Additional file 2. We note that T-score thresholds, part of the eligibility criteria in the FREEDOM study to identify postmenopausal women with osteoporosis, were not required for subjects to be eligible for enrollment in the Extension.

Statistical analysis

Subject characteristics were assessed descriptively over time in subjects who enrolled in the FREEDOM study, those who enrolled in the Extension, and those who remained in the Extension study at the end of year 8. Characteristics of subjects at the FREEDOM study baseline were also assessed descriptively in subjects who enrolled in the Extension and in subjects who did not participate in the Extension. In addition, the most frequent reasons for study discontinuation were compared descriptively between the FREEDOM study and its Extension.

The effect of denosumab on long-term nonvertebral fracture risk was assessed by Kaplan-Meier estimate of time to first nonvertebral fracture over the first 5 years of the Extension (up to 8 years of denosumab treatment). Cumulative estimates and 95% confidence intervals are reported at the yearly time points. Vertebral fractures are not included in these analyses, as they were ascertained by radiography at specified intervals and were not amenable to time-to-event analysis.

Sensitivity analyses were undertaken to assess the robustness of the observed Kaplan-Meier estimates of nonvertebral fracture incidence over time. The goal of these sensitivity analyses was to evaluate the possible impact of unknown fracture status (outcome) for subjects who withdrew from the study before experiencing an incident nonvertebral fracture. These analyses employed a KMMI approach for sensitivity analyses of time-to-event data with possibly informative censoring [9]. Informative censoring occurs when subjects who discontinued are either more or less likely to experience the specific event than the remaining individuals in the future. In the current analysis, the specific event of interest is nonvertebral fracture. The KMMI approach imputes fracture status for the discontinued subjects during their unobserved remaining time as if they continued to be followed until the end of the study. A unique feature of this KMMI approach is allowance for the incorporation of various assumed increases in nonvertebral fracture risk for discontinued subjects after study discontinuation relative to the fracture risk of subjects remaining on study when imputing fracture status. Multiple imputation data sets were analyzed individually with the conventional Kaplan-Meier method, and the results from these separate analyses were then combined using the method of Rubin [10].

We chose four different scenarios of fracture risk—increases of 0%, 20%, 50%, and 100% in fracture risk after discontinuation for the subjects who withdrew before experiencing a nonvertebral fracture compared with the subjects who remained in the trial, with the highest assumption (ie, 100%) representing a doubled fracture risk after withdrawal. As judged by baseline characteristics and Fracture Risk Assessment Tool (FRAX®), a 100% increase in fracture risk (doubling of the risk) was determined to be a reasonable "worst-case" scenario for these participants, because subjects who enrolled in the FREEDOM trial were not a particularly high-risk population [1, 11], and the subjects had few comorbid conditions. For each scenario, 50 imputations were performed.

Results

Subject disposition through extension year 5

The numbers of subjects participating in the FREEDOM study and its Extension are shown in Fig. 1. Eighty-three percent of subjects completed the FREEDOM study (6478/7808), of whom 8% (550) were ineligible to participate in the Extension; the most common reason was missing more than one dose of investigational medicine during the FREEDOM study, $n = 421$. Of those who were eligible ($n = 5928$), 1378 (23%) chose not to participate in the Extension. Thus, 77% of eligible subjects ($n = 4550$) enrolled in the Extension study. Hence, of the original 7808 subjects who participated in FREEDOM, 3258 (42%) subjects did not participate in the Extension (Extension nonparticipants). At the end of Extension year 5, 3004 subjects (66% of the Extension baseline population or 38% of the original FREEDOM population) remained enrolled in the study.

Extension enrollees vs nonparticipants

FREEDOM baseline characteristics for Extension enrollees and nonparticipants are shown in Table 1. The mean age was slightly higher for Extension nonparticipants (73.1 years) compared with Extension enrollees (71.9 years). The proportion of subjects ≥ 70 years of age was slightly higher in Extension nonparticipants (77%) compared with Extension enrollees (71%).

Figure 2a compares the observed age distribution of the Extension enrollees at Extension baseline with the projected age distribution of the entire FREEDOM population if all subjects enrolled into the Extension, and shows a considerable overlap between the age distributions of these two populations. The observed age distribution for Extension enrollees and the projected age distribution for Extension nonparticipants at Extension baseline also overlapped, although the Extension nonparticipant population included older subjects (Fig. 2b).

No substantial differences were observed for other key risk factors for fracture between the enrollees and nonparticipants. Prior nonvertebral fracture incidence was the same (30%) between the Extension enrollees and nonparticipants, while BMD at the hip was similar, albeit slightly higher, in Extension enrollees compared with nonparticipants (Table 1). The age of subjects increased in a manner generally consistent with the study length, whereby at the start of the FREEDOM study, the median age was 72.0 years; at the end of 3 years, median age was 75.0 years; and after 8 years, median age was 79.0 years (Table 2). Figure 2c compares the projected age of all Extension enrollees at the end of year 8 to the observed age of the subset of subjects who reached the end of year 8. The difference between the two age distributions reflects a small percentage loss of some of the oldest subjects from the Extension study population. Figure 2d compares the age of the population remaining at the end of year 8 with the projected age of the FREEDOM population at the end of year 8, showing that the proportion of older subjects who were lost from the study over 8 years remained relatively small. Among the 3004 subjects who remained in the study at the end of year 8, 47% were ≥ 80 years old, compared with a projected 53% of Extension enrollees or 56% of the FREEDOM subjects. When we examined the mean 10-year FRAX® probability of fracture at FREEDOM baseline, the fracture probability was similar for Extension enrollees compared with Extension nonparticipants (6.7% vs 7.4% for a hip fracture and 16.9% vs 17.7% for a major osteoporotic fracture, with femoral neck BMD included in the calculations). Similarly, the baseline FRAX® scores for subjects who completed year 8 of the Extension study were somewhat lower than those who discontinued during

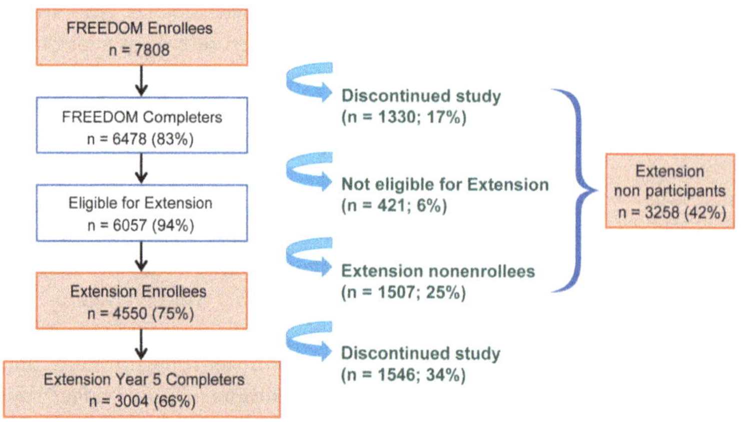

Fig. 1 Evolution of subject sample size over time

Table 1 Characteristics of Extension enrollees and nonparticipants at FREEDOM baseline

	Placebo (N = 3906)		Denosumab (N = 3902)		Combined (N = 7808)	
	Extension nonparticipants (N = 1699)	Extension enrollees (N = 2207)	Extension nonparticipants (N = 1559)	Extension enrollees (N = 2343)	Extension nonparticipants (N = 3258)	Extension enrollees (N = 4550)
Age, years						
Mean (SD)	73.1 (5.3)	71.8 (5.1)[a]	73.0 (5.4)	71.9 (5.0)[a,b]	73.1 (5.4)	71.8 (5.0)
Median (range)	73 (60–91)	72 (60–90)	73 (60–89)	72 (60–90)	73 (60–91)	72 (60–90)
Age group, n (%)						
≥ 70 years	1307 (77)	1571 (71)	1200 (77)	1672 (71)	2507 (77)	3243 (71)
≥ 75 years	612 (36)	624 (28)[a]	573 (37)	662 (28)[a,b]	1185 (36)	1286 (28)
≥ 80 years	203 (12)	143 (6)	178 (11)	144 (6)	381 (12)	287 (6)
Prior fracture, n (%)						
Prior vertebral	430 (25)	485 (23)[a]	370 (24)	559 (24)[a,b]	800 (25)	1044 (23)
Prior nonvertebral[c]	526 (31)	651 (29)	461 (30)	702 (30)[b]	987 (30)	1353 (30)
BMD T-score, mean (SD)						
Lumbar spine	−2.8 (0.7)	−2.8 (0.7)[a]	−2.8 (0.7)	−2.8 (0.7)[a,b]	−2.8 (0.7)	−2.8 (0.7)
Total hip	−2.0 (0.8)	−1.9 (0.8)[a]	−1.9 (0.8)	−1.9 (0.8)[a,b]	−2.0 (0.8)	−1.9 (0.8)
FRAX® probability,[d] %, mean (SD)						
Hip	7.4 (7.7)	6.6 (7.3)	7.5 (8.0)	6.8 (7.2)	7.4 (7.8)	6.7 (7.3)
Major osteoporotic	17.8 (9.8)	16.8 (9.7)	17.6 (9.9)	17.0 (9.6)	17.7 (9.8)	16.9 (9.6)

BMD bone mineral density, *FRAX*® Fracture Risk Assessment Tool, *SD* standard deviation
[a]Published in Papapoulos et al, 2012 [2]
[b]Published in Ferrari et al, 2015 [5]
[c]At age ≥ 55 years
[d]10-year probability of fracture calculated with femoral neck BMD

the FREEDOM or Extension studies. The subjects who discontinued had a relative increase in fracture risk of 7% to 26% (absolute increase between 1.1% and 1.8%; Additional file 3).

Reasons for early withdrawal

The most frequent reasons for study discontinuation were similar between the FREEDOM study and the Extension (Table 3). Less than 15% patients had an adverse event listed as the reason for discontinuation, and no more than 1% in either group had any particular adverse event listed as the reason for discontinuation. Subjects who experienced a fracture during the study were more likely to remain on study compared with those who did not: during the FREEDOM study, discontinuation rates in the placebo group were 12% in patients with an incident fracture and 19% in those without an incident fracture and 17% vs 16%, respectively, in the denosumab group. During the Extension, 28% of patients with an incident fracture withdrew compared with 35% of those without an incident fracture.

Kaplan-Meier estimates of nonvertebral fractures

The cumulative Kaplan-Meier estimates of incidence of nonvertebral fractures during the Extension were 2.55%, 4.45%, 6.77%, 7.84%, and 9.16% for the cross-over group and 1.49%, 2.72%, 4.48%, 5.92%, and 6.63% for the long-term group at Extension years 1, 2, 3, 4, and 5, respectively (Fig. 3 and Table 4). The results based on the KMMI approach assuming a range of increases in fracture risk after study withdrawal (0%, 20%, 50%, and 100%) for subjects who withdrew prematurely relative to the subjects with continued follow-up are presented in Table 4. When the assumed increase in fracture risk was 0%, subjects who prematurely withdrew and those who continued follow-up had the same tendency to experience a nonvertebral fracture in the future (corresponding to the observed original data results). Furthermore, the results obtained using this KMMI approach for the 20%, 50%, and 100% (or double) increased risk of fracture remained similar to the observed data for all scenarios assessed (Table 4).

Discussion

It is of concern that study subjects who choose to withdraw from participation in an osteoporosis clinical trial may have been more likely to experience an incident fracture on study, a situation often described as depletion of susceptible subjects. Preferential drop-out of susceptible study subjects, potentially resulting in retention

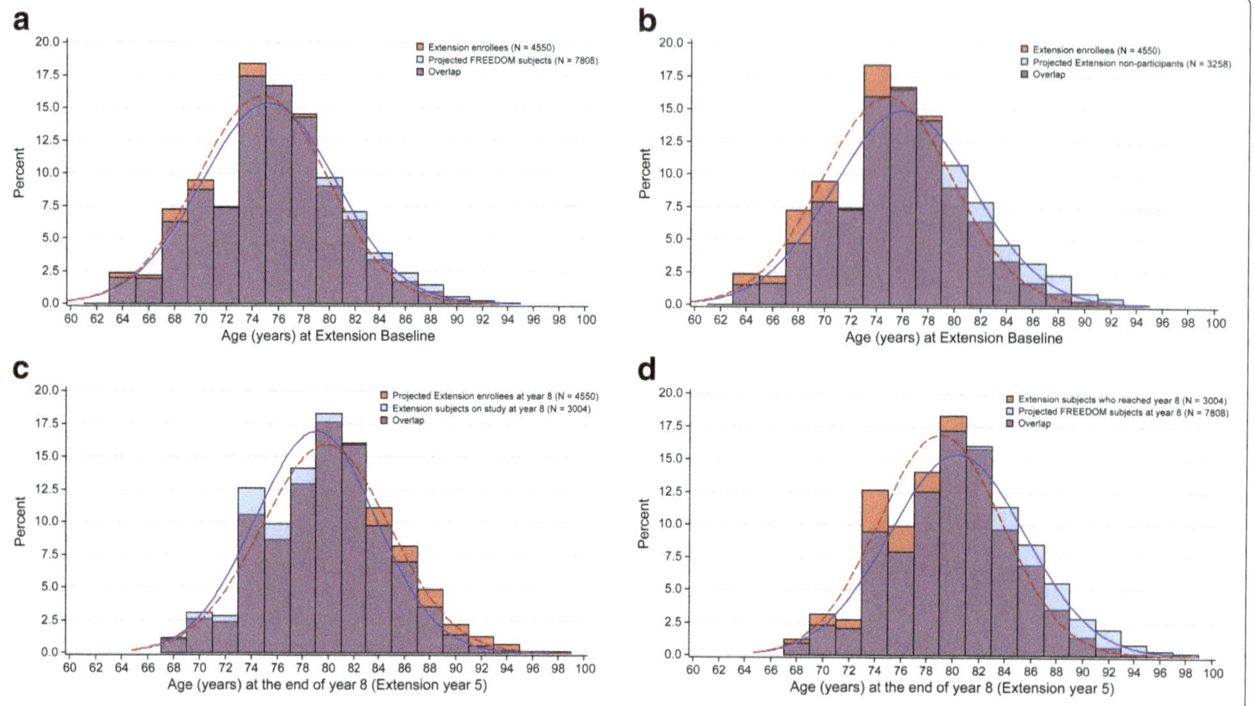

Fig. 2 Age distribution. **a** Observed age of Extension enrollees vs projected age of FREEDOM population at Extension baseline and overlap between the groups. *Lines* represent smoothed age distribution. **b** Observed age of Extension enrollees vs projected age of Extension nonparticipants at Extension baseline and overlap between the groups. *Lines* represent smoothed age distribution. **c** Projected age of Extension enrollees at year 8 vs observed age of subjects who reached year 8 and overlap between the two groups. *Lines* represent smoothed age distribution. **d** Observed age of subjects who reached the end of year 8 vs projected age of FREEDOM population at the end of year 8; overlap between the groups. *Lines* represent smoothed age distribution

Table 2 Comparison of subject characteristics over time

	FREEDOM baseline		Extension baseline		End of year 8	
	Placebo (*N* = 3906)	Denosumab (*N* = 3902)	Crossover denosumab (*N* = 2207)	Long-term denosumab (*N* = 2343)	Crossover denosumab (*N* = 1462)	Long-term denosumab (*N* = 1542)
Age, years						
Mean (SD)	72.3 (5.2)[a]	72.3 (5.2)[a]	74.8 (5.1)[b]	74.9 (5.0)[b]	79.0 (4.8)	79.1 (4.7)
Median (range)	72 (60–91)	72 (60–90)	75 (63–93)	75 (63–93)	79 (68–98)	79 (68–94)
Age group, *n* (%)						
≥ 70 years	2878 (74)	2872 (74)	1823 (83)	1974 (84)	1420 (97)	1505 (98)
≥ 75 years	1236 (32)[a]	1235 (32)[a]	1151 (52)[b]	1258 (54)[b]	1160 (79)	1255 (81)
≥ 80 years	346 (9)	322 (8)	379 (17)	407 (17)	676 (46)	737 (48)
Prior fracture, *n* (%)						
Prior vertebral	915 (23)[a]	929 (24)[a]	551 (25)[b,c]	573 (24)[b,c]	NA	NA
Prior nonvertebral[d]	1177 (30)	1163 (30)	754 (34)[c]	780 (33)[c]	NA	NA
BMD T-score, mean (SD)						
Lumbar spine	−2.8 (0.7)[a]	−2.8 (0.7)[a]	−2.8 (0.8)[b]	−2.1 (0.8)[b]	−1.9 (0.9)	−1.6 (0.9)
Total hip	−1.9 (0.8)[a]	−1.9 (0.8)[a]	−1.9 (0.8)[b]	−1.5 (0.8)[b]	−1.5 (0.8)	−1.3 (0.8)

BMD bone mineral density, *NA* not applicable (because the prior fractures cannot be defined at the end of the treatment), *SD* standard deviation
[a]Published in Cummings et al, 2009 [1]
[b]Published in Papapoulos et al, 2012 [2]
[c]Includes incident fractures during FREEDOM
[d]At age ≥ 55 years

Table 3 Top reasons for discontinuation during FREEDOM and during the Extension

	FREEDOM (Years 1–3)		Extension year 5 (Years 1–5)	
	Placebo (*N* = 3906)	Denosumab (*N* = 3902)	Crossover denosumab (*N* = 2207)[a]	Long-term denosumab (*N* = 2343)[a]
Reasons for discontinuation, *n* (%)	700 (18)	630 (16)	745 (34)	801 (34)
Consent withdrawn	403 (10)	344 (9)	325 (15)	337 (14)
Other	20 (1)	32 (1)	170 (8)[b]	184 (8)[b]
Adverse event	81 (2)	93 (2)	93 (4)	115 (5)
Death	78 (2)	62 (2)	64 (3)	80 (3)
Lost to follow-up	57 (1)	57 (1)	60 (3)	46 (2)

[a]Published in Papapoulos et al 2012 [2]
[b]Includes discontinuation after a protocol amendment to extend the Extension for an additional 5 years, which was associated with an increased discontinuation rate at the end of Extension year 2

of a cohort of "healthier" participants (a so-called "healthy cohort effect"), could influence fracture rates observed in any long-term osteoporosis study, including the Extension study. Results of the first 5 years of the Extension (up to 8 years of denosumab for the long-term group and up to 5 years for the crossover group) have shown that longer treatment with denosumab provides continued BMD gains without therapeutic plateau and sustained low fracture incidence [2, 3, 6]. The present analysis attempted to evaluate whether these results reflected continued benefit from denosumab treatment or were the result of a loss of subjects susceptible to fracture over time within the Extension study.

To further understand the implication of early withdrawal of subjects on fracture outcomes during the Extension, we employed a KMMI method for time-to-event data. This analysis was designed to assess the robustness of the nonvertebral fracture results obtained if the subjects who withdrew early before experiencing an incident nonvertebral fracture had remained on study. The KMMI approach used here is an alternative to the traditional clinical trial approach, wherein the status observed upon premature study withdrawal is analyzed (or carried forward) as the final outcome of the study.

The cumulative KMMI estimates of nonvertebral fracture incidence obtained over time remained low and similar to the observed data, even when we assumed that the subjects who withdrew early from the Extension study without an incident fracture had double the fracture risk after study withdrawal compared with the subjects who stayed on study. The baseline mean FRAX® probability for subjects who withdrew early was somewhat higher than the baseline mean FRAX® probability of subjects who continued through year 8, corresponding to a "worst-case" relative increase in fracture risk of 26%. Consequently, a 100% increase, or doubling, in fracture risk is a reasonable "worst-case" scenario for the subjects enrolled in the FREEDOM trial. Therefore, the observation of continued denosumab efficacy throughout the Extension study cannot be explained by early withdrawal of subjects with increased fracture risk.

The sensitivity analysis presented here is one potential method for estimating the impact of early withdrawals on a study outcome measure. A virtual twin analysis [12],

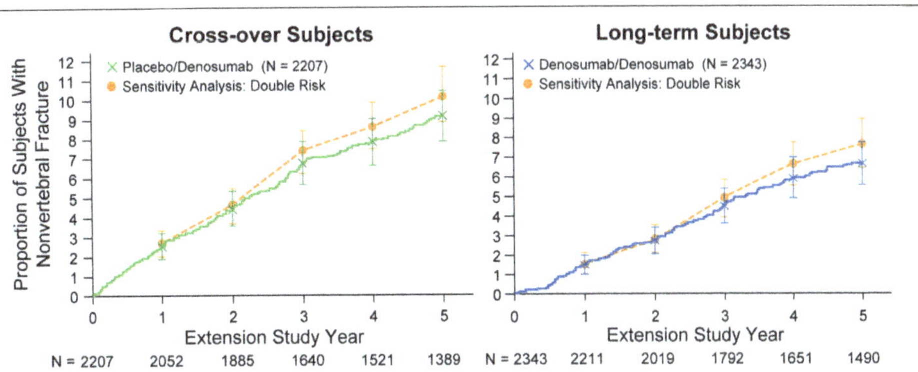

Fig. 3 Observed fracture incidence vs Kaplan-Meier estimated fracture incidence in sensitivity analyses. We compared the observed cumulative fracture incidence in crossover and long-term denosumab-treated subjects up to Extension year 5 (year 8 overall) vs the Kaplan-Meier estimated fracture incidence using a multiple imputation approach with the assumption that subjects who withdrew had double the fracture risk after study discontinuation compared with those who remained on the study. *N* is the number of subjects who remained at risk at the beginning of each year

Table 4 Sensitivity analyses for incidence of nonvertebral fractures in crossover **(a)** and long-term **(b)** subjects

a Incidence (95% CI) of nonvertebral fractures in crossover subjects

Extension	Observed in enrollees	Sensitivity analyses—estimated with multiple imputation			
		0%	20%	50%	Double Fx risk, 100%
Year 1	2.55 (1.89–3.22)	2.55 (1.89–3.22)	2.56 (1.90–3.23)	2.58 (1.91–3.25)	2.61 (1.93–3.29)
Year 2	4.45 (3.57–5.33)	4.44 (3.57–5.32)	4.47 (3.59–5.35)	4.52 (3.63–5.41)	4.59 (3.69–5.49)
Year 3	6.77 (5.67–7.88)	6.74 (5.66–7.82)	6.84 (5.75–7.93)	7.01 (5.90–8.13)	7.31 (6.15–8.47)
Year 4	7.84 (6.64–9.03)	7.79 (6.62–8.95)	7.95 (6.76–9.14)	8.20 (6.99–9.40)	8.60 (7.35–9.84)
Year 5	9.16 (7.86–10.47)	9.14 (7.87–10.41)	9.38 (8.09–10.67)	9.75 (8.41–11.09)	10.32 (8.93–11.71)

CI confidence interval, *Fx* fracture

b Incidence (95% CI) of nonvertebral fractures in long-term subjects

Extension	Observed in enrollees	Sensitivity analyses—estimated with multiple imputation			
		0%	20%	50%	Double Fx risk, 100%
Year 1	1.49 (0.99–1.98)	1.49 (0.99–1.99)	1.50 (1.00–2.00)	1.51 (1.01–2.02)	1.54 (1.02–2.05)
Year 2	2.72 (2.05–3.40)	2.73 (2.05–3.41)	2.75 (2.07–3.43)	2.79 (2.10–3.48)	2.84 (2.14–3.54)
Year 3	4.48 (3.60–5.36)	4.48 (3.60–5.37)	4.56 (3.66–5.46)	4.67 (3.76–5.59)	4.88 (3.94–5.82)
Year 4	5.92 (4.89–6.95)	5.91 (4.88–6.93)	6.04 (5.00–7.09)	6.25 (5.19–7.32)	6.61 (5.49–7.72)
Year 5	6.63 (5.54–7.73)	6.66 (5.57–7.74)	6.85 (5.74–7.95)	7.12 (5.98–8.25)	7.63 (6.42–8.85)

CI confidence interval, *Fx* fracture

A multiple imputation approach was used with varying assumptions (0, 20, 50, and 100% [ie, double]) of increased fracture risk after study discontinuation for subjects who withdrew early from the Extension relative to subjects who remained in the study. Colored boxes correspond to data plotted in Fig. 3

conducted after subjects competed 2 years of the Extension study [2], employed a completely different analytical method but led to similar conclusions. This provides further confidence that the observed low fracture incidence over time is the result of denosumab treatment.

We found that Extension nonparticipants had some very slight differences from Extension enrollees for some baseline characteristics. As anticipated, there was a loss of some of the oldest subjects (age ≥ 80 years) during the Extension because of comorbidities and mortality associated with older age. Nevertheless, nearly half of the participants at the end of year 8 were ≥ 80 years old, similar to the proportion projected if the entire FREEDOM population had remained on study through year 8 without adjustment for expected mortality. Further, we demonstrated that preferential loss of subjects who experienced an incident fracture did not occur as we had hypothesized.

Conclusions

These results show that the observed fracture incidence in the Extension study cannot be explained by depletion of susceptible subjects or, put another way, retention of a healthy cohort of participants. Rather, the results suggest that the low nonvertebral fracture incidence reflects the effect of long-term denosumab treatment, in the context of an aging population.

Additional files

Additional file 1: Design of FREEDOM and the Extension study. *Q6M* once every 6 months, *SC* subcutaneous. (DOCX 28 kb)

Additional file 2: Eligibility criteria for the Extension study. (DOC 143 kb)

Additional file 3: FREEDOM baseline FRAX® scores for subjects who continued through year 8 compared with those who did not continue through year 8. The 10-year probability of fracture calculated with femoral neck BMD. *BMD* bone mineral density, *FRAX®* Fracture Risk Assessment Tool, *SD* standard deviation. (DOC 29 kb)

Additional file 4: Institutional review boards and ethics committees for the Extension study. (DOC 120 kb)

Abbreviations

BMD: Bone mineral density; CI: Confidence interval; FRAX®: Fracture Risk Assessment Tool; Fx: Fracture; KMMI: Kaplan-Meier multiple imputation; NA: Not applicable; Q6M: Once every 6 months; SC: Subcutaneous; SD: Standard deviation

Acknowledgments
Wanda J Krall, PhD, funded by Amgen Inc., and Amy Foreman-Wykert, PhD, of Amgen Inc. assisted in the writing of this manuscript. Formatting assistance was provided by Gurpreet Kaur, CACTUS Communications, on behalf of Amgen Inc.

Funding
This work was supported by Amgen Inc. The sponsor was involved in the study design; in the collection, analysis, and interpretation of data; in the writing of report. All authors were involved in the decision to submit the article for publication.

Authors' contributions
JDA, HGB, SP, PH, MB, and SF enrolled patients in the FREEDOM study and Extension; AW and ND performed the statistical analysis; PD, CL, RW participated in the analysis conceptualization; JDA, HGB, SP, PH, MB, SF, AW, PD, CL, and RW interpreted the results and critically revised the manuscript for important intellectual content. All authors read and approved the final manuscript.

Competing interests
JDA has received consulting fees, speaker fees, and research grants from Actavis, Amgen Inc., Eli Lilly, Merck, and Novartis, and consulting fees from AgNovos. HGB has received research funding, consulting and/or speaker fees from Amgen Inc., MSD, and Shire. SP has received consulting and/or speaker fees from Amgen Inc., Axsome, Merck, Novartis, and UCB. PH received research grants, consulting fees, and speaker fees from Amgen Inc., Elli Lilly, Novartis, Pfizer, and Roche. CR is a principal investigator of clinical trials for Amgen Inc., Novartis, and Eli Lilly. MB has received research funding from Amgen Inc., Eli Lilly, and Regeneron and speaker fees from Eli Lilly and Amgen Inc. AW and RBW are employees of Amgen Inc. and hold Amgen Inc. stock. ND, PD, and CJFL were employees of Amgen Inc. while the work was conducted. SF has received consulting fees, speaker fees, and research grants from Amgen Inc., Eli Lilly, Merck, GSK, UCB, Bioiberica, and AgNovos.

Consent for publication
Not applicable.

Author details
[1]McMaster University, 501-25 Charlton Ave E., Hamilton, ON L8N 1Y2, Canada. [2]Michigan Bone and Mineral Clinic, 22201 Moross Rd, Detroit, MI 48236, USA. [3]Amgen Inc., One Amgen Ctr Dr., Thousand Oaks, CA 91320, USA. [4]Leiden University Medical Center, Albinusdreef 2, 2333, ZA, Leiden, Netherlands. [5]Krankenhaus Nordwest, Steinbacher Hohl 2-26, 60488 Frankfurt am Main, Germany. [6]United Osteoporosis Centers, 2350 Limestone Pkwy, Gainesville, GA 30501, USA. [7]Bethesda Health Research Center, 10215 Fernwood Rd Ste 40, Bethesda, MD 20817, USA. [8]Geneva University Hospital, Rue Gabrielle-Perret-Gentil 4, 1205 Genève, Switzerland.

References
1. Cummings SR, San Martin J, McClung MR, Siris ES, Eastell R, Reid IR, et al. Denosumab for prevention of fractures in postmenopausal women with osteoporosis. N Engl J Med. 2009;361(8):756–65.
2. Papapoulos S, Chapurlat R, Libanati C, Brandi ML, Brown JP, Czerwinski E, et al. Five years of denosumab exposure in women with postmenopausal osteoporosis: results from the first two years of the FREEDOM extension. J Bone Miner Res. 2012;27(3):694–701.
3. Bone HG, Chapurlat R, Brandi ML, Brown JP, Czerwinski E, Krieg MA, et al. The effect of three or six years of denosumab exposure in women with postmenopausal osteoporosis: results from the FREEDOM extension. J Clin Endocrinol Metab. 2013;98(11):4483–92.
4. Brown JP, Reid IR, Wagman RB, Kendler D, Miller PD, Jensen JE, et al. Effects of up to 5 years of denosumab treatment on bone histology and histomorphometry: the FREEDOM study extension. J Bone Miner Res. 2014;29(9):2051–6.
5. Ferrari S, Adachi JD, Lippuner K, Zapalowski C, Miller PD, Reginster JY, et al. Further reductions in nonvertebral fracture rate with long-term denosumab treatment in the FREEDOM open-label extension and influence of hip bone mineral density after 3 years. Osteoporos Int. 2015;26:2763–71.
6. Papapoulos S, Lippuner K, Roux C, Lin CJ, Kendler DL, Lewiecki EM, et al. The effect of 8 or 5 years of denosumab treatment in postmenopausal women with osteoporosis: results from the FREEDOM Extension study. Osteoporos Int. 2015;26(12):2773–83.
7. Papapoulos S, Lippuner K, Roux C, Lin CJ, Lewiecki EM, Brandi ML, et al. Effects of up to 8 years of denosumab treatment in women with postmenopausal osteoporosis: Results: from the first 5 years of the FREEDOM extension. Aust J Ageing. 2014;33 Suppl 1:[abstract] 14.
8. Adachi JD, Lin C, Ho PR, M.A. B, Bone HG, Hadji P, et al. Changes in Subject Characteristics in the Denosumab Pivotal Fracture Trial and Its Extension for up to 8 Years. http://acrabstracts.org/abstract/changes-in-subject-characteristics-in-the-denosumab-pivotal-fracture-trial-and-its-extension-for-up-to-8-years/. 2014;2014 ACR/ARHP Annual Meeting:Abstract 2254.
9. Zhao Y, Herring AH, Zhou H, Ali MW, Koch GG. A multiple imputation method for sensitivity analyses of time-to-event data with possibly informative censoring. J Biopharm Stat. 2014;24(2):229–53.
10. Rubin DB. Multiple Imputation for Nonresponse in Surveys. New York: Wiley; 1987.
11. Austin M, Yang YC, Vittinghoff E, Adami S, Boonen S, Bauer DC, et al. Relationship between bone mineral density changes with denosumab treatment and risk reduction for vertebral and nonvertebral fractures. J Bone Miner Res. 2012;27(3):687–93.
12. Vittinghoff E, McCulloch CE, Woo C, Cummings SR. Estimating long-term effects of treatment from placebo-controlled trials with an extension period, using virtual twins. Stat Med. 2010;29(10):1127–36.

Management of isolated coronal shear fractures of the humeral capitellum with Herbert screw fixation through anterolateral approach

Tengbo Yu[1], Hao Tao[1], Fenglei Xu[2], Yanling Hu[1,3*], Chengdong Zhang[1] and Guangjie Zhou[1]

Abstract

Background: Due to the intraarticular and complex nature of the coronal shear fracture of the humeral capitellum and its rarity, it has been difficult to formulate a universally accepted method of surgical management. The purpose of this study is to retrospectively evaluate the clinical outcomes of 15 patients with isolated coronal shear fractures of the capitellum treated by Herbert screw fixation through anterolateral approach, and to address the safety and tips for this surgical procedure.

Methods: This retrospective study included 15 isolated coronal shear fractures of the capitellum without posterior involvement, which were classified according to the Dubberley classification as 11 type 1A fractures and 4 type 3A fractures. All fractures were treated with Herbert screws fixation via the anterolateral approach. Clinical and radiographic evaluation was performed regularly, with a mean follow-up of 29 months.

Results: The mean operative time was 81 min. There were no wound healing problems or infection. One incomplete posterior interosseous nerve injury occurred, which recovered soon without residual compromise. All fractures healed well. At the final follow-up, the average range of motion was 134°in flexion-extension and 172°in supination-pronation. There was no significant difference between the affected and the unaffected elbows with regard to motion in flexion-extension or flexion-extension. The average Mayo Elbow Performance Index Score was 93 with 11 excellent and 4 good. No evidence of avascular necrosis, posttraumatic osteoarthritis, or heterotrophic ossification was found.

Conclusion: Open reduction and internal fixation using Herbert screws through a anterolateral approach is a reliable and effective treatment for coronal shear fractures of capitellum, and able to achieve stable fixation and restoration of a functional range of motion.

Keywords: Capitellum, Fracture, Internal fixation, Anterolateral approach, Herbert screw

Background

Fractures of the humeral capitellum are rare injuries, accounting for nearly 1% among all elbow fractures [1]. These fractures are usually a result of axial loading to the capitellum and occasionally to the trochlea transmitted through the radial head.

* Correspondence: huyanlingqy@126.com
[1]Department of Orthopaedic Surgery, Affiliated Hospital of Qingdao University, Qingdao, Shandong 266000, People's Republic of China
[3]Department of Orthopaedic Surgery, Affiliated Hospital of Qingdao University, 59 Haier Road, Qingdao City 266003, Shandong Province, China

Treatment strategies for these injuries have evolved from conservative management to surgical management. Currently, open reduction and internal fixation with an aim to provide stable and congruent joint has been regarded as preferred treatment [2–8], whereas the intraarticular and complex nature of these fractures makes optimal surgical exposure and fixation method debatable. For coronal shear fracture of capitellum without involvement of posterior aspect, the most commonly used approach is the lateral approach of elbow joint [2–8]. Though favorable outcomes have been reported, exposure of the radiocapitellar compartment and visualization of the trochlea and medial articular extension is inadequate through this approach. Several studies have adopted the anterolateral approach to the elbow joint to treat this type of fracture, which is superior to the lateral approach for exposure range of the anterior aspect of the elbow joint [9–11]. As regard to articular surface reconstruction, various implants including Kirschner wires, headleass compression screws, Herbert screws, mini-fragment screws, and bioabsorbable implants have been adopted. Herbert screw fixation is a good option due to excellent compression at the fracture site, stable fixation, and nonprominence of the implant intra-articularly [12].

Given the intraarticular and complex nature of the coronal shear fracture of the humeral capitellum and its rarity, it has been difficult to formulate a universally accepted method of surgical management. The purpose of this study is to present the clinical outcomes of a retrospective study of 15 cases with isolated coronal shear fractures of the capitellum treated by Herbert screw fixation through anterolateral approach, and to address the safety and tips for this surgical procedure. We hypothesized that open reduction and Herbert screws fixation through anterolateral approach is a reliable and effective management for coronal shear fractures of capitellum.

Methods

Patients

From January 2009 to June 2015, 18 consecutive patients with isolated coronal shear fractures of the capitellum without posterior condyle involvement were treated with open reduction and Herbert screw fixation through the anterolateral approach within 2 weeks after the injury. Two patients were lost to follow-up, and 1 died of unrelated illness. This study was approved by the Institutional Review Board of the affiliated hospital of Qingdao University, and 15 patients consented to participate in the study. Nine patients were female, and 6 were male. The mean age (and standard deviation) was 42 ± 13 years (range, 19 to 64 years). Ten patients occurred after a fall, and 5 occurred in road traffic accidents. The mean time from presentation to surgical treatment was 4 ± 1 days (range, 1 to 7 days). The mean duration of follow-up was 29 ± 4 months (range, 24 to 36 months) (Table).

Plain radiographs were performed routinely. All patients underwent computed tomography (CT) scans with a 3D reconstruction for better definition of the fracture line and to rule out associated injuries, such as the coronoid process fractures, a dislocation or injury to the radial head, epicondylar avulsion fractures or elbow dislocations. Only isolated coronal shear fractures were included in this study.

Fractures in this study were classified according to the Dubberley classification system [2].Type 1 is a fracture involving primarily the capitellum with or without the lateral trochlear ridge. Type 2 is a fracture involving the capitellum and the trochlea as one piece. Type 3 is a fracture involving both the capitellum and the trochlea as separate fragments. These fractures were further classified as type A and type B based on the absence or presence of posterior condylar comminution. All fractures in the current series were coronal shear fractures without posterior comminution. Eleven patients sustained type 1A fracture, 4 were type 3A.

Surgical technique

All the patients were administered a brachial plexus anesthesia and placed in the supine position with a tourniquet on the upper arm. Varus and valgus stress examination under anesthesia was performed to rule out concomitant ligamentous injury.

A curved incision began 5 cm above the elbow flexion crease in the supinated forearm, and followed the lateral border of the biceps distally, but curved laterally at the elbow joint level to avoid crossing a flexion crease at 90°. Then it extended distally in the forearm along the medial border of brachioradialis. The interval was made between the brachialis and brachioradialis. The forearm lateral cutaneous nerve need to be protected in the superficial plane. In the deeper plane, the radial nerve need to be identified and protected (Fig. 1a). The brachioradialis and the radial nerve were retracted laterally and the biceps medially to expose the anterior capsule of the elbow joint. The capsule was incised to expose the capitellum (Fig. 1b).

The fracture site was debrided by removing blood clots, loose pieces of bone, and any interposed tissue. Saline irrigation was used to achieve greater clarity. The fracture was reduced by matching the articular fracture lines. Provisional fixation was performed with 2 or 3 guidewires for the Herbert screw. The guidewires were passed across the fracture site where the planned screw track was to be inserted. After anatomic reduction was confirmed with fluoroscopy, Herbert screws were inserted over the guidewires in anterior to posterior direction to achieve definitive fixation. The screws were buried beneath the articular surface. Upon fixation, the elbow was made to go through the full flexion-extension and rotation arc to check for the stability of fixation. Final reduction and position of the implant was checked with fluoroscopy. The closure of the wound was done in layers over a drain.

Postoperative care

A long arm posterior plaster splint was applied routinely with the elbow at approximately 90° of flexion, which was kept for 2 week. Active range of motion (ROM) was started when the splint was removed.

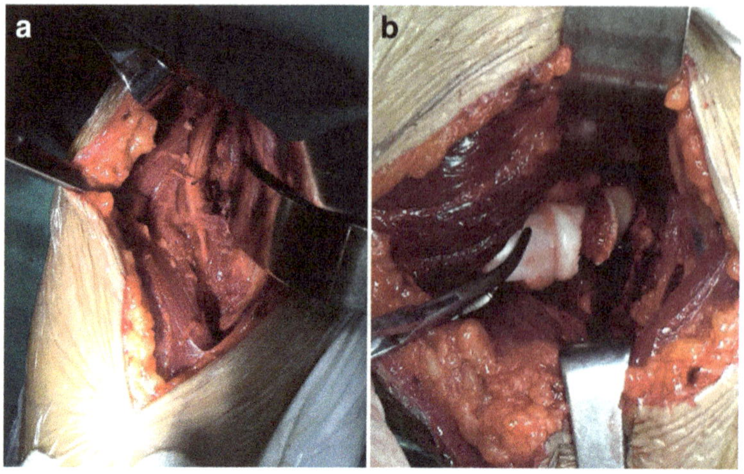

Fig. 1 Dissection of anterolateral approach to the elbow joint. **a**: The dissection of radial nerve. **b**: The exposure of fracture fragment

Operation time, wound healing complication and nerve injury were recorded. Clinical and radiographic evaluation was performed postoperatively at approximately 1, 2, 3, 6, 12 months. Then patients were called back for evaluation for the purposes of this study. At each follow-up, Pain, ROM and stability of the elbow joint was assessed by clinical examination, which enabled calculation of the Mayo Elbow Performance Index (MEPI) Score. The MEPI consists of four parts: pain (with a maximum score of 45 points), ulnohumeral motion (20 points), stability (10 points) and the ability to perform five functional tasks (25 points). If the total score is included between 90 and 100 points, it can be considered excellent; between 75 and 89 points, good; between 60 and 74 points, fair; and less than 60 points, poor. In addition, radiographic examination was performed to evaluate the status of the bony union, heterotopic ossification, incidence of posttraumatic osteoarthritis and avascular necrosis.

Statistical analysis

The paired t-test was used for statistical comparisons with regard to ROM between the affected and the unaffected elbow with SPSS for Windows 15.0 (SPSS, USA). Differences were considered to be significant if $p < 0.05$.

Results

The mean operative time was 81 ± 12 min (range, 65 to 105 min). There were no wound healing problems and infection. One patient sustained incomplete posterior interosseous nerve palsy, who presented with extension deficit of his ring finger and little finger at the metacarpophalangeal joint level. It recovered completely in 4 weeks without residual compromise. All fractures healed well in their normal anatomic position as seen on radiographs.

At the final follow-up, three patients reported mild pain and one described moderate ache during activity without restriction in activities of daily living. No patient had any subjective complaints of instability of the elbow. The average loss of ROM of the affected elbows was 10° of flexion-extension and 7° of supination-pronation compared with the unaffected elbows. But the average ROM of the affected and unaffected elbows did not differ significantly with respect to flexion-extension ($134° \pm 10°$ and $144° \pm 4°$ respectively; $p = 0.066$), and supination-pronation ($172° \pm 11°$ and $179° \pm 2°$ respectively; $p = 0.083$). The average MEPI Score was 93 ± 8 (range, 75 to 100) with 11 excellent and 4 good. All patients were satisfied with the operative outcome and returned to their previous activity levels. No evidence of avascular necrosis, posttraumatic osteoarthritis, or heterotrophic ossification was found (Table 1). An illustrative case was shown in Fig. 2.

Discussion

Surgical approaches are usually based on fracture type and complexity, comfort of the orthopedic surgeon, and protection of the blood supply. For coronal shear fracture of capitellum without posterior condyle involvement, the surgical approaches include the lateral approach and anterolateral approach to the elbow joint. The most commonly used approach in the literature is the lateral approach, which allows exposure to the elbow joint by elevation of the common extensor origin from the lateral epicondyle [2–8]. Nevertheless, its disadvantage is inadequate exposure of the capitulum and trochlea, which can limit visualization of accurate reduction of the fracture fragment, and make it relatively difficult to insert the screws perpendicular to the fracture site, especially for those capitellar fractures that extend to the trochlea. Dubberley et al. suggested that a flexor-pronator split or sectioning of the lateral collateral ligament should be performed if the medial aspect of the trochlea can not

Table 1 Demographics and clinical outcomes of reported patients

Patient	Gender	Age (year)	Mechnism	Dubberley classification	Follow-up (month)	ROM in flexion / extension (degree)	ROM in supination / pronation (degree)	MEPI Score
1	F	26	Fall	1A	24	145	180	100
2	M	48	Fall	1A	30	140	180	95
3	F	64	RTA	3A	36	130	160	85
4	F	35	Fall	1A	34	135	180	100
5	M	51	RTA	3A	28	125	155	85
6	M	28	Fall	1A	36	145	180	100
7	F	52	RTA	3A	31	120	155	85
8	M	19	RTA	1A	33	150	180	100
9	F	56	Fall	1A	29	130	175	95
10	M	60	Fall	1A	25	125	160	90
11	F	43	Fall	1A	24	130	175	95
12	F	39	Fall	1A	26	130	180	95
13	F	57	Fall	3A	27	120	155	75
14	F	33	Fall	1A	24	145	180	100
15	M	23	RTA	1A	24	145	180	100

ROM range of motion, *MEPI* Mayo Elbow Performance Index, *F* female, *Fall* ground level fall, *M* male, *RTA* road traffic accident

be seen adequately or reduction can not be confirmed from the lateral approach [2]. The anterolateral approach can expose the capitellum and trochlea widely enough to facilitate the reduction and fixation of the intra-articular fragments by directly approaching the anterior aspect of the elbow [9–11]. In addition, the anterolateral approach avoids the release of the common extensor origin, which may lead to postoperative extensor lag. So the use of anterolateral approach can circumvent the disadvantages of lateral approach. Based on our experience, the anterolateral approach was characterized by sufficient visualization of the joint including the medial articular surface, ease of achieving anatomic reduction and perpendicular fixation with screws in anterior to posterior direction.

The disadvantage for anterolateral approach is the plane of dissection much closer to the important neurovascular structures in the elbow, which carries a risk of iatrogenic injury to the radial nerve. In two research reports about anterolateral approach, no nerve injury occurred. Whereas Vaishya R et al. [11] reported one patient in their case series sustained postoperative posterior interosseous nerve palsy that recovered completely. In this case series, one incomplete posterior interosseous nerve injury occur, which recovered soon without residual compromise. In our opinion, the radial nerve dissected in this approach can be easily retracted and protected. The incidence of radial nerve injury is very small with direct visualization and careful retraction.

Fractures of elbow are usually associated with ligamentous injuries which can lead to elbow instability. Coronal shear fractures of the capitellum combined with elbow dislocation have been reported by Giannicola et al. as a potential pattern of complex elbow instability

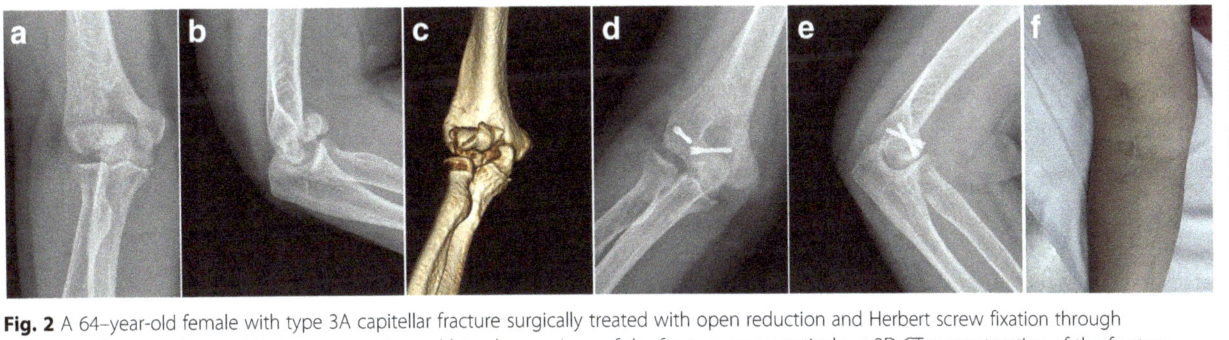

Fig. 2 A 64-year-old female with type 3A capitellar fracture surgically treated with open reduction and Herbert screw fixation through anterolateral approach. **a** and **b**: Anteroposterior and lateral x-ray views of the fracture preoperatively. **c**: 3D CT reconstruction of the fracture preoperatively. The fragments were displaced anteriorly and superiorly. **d** and **e**: Anteroposterior and lateral x-ray views 12 months postoperatively showed union of the capitellar fracture which was fixed with 2 Herbert screws in an anterior to posterior fashion. **f**: Incision appearance of anterolateral approach

where eventual associated injuries of the lateral collateral ligament (LCL) and medial collateral ligament (MCL) should be assessed [13]. In the study of Mighell et al., Dubberley type 1A capitellar fractures were not associated with LCL injury, and two LCL injuries were found in five type 2A capitellar fractures [3]. Are A et al. reported no evidence of any LCL or MCL injury for isolated type 1A capitellar fractures [5]. In this series, no concomitant LCL or MCL injuries were found. In our opinion, ligamentous injuries occur in capitellar fractures combined with elbow dislocations. Examination under anesthesia should be done as a routine to rule out potential ligamentous instability. For coronal capitellar fractures with LCL injury diagnosed intraoperatively, lateral approach is preferred because the LCL injury and fracture can be treated through one lateral incision.

The method of fracture fixation is also an issue of interest for fracture management. Kirschner wires, metallic screws, bioabsorbable implants and fibrin glue have been reported for reconstruction of capitellar fractures [12]. Metallic screw fixation was the most commonly used technique. Biomechanical studies have demonstrated that metallic screws can provide favourable stability for constructed capitellum fractures [14, 15]. Although several different types of screw (cannulated, cortical lag, cancellous, headless, and Herbert screws) were used, no direct comparison between the different screws could be made due to the heterogeneous reporting of clinical outcomes. Nowadays, Herbert screws fixation has become popular for capitellar fractures and good clinical results have been published because the advantages offered by these screws include excellent compression at the fracture fragments, stable fixation, and nonprominence of the implant intraarticularly [7, 16].

In the present study, good-to-excellent outcomes were achieved according to MEPI Score for all the shear fractures of capitellum without involvement of posterior aspect. These results were similar to those previously published [4, 6, 17]. Although four patients reported mild or moderate pain during activity, all patients were satisfied with the operative outcomes and returned to their previous levels of activity. Furthermore, no avascular necrosis or posttraumatic osteoarthritis occurred in this case series, which is in accordance with several studies [5, 7, 9–11]. In our opinion, protection of capitellar soft tissue attachment, anatomical reduction and stable fixation with minimal damage to articular cartilage can minimize the incidence of both complications. In general, satisfactory outcomes for coronal shear fractures of capitellum can be expected by accurate reduction, adequate fixation and early functional exercises. All of these can be easily achieved by the use of Herbert screw fixation through anterolateral approach to the elbow joint.

The limitation of this study was the small number of patients and short-term follow-up period. The larger numbers of patients and longer follow-up period is necessary to determine the true incidence of osteonecrosis and posttraumatic arthritis.

Conclusion

Our findings suggest that open reduction and Herbert screw internal fixation through the anterolateral approach is a reliable and effective treatment for coronal shear fractures of capitellum, and able to achieve stable fixation and restoration of a functional range of motion.

Abbreviations

LCL: Lateral collateral ligament; MCL: Medial collateral ligament; MEPI: Mayo elbow performance index; ROM: Active range of motion

Acknowledgements

We would like to thank all the staff in Department of Orthopaedic Surgery, Affiliated Hospital of Qingdao University for their help on this study.

Funding

We received no external funding for this study.

Authors' contributions

TB Y, YL H, HT and FL X made substantial contributions to the design of this study, acquisition of data, analysis and interpretation of data, and drafting of the manuscript; CD Z and GJ Z participated in the design of the study, and assisted with drafting the manuscript. All authors read and approved the final manuscript.

Consent for publication

Not applicable.

Competing interests

The authors declare that they have no competing interests.

Author details

[1]Department of Orthopaedic Surgery, Affiliated Hospital of Qingdao University, Qingdao, Shandong 266000, People's Republic of China. [2]Department of Radiology, Affiliated Hospital of Qingdao University, Qingdao, Shandong 266000, People's Republic of China. [3]Department of Orthopaedic Surgery, Affiliated Hospital of Qingdao University, 59 Haier Road, Qingdao City 266003, Shandong Province, China.

References

1. Bryan RS, Morrey BF. Fractures of the distal humerus. In: Morrey BF, edtior. The elbow and its disorders. 3rd Philadelphia, PA: WB Saunders; 1985. p 325–333.

2. Dubberley JH, Faber KJ, Macdermid JC, Patterson SD, King GJ. Outcome after open reduction and internal fixation of capitellar and trochlear fractures. J Bone Joint Surg Am. 2006;88(1):46–54.
3. Mighell M, Virani NA, Shannon R, Echols EL Jr, Badman BL, Keating CJ. Large coronal shear fractures of the capitellum and trochlea treated with headless compression screws. J Shoulder Elb Surg. 2010;19(1):38–45.
4. Ruchelsman DE, Tejwani NC, Kwon YW, Egol KA. Open reduction and internal fixation of capitellar fractures with headless screws. J Bone Joint Surg Am. 2008;90(6):1321–9.
5. Are A, Tornatore I, Theodorakis E. Operative management of a shear fracture of the bilateral capitellum: a case report and review of the literature. Chin J Traumatol. 2016;19(4):231–4.
6. Ashwood N, Verma M, Hamlet M, Garlapati A, Fogg Q. Transarticular shear fractures of the distal humerus. J Shoulder Elb Surg. 2010;19(1):46–52.
7. Singh AP, Singh AP, Vaishya R, Jain A, Gulati D. Fractures of capitellum: a review of 14 cases treated by open reduction and internal fixation with Herbert screws. Int Orthop. 2010;34(6):897–901.
8. Patterson SD, Bain GI, Mehta JA. Surgical approaches to the elbow. Clin Orthop. 2000;370:19–33.
9. Cornelius AL, Bowen TR, Mirenda WM. Anterolateral approach for an unusual pediatric capitellar fracture: a case report and review of the literature. Iowa Orthop J. 2012;32:215–9.
10. Imatani J, Morito Y, Hashizume H, Inoue H. Internal fixation for coronal shear fracture of the distal end of the humerus by the anterolateral approach. Shoulder Elbow Surg. 2001;10(6):554–6.
11. Vaishya R, Vijay V, Jha GK, Agarwal AK. Open reduction and internal fixation of capitellar fracture through anterolateral approach with headless double-threaded compression screws: a series of 16 patients. J Shoulder Elb Surg. 2016;25(7):1182–8.
12. Trinh TQ, Harris JD, Kolovich GP, Griesser MJ, Schickendantz MS, Jones GL. Operative management of capitellar fractures: a systematic review. J Shoulder Elb Surg. 2012;21(11):1613–22.
13. Giannicola G, Sacchetti FM, Greco A, Cinotti G, Postacchini F. Management of complex elbow instability. Musculoskelet Surg. 2010;94(Suppl 1):S25–36.
14. Koslowsky TC, Zilleken C, Dargel J, Thelen U, Burkhart KJ, Heck S, et al. Reconstruction of a Bryan and Morrey type I capitellar fracture in a sawbone model with four different fixation devices: an experimental study. Injury. 2012;43(3):381–5.
15. Elkowitz SJ, Polatsch DB, Egol KA, Kummer FJ, Koval KJ. Capitellum fractures: a biomechanical evaluation of three fixation methods. J Orthop Trauma. 2002;16(7):503–6.
16. Sano S, Rokkaku T, Saito S, Tokunaga S, Abe Y, Moriya H. Herbert screw fixation of capitellar fractures. J Shoulder Elb Surg. 2005;14(3):307–11.
17. Tarallo L, Mugnai R, Adani R, Zambianchi F, Costanzini CA, Catani F. Shear fractures of the distal humerus: is the use of intra-articular screws a safe treatment? Musculoskelet Surg. 2015;99(3):217–23.

5

Treatment of thoracic or lumbar burst fractures with Balloon Assisted Endplate Reduction using Tricalcium Phosphate cement: histological and radiological evaluation

Joep Kitzen[1*], Martijn G. M. Schotanus[1], Herbert S. W. Plasschaert[2], Frans-Jan H. Hulsmans[3] and Pieter B. J. Tilman[1]

Abstract

Background: Short-segment pedicle-screw instrumentation is frequently used to stabilize thoracolumbar burst fractures. A recognized disadvantage of this procedure is recurrent kyphosis from intervertebral disc creep into the fractured central endplate. Balloon Assisted Endplate Reduction (BAER) using Tricalcium Phosphate bone cement (TCP) enables elevation of the centrally depressed endplate. Our objective was to evaluate the bone-tissue response to TCP and to analyse whether BAER using TCP can prevent recurrent kyphosis after removal of the instrumentation.

Methods: Fourteen patients with traumatic thoracolumbar burst fractures were operated with BAER using TCP in combination with short-segment instrumentation. Nine months after surgery, instrumentation was removed and transpedicular biopsies were taken for histological and histochemical analysis. Roentgenograms pre- and postoperatively and at latest follow-up after removal of the instrumentation were evaluated.

Results: Average follow-up was 2.6 years. Analysis of the biopsies showed a variable degree of bone remodelling with incorporation of TCP into newly formed bone matrix. No extensive foreign body reactions, inflammation, granulomatous responses or tissue necrosis were observed. Wedge-angle, kyphosis-angle and both the anterior-posterior and central-posterior vertebral body height ratios improved significant postoperatively ($p < 0.001$). After removal of the instrumentation no significant differences in wedge-angle or height ratios were seen ($p = 0.12$). The kyphosis-angle increased four degrees ($p = 0.01$).

Conclusion: TCP showed good histological osseointegration with no adverse events. TCP can therefore be safely used and could be beneficial in treatment of thoracolumbar burst fractures. BAER with TCP in combination with short-segment instrumentation might reduce recurrence of deformity even after removal of the instrumentation in comparison to short-segment instrumentation alone.

Keywords: Kyphoplasty, TCP, BAER, Biocompatibility, Recurrent kyphosis

* Correspondence: joep.kitzen@gmail.com
[1]Department of Orthopaedic Surgery, Zuyderland Medical Centre, Postbus 5500, 6130 MB Sittard-Geleen, the Netherlands
Full list of author information is available at the end of the article

Background

The best treatment option for thoracic- and lumbar burst fractures without neurological deficits is unclear. Several operative methods exist, but none has proven to be superior in terms of patient outcome. Treatment objectives after thoracic- and lumbar burst fractures are to stabilize the spine, prevent neurological deterioration, restore sagittal balance, retain as much segmental mobility as possible with the least operative tissue trauma and to mobilize the patient as quickly as possible.

Short-segment pedicle-screw instrumentation is widely used and can be done minimally invasive. However a recognized disadvantage of this procedure is early instrumentation failure [1, 2] and recurrent kyphosis [3]. Presumably because the posterior instrumentation alone does not provide sufficient support to allow the fractured vertebral body to heal without supplemental load-sharing through anterior column reconstruction. This anterior column insufficiency results form collapse of disc space and not from collapse of the fractured vertebral body [4, 5]. Öner et al. demonstrated that this collapse of disc space results from creep of the intervertebral disc into the fractured central endplate [6–8].

Posterior spinal fusion has been used to augment the stability of posterior implants. Several studies recommend posterior fusion, [9, 10] but others have claimed that it affords no benefit [11, 12]. A recent randomized trial of Jindal et al. [13] compared short-segment pedicle screw fixation with or without fusion of the affected segment. They showed a significant longer duration of surgery and higher peri-operative blood transfusion requirements in the fusion group. Whereas there were no clinical or radiological differences between the two groups.

Several studies evaluated the use of transpedicular vertebral body fracture reduction with Balloon Assisted Endplate Reduction (BAER) using Tricalcium Phosphate bone cement (TCP) and short-segment pedicle-screw instrumentation in thoracic- or lumbar burst fractures [14–17]. These studies demonstrated substantial reduction of the segmental kyphosis, presumably because BAER in combination with TCP cement prevents intervertebral disc creep by enabling elevation of the centrally depressed endplate. None of these studies reported on maintaining reduction after removal of the instrumentation. Removal of the instrumentation seems favourable in the lumbar spine since in non-fused segments without traumatic disc injury, segmental mobility presumably returns after the instrumentation is removed. Yurac et al. demonstrated residual mobility in these segments after the instrumentation was removed approximately 11 months after the initial posterior stabilisation for thoracolumbar burst fractures [18].

TCP cement rather than polymethylmethacrylate cement (PMMA) was used in the previously mentioned studies [14–17], because of its biocompatible properties shown in animal models [19, 20]. Biomechanically, TCP- and PMMA reinforced vertebrae have demonstrated nearly identical failure loads under compression [21, 22]. The use of the biocompatible TCP cement seems favourable. To our knowledge no studies on the biocompatibility of TCP cement for kyphoplasty in the human spine have been reported.

The main objectives of this retrospective cohort study were to evaluate the bone-tissue response of TCP cement in the human spine and to analyse whether BAER using TCP in combination with short-segment instrumentation for traumatic thoracic- or lumbar burst fractures can prevent recurrent kyphosis after removal of the instrumentation.

Methods

The current study was approved by the Zuyderland medical ethics committee (13 N31) and registered at the Dutch Trial Registry (NTR3498). Informed consent was acquired in all patients. Medical records of patients who sustained an acute traumatic thoracolumbar burst fracture. (AO-type A.3 or B.1) between 2003 and 2010 were reviewed. The fractures were classified on CT-scan according to the AO-Magerl classification [23] and the load sharing classification (LSC) [1]. In 14 patients a BAER with TCP and short-segment pedicle-screw instrumentation was performed and consequently were included for analysis.

Patients

The study group included eight female and six male patients with an average age of 41 years (range 23 to 61 years). The mean follow up was 29 months (range 9 to 100 months). All patients were operated between 0 to 21 days post injury (average 5 days). The mechanisms of injury were a fall from a height (N = 6), a traffic accident (N = 3) and domestic trauma (N = 5). The level of spinal involvement and type of fracture are listed in Table 1.

Two patients had a spinal involvement of two levels. One patient sustained a burst fracture in both L1 and L2. The second patient sustained a burst fracture of L2 combined with a small compression fracture of L3 (AO-type A1.1). None of these patients had neurological deficits, pre-existing spinal deformity, spinal stenosis, osteoporosis (criteria WHO) or previous spinal surgery.

Surgical procedure

All patients were operated on by the senior author (PT). Surgical procedures were performed with the patients under general anaesthesia with endotracheal intubation. Patients were placed in a prone position. Pedicle screws were placed into the non-fractured vertebrae one above and one below the fractured vertebrae. Consequently in the patients with 2 levels of spinal involvement, 3 instead of 2 segments were

Table 1 Level of spinal involvement, fracture classification and type of procedure

Patient	Level of spinal involvement	Fracture classifaction[1]	Load sharing classification[3]	Type of procedure
1	L1 and L2	A3.1 and A3.2[2]	5 and 7[2]	Open procedure
2	L2 and L3	A3.2 and A1.2[2]	8 and 3[2]	Open procedure
3	L1	A3.1	5	Open procedure
4	L2	A3.2	7	Open procedure
5	L1	A3.3	9	MIS[4]
6	T12	A3.1	5	MIS[4]
7	L1	A3.1	5	MIS[4]
8	L4	A3.3	7	MIS[4]
9	L2	A3.2	7	MIS[4]
10	L2	A3.1	5	MIS[4]
11	L1	A3.1	7	MIS[4]
12	L3	A3.2	6	MIS[4]
13	Th11	A3.2	8	MIS[4]
14	L2	B1.2	7	MIS[4]

[1]AO-Magerl classification
[2]Respectively
[3]McCormack load sharing classification
[4]Minimally invasive surgery

stabilised. Subsequently reduction of the kyphosis was achieved by inflation of the Kyphon® balloon-kyphoplasty in the fractured vertebrae (Medtronic, Minneapolis, Minnesota, USA). In the patient with a burst fracture in both L1 and L2, balloon-kyphoplasty was applied in both vertebrae. Stabilisation was achieved with an open procedure without fusion in the first 4 consecutive patients. Subsequently a percutaneous procedure was performed in the following 10 patients. The Monarch polyaxial spinal fixation device® and the Expedium Viper minimally invasive pedicle screw system® (Depuy, Warsaw, Indiana, USA) were used (Table 1). No distraction over the instrumentation was applied to achieve fracture reduction. For the cement augmentation, Calcibon® (Biomet, Warsaw, Indiana, USA) was used in the first 8 patients. In the subsequent 6 patients Kyphos® (Medtronic, Minneapolis, Minnesota, USA) was applied. The volume of injected TCP per vertebra ranged from 3 to 6 mL.

In 12 patients transpedicular biopsies from the bone-cement interface were taken during removal of the instrumentation using a Jamshidi needle. Two patients refused a biopsy. Instrumentation was removed on average 9 months (range 6 to 14 months) after the initial surgery. At that time-point consolidation of the fractured vertebra was expected based on radiological evaluation.

Histological and histochemical analysis

Analysis of the biopsies was performed by a single pathologist (HP). The biopsies were fixated using 4% buffered formalin and subsequently decalcified with Ethylenediaminetetraacetic Acid. After paraffin embedding, histological slices were cut and stained with haematoxylin and eosin. Goldner, elastica von Gieson, Giemsa, periodic acid shift and/or reticulin stains were used to visualize the osteoid formation, the amount of fibrosis or to identify the cell population present in the biopsies. One additional sample consisting only of cement was processed in the same way as the biopsies for histological examination. The decalcified remnants of the cement were compared with the bone biopsies and used to identify the remnants of cement in the samples. The biopsies were scored for the presence of osteoid formation, woven bone, osteoclasts and osteoblasts using a score of one to three. One stands for a little amount or near absence of the features, two representing medium changes and three for a large amount or obvious features. The sum of these two results was made to determine the amount of bone remodeling (score of two to six). Finally, the amount of haematopoietic tissue present was measured (score of one to three).

Radiological evaluation

For study purposes standing anteroposterior and lateral roentgenograms pre- and approximately 9 months postoperatively and at latest follow-up after removal of the instrumentation were analysed (3 to 91 months after removal of the instrumentation). In eight out of the 12 patients with lumbar fractures, flexion-extension roentgenograms were available at latest follow-up. All roentgenograms were evaluated by two independent observers who were not involved in patient care (JK, FH). Mean values of their measurements were calculated. Interclass correlation coefficient was used to determine the conformity between the two observers. The wedge angle (WA, Fig. 1a), the segmental kyphosis angle (KA, Fig. 1b) and the ratios between both the anterior- and the posterior vertebral body height (APVBHr, Fig. 1c) and the central- and posterior vertebral body height (CPVBHr, Fig. 1c) were determined. Residual mobility was reported when both observers noted more than three degrees of range of motion between the flexion and extension roentgenograms in either the proximal or distal adjacent segment. Range of motion was defined as described by Tanz et al. [24] CT-scans were taken before and after the initial surgery to evaluate spinal canal encroachment, cement leakage and malposition of the instrumentation in all patients except for one.

Patient reported outcome

After removal of the instrumentation at latest follow-up, back pain intensity was recorded on the basis of a Pain Visual Analog Scale (VAS, 10 point scale). Functional outcome after surgery was evaluated using the Short Form-36 survey (SF-36, domains physical function and bodily pain) and the

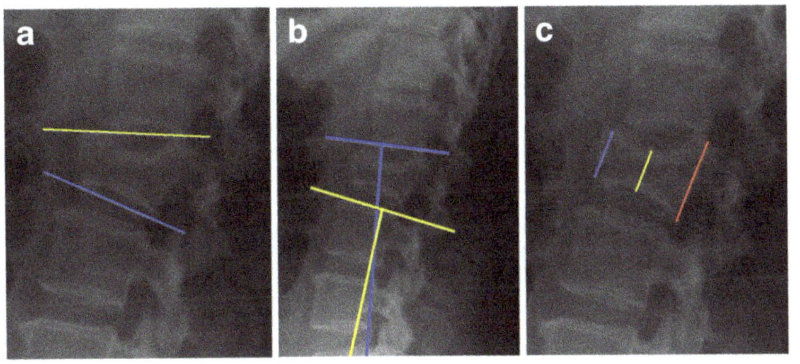

Fig. 1 a *WA:* Angle between the superior- and inferior endplate of the fractured vertebra. **b** *SK:* Angle between the adjacent vertebral endplates of the fractured vertebra. **c** *APVBHr resp. CPVBHr:* Ratios between the anterior- resp. central vertebral height in relation to the posterior vertebral height

Roland Morris Disability Questionnaire score (RDQ). Younger patients might show better compensation mechanisms after thoracolumbar fractures. A comparison between patients older than 40 years was made.

Data analysis

Statistical analysis was performed with use of SPSS (Version 23.0). The non-parametric Wilcoxon Signed-Rank test was used for changes of each radiographic parameter. The level of significance was set at $p < 0.05$.

Results

Histological and histochemical analysis

Twelve bone biopsies, taken 6 to 14 months after the initial surgery, were processed for histological examination. One sample was lost due to technical failure. In all of the 11 remaining biopsies, remnants of the cement were easily identified (Table 2). The presence of newly formed bone in the biopsies was striking (Figs. 2 and 3). This newly formed bone is deposited around cement particles with multiple osteoclasts and osteoblasts surrounding the particles. Thus producing islands and strands of bone, illustrating the osteoconductive properties of the TCP.

As shown in Table 2, there is no clear correlation between the time of biopsy and the degree of bone remodelling. Extensive remodelling (score of 6) was found at 6 months and at 9 months (Fig. 4). On the other hand no remodelling (score of 2) was found in other biopsies taken at 7 or 9 months. No histological differences between the two types of cement (Calcibon and Kyphos) were observed.

The hematopoietic tissue situated in between the bony trabeculae and between the trabeculae and the remnants of the cement showed no striking aberrations (Table 2). No cellular discrepancies were identified when examining the megakaryopoiesis, myelopoiesis and erythropoiesis. One biopsy showed a marked but localized histiocytic giant cell reaction with ingestion of some debris in the multinucleated cells indicative for the resorption of TCP (Fig. 5). In all other biopsies extensive foreign body reactions, inflammation, granulomatous responses or tissue necrosis were absent.

Table 2 Histological and histochemical analysis of the transpedicular biopsies from the bone-cement interface

Patient	Elapsed time (in months)[a]	Osteoid formation[b]	Osteoclasts & osteoblasts[b]	Combined[c]	Residual cement[b]	Haematopo-ietic tissue[b]
1	6	3	3	6	1	1
2	6	2	2	4	2	3
3	7	2	1	3	1	1
4	7	2	2	4	3	2
5	8	2	2	4	3	1
6	8	3	3	6	3	1
7	8	2	1	3	2	3
8	9	3	3	6	3	1
9	9	2	2	4	1	1
10	9	1	1	2	3	1
11	14	2	3	5	3	1

[a]Elapsed time between the initial surgery and the removal of the instrumentation
[b]Score of 1 to 3
[c]Score of 2 to 6

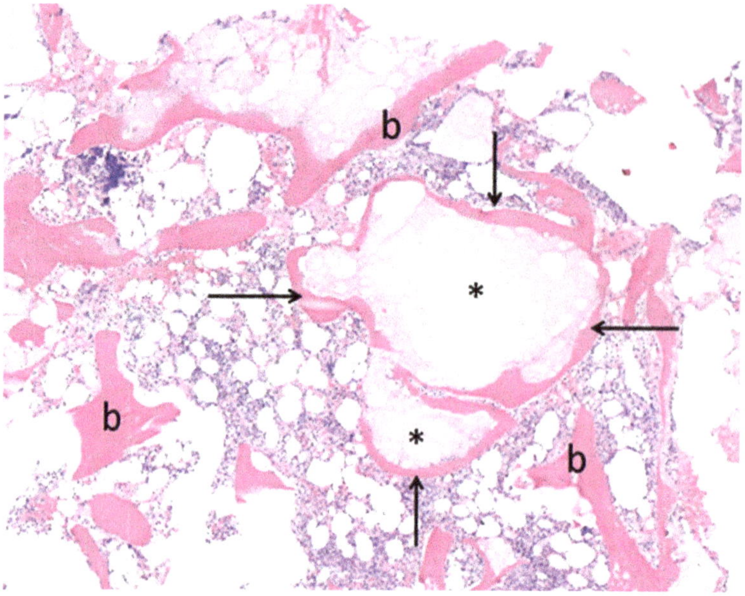

Fig. 2 Island of bone (arrows) surrounding remnants of cement (*), compared to the usual bone trabeculae (b)

Radiological evaluation

The mean values for the reduction of the segmental kyphosis angle and restoration of the central endplates pre- and postoperatively and after removal of the instrumentation are displayed in Table 3. Interclass correlation coefficient for all angles and ratios measured between two observers (JK, FH) ranged between 0.83 and 0.95. Preoperative wedge- and segmental kyphosis angle as well as both the APVBHr and CPVBHr improved significantly ($p < 0.001$) after the initial surgery. No signs of spinal canal encroachment, cement leakage or malposition of the instrumentation were seen on CT-scan. Convection was similar among patients with a percutaneous- or open posterolateral procedure.

After removal of the instrumentation the wedge angle as well as both height ratios were preserved. The segmental kyphosis angle increased significantly with a mean of four degrees (Table 3). However a

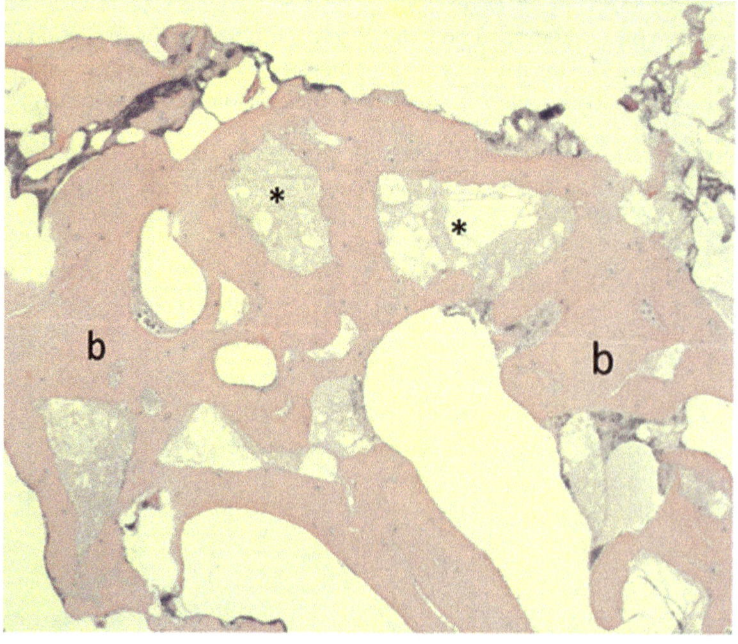

Fig. 3 The result of bone remoddeling is shown in this picture, with remnants of the cement (*) and very broad bony trabeculae(b)

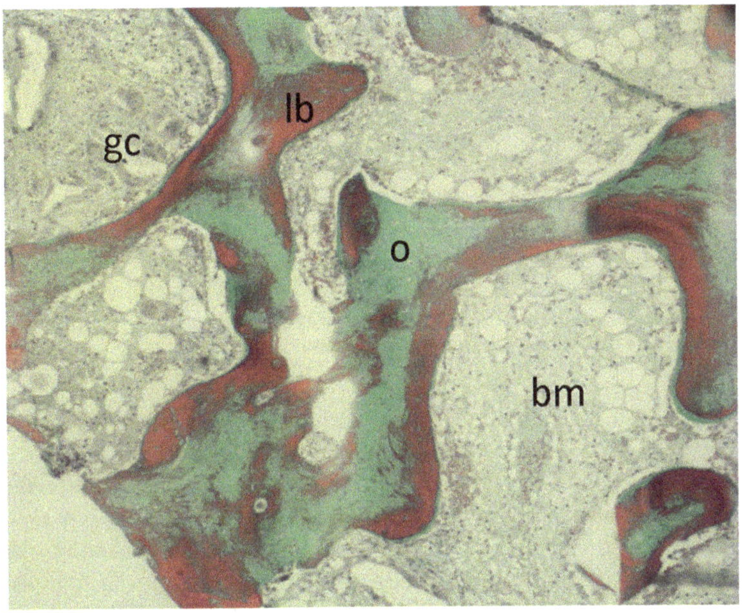

Fig. 4 Goldner staining: Osteid (newly formed bone) colours green (o), mineralised bone stains red (b). The bone marrow in between is not stained (bm), although some giant cell reaction can be seen (gc). This is illustrated in more detail in fig. 5

significant reduction of five degrees ($p = 0.01$) was maintained in comparison to the preoperative kyphosis angle.

On roentgenograms at latest follow-up no spontaneous fusion was observed. However residual mobility (Fig. 6) was observed in six patients out of the eight patients in whom flexion-extension radiographs were obtained. This residual mobility was most pronounced in the distal adjacent segment, although as seen in Fig. 6 it was present at the proximal adjacent segment as well.

Patient reported outcome

Average VAS pain scale after removal of the instrumentation was 2.8 (SD, 2.3). The SF-36 score and the RDQ score were respectively 72 (SD, 21) and 5.3 (SD, 5.9). When the patients older than 40 years ($n = 7$) in our group were

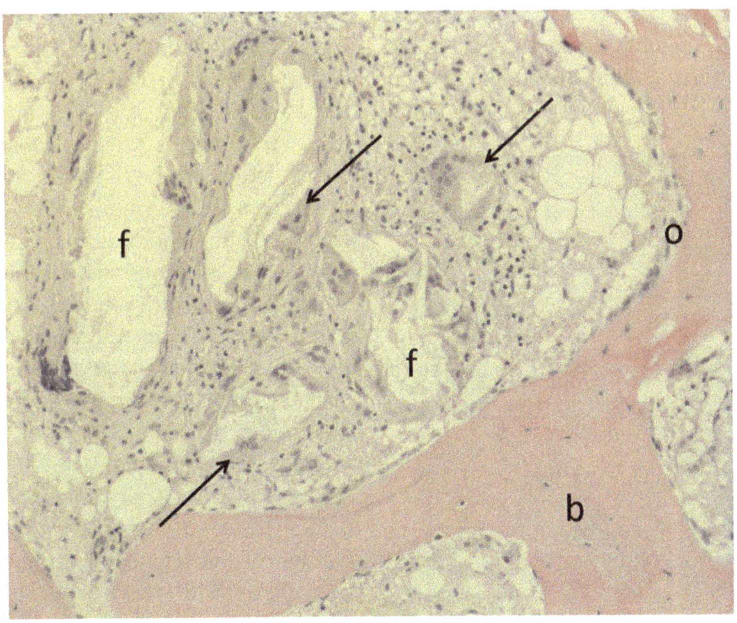

Fig. 5 Focal giant cell reaction (arrow), the multinucleated giant cells form aggregates and engulf some foreign body material (f), presenting as empty space in the histology. Osteoblastic rimming (o) of a bone lamella (b) is seen next to it

Table 3 Mean values for the reduction of the segmental kyphosis angle and restoration of the central endplates pre- and postoperatively and after removal of the instrumentation

	Before surgery (n = 14)	Before removal instrumentation (n = 14)	P-value[1]	After removal instrumentation (n = 14)	P-value[2]
Wedge Angle (in degrees)	19 (8.8)	9 (6.2)	0,000	10 (6.8)	0.25
Segmental kyphosis angle (in degrees)	9 (6.8)	0 (7.8)	0,000	4 (7.9)	0.01
Central-posterior vertebral body height ratio	0.4 (0.2)	0.8 (0.1)	0,001	0.8 (0.1)	0.26
Anterior-posterior vertebral body height ratio	0.6 (0.2)	0.8 (0.1)	0,000	0.8 (0.1)	0.12

All values are shown as average (standard deviation)
[1]findings after the initial surgery compared with those before removal of the instrumentation
[2]findings after the initial surgery compared with those after removal of the instrumentation

compared to those younger (n = 7) no significant changes in VAS- (p = 0.33), RDQ- (p = 0.36) and SF-36 score (p = 0.44) were seen. With the exception of screw breakage in one patient, no other complications occurred (Table 1, patient 8). It must be noted that the patient with the screw breakage was a drug addict. In terms of both functional outcome and reduction of the segmental kyphosis this patient performed less.

Discussion

In the current study the biocompatible properties of the TCP cement in the human spine were studied. In addition we evaluated if BAER using TCP cement in combination with short-segment instrumentation, could prevent recurrent kyphosis after removal of the instrumentation in patients with thoracic- or lumbar burst fractures.

Recurrence of deformity after short-segment instrumentation for thoracic- or lumbar burst fractures may result from intervertebral disc creep into the fractured central endplate [6–8]. A cadaver study by Verlaan et al. demonstrated that BAER with TCP cement significantly decreases the impression of the central endplate [25]. Indirect reduction of the fractured vertebral body by distraction using pedicle-screw instrumentation alone, leads to an insufficient reduction of the centrally depressed endplate [26]. Mermelstein et al. provided biomechanical evidence that in lumbar burst fractures, short-segment instrumentation in combination with transpedicular vertebral body reconstruction with TCP cement reduced pedicle screw-bending moments and increased the overall stiffness of the construct [27].

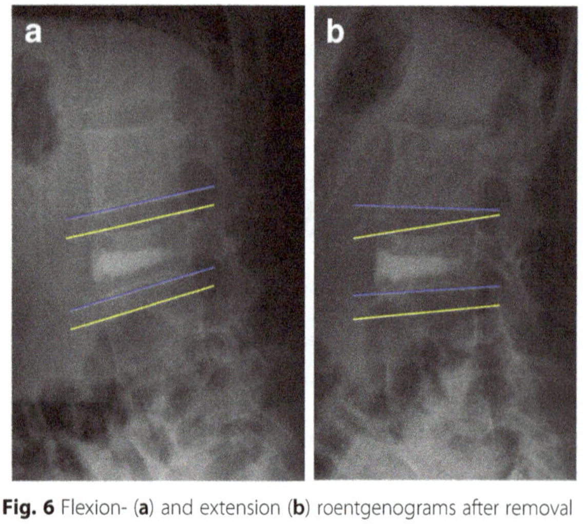

Fig. 6 Flexion- (**a**) and extension (**b**) roentgenograms after removal of the instrumentation visualizing residual mobility

Several clinical studies evaluated the use of TCP for the reconstruction of osseous defects of the vertebral body, the distal part of the radius and the proximal part of the tibia and femur [16, 25, 28–30]. Verlaan et al. published a favourable histological bone response to TCP cement after vertebroplasty in goats [20]. The biopsies in our population showed comparable incorporation of the TCP cement into newly formed bone matrix, indicative for the biocompatible properties of the TCP cement. Extensive foreign body reaction, inflammation, granulomatous response or tissue necrosis were not seen. These findings are consistent with the study of Ooms et al. [19]. In this study calcium phosphate cement was injected as a paste into tibia cortical bone defects in goats. After histological evaluation they concluded that the material had good biocompatible properties. Furthermore TCP cement in contrast to PMMA is an endothermic reaction when it hardens. Exothermic reactions of the cement might induce necrosis and consequently degeneration of the discus [31].

Our study demonstrates a significant reduction of the segmental kyphosis after restoration of the central endplates when, in addition to the short-segment instrumentation, BAER with TCP was performed. These findings are consistent with other recently conducted studies [14–17]. A systematic review of Verlaan et al. demonstrated an average recurrent kyphosis (loss of reduction of the segmental kyphosis angle) of ten degrees in patients with thoracic or lumbar fractures treated with short-segment pedicle-screw instrumentation alone [3]. In the study of Jindal et al. [13] an average recurrent kyphosis of 5.5° was seen in the fusion group compared to 3.6° in the non-fusion group. The segmental kyphosis angles at latest follow-up were respectively 9.9° and 7.9°.

None of the previously mentioned studies report on the effects after removal of the instrumentation. A study by Öner et al. demonstrates a recurrent kyphosis of 10 degrees after removal of the instrumentation in patients with thoracolumbar fractures managed with posterior reduction and fusion [6]. In our series the restoration of the central impression of the endplates was maintained after removal of the instrumentation. A recurrent kyphosis of four degrees was observed after removal of the instrumentation. This loss of reduction occurred therefore probably in the discus space and was to our opinion not substantial, especially when compared to patients managed without BAER or with fusion of the affected segments.

Although in 6 out of 8 patients residual mobility was clearly observed, it is difficult to draw definitive conclusions since in only eight out of the 12 patients with lumbar fractures, flexion-extension roentgenograms were available. However this may speak in favor for removal of the material especially when the recurrent kyphosis afterwards is not substantial.

Based on the VAS scale, SF-36- and RDQ-score, functional outcome after removal of the instrumentation was good and comparable with the literature [14, 15]. Unfortunately no patient reported outcome measurements were obtained before removal of the instrumentation. It would have been interesting to be able to investigate if removal of the instrumentation is beneficial on functional outcome. With the exception of screw breakage and recurrence of deformity in one patient, there were no complications. This non-compliant patient had an LSC score of 7 and an AO-type A3.3 fracture, whereas most of the other patients sustained either an AO-type A3.1 or A3.2 fracture. Retrospectively a circumferential spondylodesis would have been a better treatment option when considering his compliance in relation to the severity of his fracture. McCormack et al. stated that spine fractures with low LSC scores (3 to 6 points) can be managed with short-segment posterior stabilization alone; whereas burst fractures with high LSC scores (7 to 9 nine points) require anterior stabilization to prevent early instrumentation failure [1]. In our series 9 out of the 14 patients had a LSC score of 7 or higher and only one non-compliant patient had early instrumentation failure. It seems that BAER gives sufficient support to the anterior column without supplemental anterior stabilisation. The main limitation of the current study is its retrospective nature and its small number of patients in combination with the heterogeneity of the population their follow-up.

Conclusion

TCP cement showed histological osseointegration without adverse histological findings. TCP can therefore be safely used in treatment of thoracolumbar burst fractures. In addition this study indicates that BAER with TCP cement in combination with short-segment instrumentation might reduce the recurrence of deformity of the fractured vertebrae even after removal of the instrumentation when compared to short-segment instrumentation alone.

Abbreviations

APVBHr: Anterior vertebral body height ratio; BAER: Balloon Assisted Endplate Reduction; CPVBHr: Central vertebral body height ratio; KA: Segmental kyphosis angle; LSC: Load sharing classification; MIS: Minimally invasive surgery; PMMA: Polymethylmethacrylate cement; RDQ: Roland Morris Disability Questionnaire score; SD: Standard deviation; SF-36: Short Form-36 survey; TCP: Tricalcium Phosphate bone cement; VAS: Pain Visual Analog Scale; WA: Wedge angle

Acknowledgements

Not Applicable.

Authors' contributions

Author contributions to the manuscript preparation include the following: JK and MS drafted the manuscript. JK, HP and FH participated in interpretation and acquisition of data. PB performed the surgical procedure on all patients. All authors read and approved the final manuscript.

Consent for publication

Not applicable.

Competing interests

The authors declare that they have no competing interests. The content of this manuscript has not been published, or submitted for publication elsewhere. All authors have approved the manuscript for submission.

Author details

[1]Department of Orthopaedic Surgery, Zuyderland Medical Centre, Postbus 5500, 6130 MB Sittard-Geleen, the Netherlands. [2]Department of Pathology, Zuyderland Medical Centre, Sittard-Geleen, the Netherlands. [3]Department of Radiology, Zuyderland Medical Centre, Sittard-Geleen, the Netherlands.

References

1. McCormack T, Karaikovic E, Gaines RW. The load sharing classification of spine fractures. Spine (Phila Pa 1976). 1994;19(15):1741–4.
2. McLain RF, Sparling E, Benson DR. Early failure of short-segment pedicle instrumentation for thoracolumbar fractures. A preliminary report. J Bone Joint Surg Am. 1993;75(2):162–7.
3. Verlaan JJ, Diekerhof CH, Buskens E, van der Tweel I, Verbout AJ, Dhert WJ, Oner FC. Surgical treatment of traumatic fractures of the thoracic and lumbar spine: a systematic review of the literature on techniques, complications, and outcome. Spine (Phila Pa 1976). 2004;29(7):803–14.
4. Leferink VJ, Zimmerman KW, Veldhuis EF, ten Vergert EM, ten Duis HJ. Thoracolumbar spinal fractures: radiological results of transpedicular fixation combined with transpedicular cancellous bone graft and posterior fusion in 183 patients. Eur Spine J. 2001;10(6):517–23.
5. Speth MJ, Oner FC, Kadic MA, de Klerk LW, Verbout AJ. Recurrent kyphosis after posterior stabilization of thoracolumbar fractures. 24 cases treated with a Dick internal fixator followed for 1.5-4 years. Acta Orthop Scand. 1995;66(5):406–10.
6. Oner FC, van der Rijt RR, Ramos LM, Dhert WJ, Verbout AJ. Changes in the disc space after fractures of the thoracolumbar spine. J Bone Joint Surg Br. 1998;80(5):833–9.

7. Oner FC, van Gils AP, Dhert WJ, Verbout AJ. MRI findings of thoracolumbar spine fractures: a categorisation based on MRI examinations of 100 fractures. Skelet Radiol. 1999;28(8):433–43.
8. Oner FC, vd Rijt RH, Ramos LM, Groen GJ, Dhert WJ, Verbout AJ. Correlation of MR images of disc injuries with anatomic sections in experimental thoracolumbar spine fractures. Eur Spine J. 1999;8(3):194–8.
9. McNamara MJ, Stephens GC, Spengler DM. Transpedicular short-segment fusions for treatment of lumbar burst fractures. J Spinal Disord. 1992;5(2):183–7.
10. Parker JW, Lane JR, Karaikovic EE, Gaines RW. Successful short-segment instrumentation and fusion for thoracolumbar spine fractures: a consecutive 41/2-year series. Spine (Phila Pa 1976). 2000;25(9):1157–70.
11. Dai LY, Jiang LS, Jiang SD. Posterior short-segment fixation with or without fusion for thoracolumbar burst fractures. A five to seven-year prospective randomized study. J Bone Joint Surg Am. 2009;91(5):1033–41.
12. Wang ST, Ma HL, Liu CL, Yu WK, Chang MC, Chen TH. Is fusion necessary for surgically treated burst fractures of the thoracolumbar and lumbar spine?: a prospective, randomized study. Spine (Phila Pa 1976). 2006;31(23):2646–52. discussion 2653
13. Jindal N, Sankhala SS, Bachhal V. The role of fusion in the management of burst fractures of the thoracolumbar spine treated by short segment pedicle screw fixation: a prospective randomised trial. J Bone Joint Surg Br. 2012;94(8):1101–6.
14. Korovessis P, Hadjipavlou A, Repantis T. Minimal invasive short posterior instrumentation plus balloon kyphoplasty with calcium phosphate for burst and severe compression lumbar fractures. Spine (Phila Pa 1976). 2008;33(6):658–67.
15. Marco RA, Kushwaha VP. Thoracolumbar burst fractures treated with posterior decompression and pedicle screw instrumentation supplemented with balloon-assisted vertebroplasty and calcium phosphate reconstruction. J Bone Joint Surg Am. 2009;91(1):20–8.
16. Oner FC, Verlaan JJ, Verbout AJ, Dhert WJ. Cement augmentation techniques in traumatic thoracolumbar spine fractures. Spine (Phila Pa 1976). 2006;31(11 Suppl):S89–95. discussion S104
17. Verlaan JJ, Dhert WJ, Verbout AJ, Oner FC. Balloon vertebroplasty in combination with pedicle screw instrumentation: a novel technique to treat thoracic and lumbar burst fractures. Spine (Phila Pa 1976). 2005;30(3):E73–9.
18. Yurac R, Marre B, Urzua A, Munjin M, Lecaros MA. Residual mobility of instrumented and non-fused segments in thoracolumbar spine fractures. Eur Spine J. 2006;15(6):864–75.
19. Ooms EM, Wolke JG, van de Heuvel MT, Jeschke B, Jansen JA. Histological evaluation of the bone response to calcium phosphate cement implanted in cortical bone. Biomaterials. 2003;24(6):989–1000.
20. Verlaan JJ, Oner FC, Slootweg PJ, Verbout AJ, Dhert WJ. Histologic changes after vertebroplasty. J Bone Joint Surg Am. 2004;86-A(6):1230–8.
21. Perry A, Mahar A, Massie J, Arrieta N, Garfin S, Kim C. Biomechanical evaluation of kyphoplasty with calcium sulfate cement in a cadaveric osteoporotic vertebral compression fracture model. Spine J. 2005;5(5):489–93.
22. Rotter R, Pflugmacher R, Kandziora F, Ewert A, Duda G, Mittlmeier T. Biomechanical in vitro testing of human osteoporotic lumbar vertebrae following prophylactic kyphoplasty with different candidate materials. Spine (Phila Pa 1976). 2007;32(13):1400–5.
23. Magerl F, Aebi M, Gertzbein SD, Harms J, Nazarian S. A comprehensive classification of thoracic and lumbar injuries. Eur Spine J. 1994;3(4):184–201.
24. Tanz SS. Motion of the lumbar spine; a roentgenologic study. Am J Roentgenol Radium Therapy, Nucl Med. 1953;69(3):399–412.
25. Verlaan JJ, van Helden WH, Oner FC, Verbout AJ, Dhert WJ. Balloon vertebroplasty with calcium phosphate cement augmentation for direct restoration of traumatic thoracolumbar vertebral fractures. Spine (Phila Pa 1976). 2002;27(5):543–8.
26. Fredrickson BE, Edwards WT, Rauschning W, Bayley JC, Yuan HA. Vertebral burst fractures: an experimental, morphologic, and radiographic study. Spine (Phila Pa 1976). 1992;17(9):1012–21.
27. Mermelstein LE, McLain RF, Yerby SA. Reinforcement of thoracolumbar burst fractures with calcium phosphate cement. A biomechanical study. Spine (Phila Pa 1976). 1998;23(6):664–70. discussion 670-661
28. Cassidy C, Jupiter JB, Cohen M, Delli-Santi M, Fennell C, Leinberry C, Husband J, Ladd A, Seitz WR, Constanz B. Norian SRS cement compared with conventional fixation in distal radial fractures. A randomized study. J Bone Joint Surg Am. 2003;85-A(11):2127–37.
29. Lobenhoffer P, Gerich T, Witte F, Tscherne H. Use of an injectable calcium phosphate bone cement in the treatment of tibial plateau fractures: a prospective study of twenty-six cases with twenty-month mean follow-up. J Orthop Trauma. 2002;16(3):143–9.
30. Mattsson P, Alberts A, Dahlberg G, Sohlman M, Hyldahl HC, Larsson S. Resorbable cement for the augmentation of internally-fixed unstable trochanteric fractures. A prospective, randomised multicentre study. J Bone Joint Surg Br. 2005;87(9):1203–9.
31. Urrutia J, Bono CM, Mery P, Rojas C. Early histologic changes following polymethylmethacrylate injection (vertebroplasty) in rabbit lumbar vertebrae. Spine. 2008;33(8):877–82.

6

Validity of humerus fracture classification in the Swedish fracture register

David Wennergren[*†], Stina Stjernström[†], Michael Möller, Mikael Sundfeldt and Carl Ekholm

Abstract

Background: The ability to correctly classify fractures is of importance for choosing the appropriate treatment and for providing appropriate data for research and quality registers. In the Swedish Fracture Register (SFR) fractures of all types are registered by the attending physician, often a junior doctor. For the majority of fractures, a modified AO/OTA classification is used. This study aimed to validate the accuracy of classification of humerus fractures in the SFR and also at providing insight into inherent classification uncertainties.

Methods: One hundred and sixteen humerus fractures (among them 90 proximal) were retrieved by computer randomisation from the SFR and reassessed independently at two occasions, 6 weeks apart, by three senior orthopaedic surgeons blinded to patient information and a consensus "gold standard" classification was established. This was compared with the classifications that had been entered into the register.

Results: The agreement between gold standard classification and original classification in the SFR was kappa = 0.57 for all humerus fractures. For proximal humerus fractures kappa-coefficient for intra-observer agreement was 0.593, 0.599 and 0.752 for the three observers respectively. Taking into account the similarities between certain fracture groups, a modified calculation of agreement was performed. With this modification the intra-observer agreement was 0.910-0.974 and inter-observer agreement was 0.912.

Conclusion: The classification of humerus fractures in the Swedish Fracture Register was just as accurate as in previous studies, i.e. moderate as defined by Landis and Koch. However, when we introduced a modified analysis, that takes into account the similarities between certain fractures, the accuracy was "near perfect".

Keywords: Fracture classification, Validity, Agreement, Accuracy, Humerus fracture, Fracture register

Background

Understanding fracture morphology is an essential step in assessing fractures for appropriate treatment. Regardless of the classification system that is used, inter- and intra-observer agreement have been poor to moderate using plain radiographs [1, 2]. Previous studies of the reliability of fracture classification have been performed using a selection of fractures in a test situation.

Classifying fractures means clustering fracture patterns into different sets. Although the boundaries of the sets may be fairly well defined, the fractures that are going to be classified are part of a continuum. Fractures may display features of two different fracture sets to a varying degree and, to some degree, the assessment by the person working with the system is subjective. Furthermore, in fracture classification, there are no absolutely correct answers but rather degrees of agreement between different assessors.

The Swedish Fracture Register (SFR) is an on-line national fracture registration system in which the individual doctor, who sees the patient at the emergency department and later during treatment, enters data relating to the fracture: fracture date, trauma mechanism, fracture localisation and fracture classification, including multiple fractures [3]. Treatment is registered, primary treatment including non-surgical treatment, as well as secondary procedures. Questionnaires (Eq5D, SMFA) are mailed to the patient 1 year after the injury for follow-up to be compared with the ones completed by the patient at the time of injury regarding his/her pre-injury health (recall technique). In the context of the

* Correspondence: david.wennergren@vgregion.se
[†]Equal contributors
Department of Orthopaedics, Sahlgrenska University Hospital, SE-413 45 Gothenburg, Mölndal, Sweden

present study, it should be pointed out that junior doctors who are not specifically trained for this work do the majority of the classification work.

Fracture classification is carried out by indicating the fracture location on the image of a skeleton (with courtesy of AO foundation), e.g. on the left proximal humerus. This image expands to display a grid with the different fracture groups and the one corresponding to the relevant fracture is chosen. For the SFR, the AO/OTA system has been used as it is a comprehensive classification system that covers most body regions [4]. Slight modifications have been made by selecting fracture subgroups from a more detailed level in order to improve the logic of the system e.g. in the SFR, for proximal humerus fractures in addition to the nine AO/OTA groups (A1-C3), there are three subgroups to enable the classification of unifocal fractures with dislocation (A1.3), head split fractures (C2.3) and pure anatomical neck fractures (C3.1), fracture types not found at group level (Fig. 1). When possible, the similarities between other frequently used classification systems, Neer, and the AO/OTA system have been highlighted to make it more "friendly" to the user [5]. Still the quality and usefulness of the data in a register such as the SFR is dependent on the accuracy of the classification of fractures. Previous studies on accuracy of the classification of tibia and ankle fractures have shown moderate to substantial accuracy [6, 7]. A study on the epidemiology of humerus fractures based on data from the SFR was recently published [8].

The aim of this study was to analyse the accuracy of the classification of humerus fractures as it is used in daily practice in the SFR. Our second aim, while analysing the subgroup of proximal humeral fractures, was to get a deeper understanding of the generally low reliability of fracture classification using concepts from "fuzzy logic" [9].

Ethics

The study was approved by the Central Ethical Review Board, Gothenburg (ID 999–13).

Methods

In January 2014, 116 humerus fractures (among them 90 proximal humeral fractures) were selected by computerised randomisation from the 1772 humerus fractures (1374 proximal humeral fractures) registered in 2011 and 2012 in the Swedish Fracture Register at Sahlgrenska University Hospital (Fig. 2). One of the authors (SS) acquired all the radiological investigations that

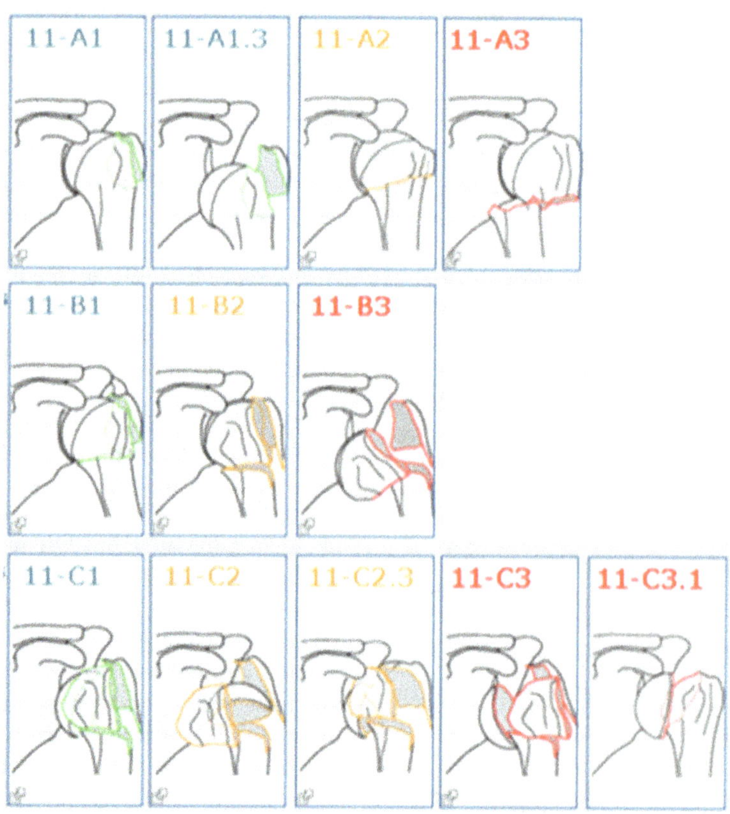

Fig. 1 Fracture groups as presented in the SFR

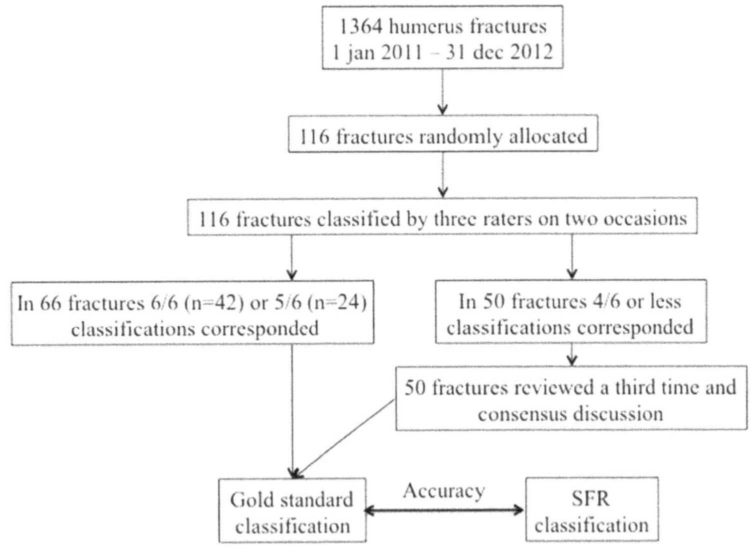

Fig. 2 Flow chart of how the study was conducted

were available for each patient at the time of registration in the SFR. The patients with proximal humeral fractures were all investigated with a standard radiographic series of three planes, i.e. anterior-posterior, lateral, and axial view except in 23 patients where the axial view was not done. 12 of the 116 patients were investigated with a CT-scan – 7/90 of the proximal humeral fractures, 5/11 of the distal humeral fractures and none of the diaphyseal humeral fractures. On two occasions, 6 weeks apart, all the images were presented to the three observers (two senior trauma surgeons and one trauma/shoulder surgeon) for independent assessment and fracture classification. No information about the patients' age, gender or subsequent treatment was given. On all occasions, handouts and the drawings used in the SFR were available, with a detailed description of the classification system. In this way all fractures were classified six times. In cases where five or six out of six classifications corresponded this classification was considered the true classification of the fracture i.e. the gold standard classification. Once the compilation of the data was completed, a third classification session took place for the fractures for which complete agreement had not been reached. Remaining disagreement was resolved after an open discussion between the three observers and the final result was named the gold standard. The original classification in the SFR was then compared with the gold standard classification.

For the proximal humerus fractures the classification system was further analysed. The 12 fracture groups can be defined by eight Boolean questions (yes/no) (Table 1) and one question to determine the segment, similar to the work by Shrader et al. [10]. To understand the grounds for classification disagreement, the possible relationship between fracture groups was analysed. Fracture groups or subgroups separated by only one question were regarded as "related", with the exception of "glenohumeral dislocation". Fractures differing in two or more

Table 1 Question answered yes/no (1/0) defining the fracture groups of proximal humerus fractures. The "0"s have been omitted for clarity

	A1	A1.3	A2	A3	B1	B2	B3	C1	C2	C2.3	C3	C3.1
Two-part extra-articular	1	1	1	1								
Tuberosity only	1											
Three-part, extra-articular – bifocal					1	1	1					
Four-part, articular								1	1	1	1	
Glenohumeral dislocation		1					1				1	
Metaphyseal impaction/stable			1		1			1				
Anatomical neck only												1
Head split									1			
Proximal segment (inside the square)	1	1	1	1	1	1	1	1	1	1	1	1

questions are regarded as being unrelated. "Related" fractures differ by only one question and one could be mistaken for the other if the defining fracture line is vague (e.g. whether or not there is a fracture of the greater tuberosity, or whether or not the fracture is impacted/stable).

Statistical analysis

Sample size calculations were made based on kappa statistics from previous studies [1, 2, 10–14]. Based on the kappa values in these previous studies an approximate kappa value of 0.5 was expected. In order to achieve a 95% confidence interval that did not span more than one category on the scale defined by Landis and Koch, a relative error of 20% corresponding to kappa ±0.1 was accepted [15]. Intra- and inter-observer agreement analysis was performed, calculating the kappa coefficients and confidence intervals using SAS software. For the fracture groups that were regarded as "related" fractures, an intermediate fracture group was created, e.g. for the fractures assessed as "A2" in one instance and as "B1" in another, the intermediate group "A2-B1" was constructed to classify these fractures (Table 2). In this way, ten intermediate groups were constructed.

Results

Age and gender distribution for all humerus fractures is presented in Table 3. Accuracy, defined as agreement between the classification in the SFR and gold standard classification, for all humerus fractures was kappa 0.57 for AO/OTA group (four signs) and 0.66 for AO/OTA type (three signs) (Table 4).

Proximal humerus fractures

The distribution of proximal humerus fractures between the fracture groups as determined by the gold standard classification is similar to the distribution described by Court-Brown et al. for an Edinburgh population (Table 5) [16].

Table 2 Intermediate fracture groups, constructed on the boundary between "related" groups, i.e. groups separated by only one of the defining questions listed in Table 1

A1-B1
A1.3-B3
A2-A3
A2-B1
B1-B2
B1-C1
B2-C2
B2-C2.3
C1-C2
C2-C2.3

Table 3 Distribution of patients according to age, gender and fracture segment (proximal humerus, diaphyseal humerus and distal humerus) as defined by gold standard classification

	Women	Men	Total
Median age (range)	71 (19–102) *n* = 81	50 (16–92) *n* = 35	67,5 (16–102) *n* = 116
Median age (range) among proximal humeral fractures (AO/OTA 11XX)	71 (19–102) *n* = 67	58,5 (17–92) *n* = 22	69 (17–102) *n* = 89
Median age (range) among diaphyseal humeral fractures (AO/OTA 12XX)	82 (30–90) *n* = 8	34,5 (18–72) *n* = 8	54,5 (18–90) *n* = 16
Median age (range) among distal humeral fractures (AO/OTA 13XX)	67 (48–93) *n* = 6	37 (16–82) *n* = 5	60 (16–93) *n* = 11

Full intra-observer agreement for the three observers was seen in 71, 58 and 56 respectively of the 90 cases of proximal humerus fractures. The kappa values of the intra-observer analysis are given in Table 6. When inter-observer agreement between the SFR and the gold standard classification was tested, complete agreement was seen in 57 of the 90 cases.

If the ten intermediate groups were included, complete intra-observer agreement was seen in 89, 86 and 81 of the 90 cases. When comparing the SFR with the gold standard classification with the ten intermediate groups included, 27 fractures could be classified as belonging to one of these. As a result, complete agreement was seen between the SFR and the gold standard classification in 84 of the 90 tested cases. The kappa values are given in Table 7.

Discussion

This paper has two aims: to analyse the reliability of fracture classification as it is used in daily practice and to understand the limitations of fracture classification validity. When the accuracy of classification in the SFR, as carried out by junior doctors at an emergency department, was tested against the senior consensus group, the

Table 4 Percentage of agreement (PA) and Cohen's Kappa coefficient with 95% confidence interval for accuracy, defined as SFR classification compared with gold standard classification (GS) for all humerus fractures

	Accuracy SFR vs GS	
	PA	Kappa (95% CI)
AO/OTA group (4 signs)	61%	0.57 (0.47-0.67)
AO/OTA type (3 signs)	75%	0.66 (0.55-0.76)

AO/OTA group – 4 signs refer to a full AO/OTA classification with 4 signs e.g. 11A1. AO/OTA type – 3 signs refer to a simplified AO/OTA classification with 3 signs only e.g. 11A

Table 5 Comparison of the relative distribution (%) of proximal humeral fractures by AO/OTA groups in the SFR assessed by the gold standard and the Edinburgh population [16]

AO/OTA group	SFR	Court-Brown et al.
A1	10,4	14
A1.3	4.6	5
A2	24.2	27
A3	18.4	20
B1	23.0	19
B2	15.0	7
B3	1.2	0.6
C1	1.2	1.1
C2	0	2.4
C3	1.2	2.3

kappa value was in the range of previous studies (0.57) [1, 2, 10–14]. Although this result corresponds to moderate agreement, according to the criteria formulated by Landis and Koch, we suggest that this result is as good as could be expected, considering that the registering doctors were under the time pressure of the emergency ward and that they were not specifically trained for the task and perhaps not even completely motivated [15]. The results are in accordance with similar studies on tibia and ankle fractures in the SFR [6, 7]. The fact that there was a considerable resemblance between the epidemiology of the randomly acquired cases and that of the incidence analysis from Edinburgh supports our notion that the classification as used in the SFR has good validity and that the selected cases are representative of the normal fracture population [16]. Conversely, it also supports the data in the report by Court-Brown et al., although only one person carried out their classification, without intra-observer error being tested.

Systems for classifying proximal humeral fractures have been developed, based on the four segments of epiphyseal union as defined by Codman and subsequently modified by Neer [5]. Another modification has been proposed by Hertel [17, 18]. These systems comprise up to 16 different fracture groups. A slightly different system has been introduced by AO/OTA, based on the generalised system for classifying fractures in the proximal or distal segment of long bones but adapted for the shoulder, which is used in the SFR.

It has been suggested that the poor inter- and intra-observer agreement that has been observed using any classification system is due to the surgeons' inability to accurately interpret the fracture. Despite the use of CT imaging in some studies, it has not been shown to improve the results uniformly [2, 11–13, 19]. The kappa values obtained from these studies improve only slightly or not at all, when the classification systems were simplified or reduced to two options, displaced or undisplaced [1, 14, 20]. However, it has been suggested in one study that the use of CT-based stereo visualisation may substantially improve classification reliability, which has also been seen in tibial plateau fractures [21, 22].

We believe that, regardless of imaging methods or classification protocol, there is always going to be some degree of disagreement between observers. Any classification system basically attempts to divide a continuum of all the different fracture types into discreet groups. Regardless of system or imaging methods, there are always going to be boundary problems for fractures with the characteristics of two or more fracture groups. Boundaries between fracture groups could be defined by Boolean questions to be answered "yes" or "no" and a list of these questions could be used as an analytical pathway [10]. Fractures on either side of a boundary, separated by only one question, could be regarded as related and deviating assessments are possible depending on how subtle the differentiating feature is.

This is similar to the reasoning behind "fuzzy sets". A "fuzzy set" is "a class with a continuum of grades of membership" [9]. In recent years, mathematics and the understanding of sets with imprecise properties have been developed and have found applications in numerous fields, such as the automated determination of vertebral column disorders and weed classification for precision herbicide application [23–25]. When dealing with the imprecise nature of fracture classification, it should also be pointed out that there is no "perfect truth" – it is instead a question of weighing "expert" opinions.

Rather than describing "grades of membership" for individual fractures that did not perfectly fit the definition of one fracture group alone, we introduced intermediate

Table 6 Intra-observer kappa values with upper and lower confidence interval (CI) for proximal humerus fractures, calculated with or without taking "related" fractures into account (intermediate groups)

	Without intermediate groups		With intermediate groups	
	Mean kappa value	95% CI	Mean kappa value	95% CI
Rater 1	0.752	0.652 – 0.853	0.974	0.939 – 1.000
Rater 2	0.599	0.481 – 0.717	0.910	0.846 – 0.974
Rater 3	0.593	0.478 – 0.707	0.914	0.853 – 0.975

Table 7 Inter-observer kappa values with upper and lower confidence interval (CI) for proximal humerus fractures, calculated with or without taking "related" fractures into account (intermediate groups)

	Without intermediate groups		With intermediate groups	
	Mean kappa value	95% CI	Mean kappa value	95% CI
Gold vs SFR	0.577	0.457 – 0.697	0.912	0.850 – 0.974

groups where appropriate, to comprise fractures with the features of two adjoining groups. Having introduced the intermediate groups, the kappa value rose from 0.0577 to 0.912, when the SFR was compared with the "gold standard", and from 0.593–0.752 to 0.910–0.974 for the intra-observer comparisons. Another way to describe this is that in most of the cases where there is disagreement, the disagreement is between "related fracture groups". The unadjusted kappa values correspond to what has previously been published. On the other hand the adjusted kappa values are exceedingly high and have to be interpreted with caution. The high, adjusted kappa values may represent a near upper limit of agreement when the boundary problem is taken into account. Two surgeons with a divergent view of slight details that may change the classification are still likely to perceive the fracture in the same way, as long as the fracture groups are "related". This may explain the higher agreement for treatment recommendations than for the fracture classification [26].

Strengths and limitations of the present study

Although sample size calculations were made the 116 randomly allocated humerus fractures included only 16 diaphyseal and 11 distal humerus fractures. However the statistical analysis was done on all humerus fractures and proximal humerus fractures respectively and the low numbers of diaphyseal and distal humerus fractures therefor should not affect the reliability of results. The current study has the same design and similar results as the previous studies on the validity of tibia fracture and malleolar fracture classification in the SFR [6, 7]. With the AO/OTA classification system classifying the correct segment could pose a problem, e.g. whether the fracture belongs to segment 1 (proximal) or segment 2 (diaphysis). In the current study there was disagreement regarding to what segment a fracture should be assigned in seven cases (in three cases between gold standard and the SFR and in four cases within the consensus group). We therefor find it important to study the whole of humerus. We also think it is important that the studies on validity of fracture classification in the SFR are of the same design. The inter-observer variation that was tested used data extracted from the SFR, against the "gold standard". We have therefore tested the accuracy of the classification system as used in real life, by doctors not specifically trained and not with the mind-set of a test situation. The introduction of "intermediate groups" has several limitations. The purpose of this is not to introduce a new classification system to be used in clinical practice. The purpose is merely to introduce a new way of analysing agreement in fracture classification that shows that most disagreements are between the "related fracture groups". The test was carried out on a fairly large number (n = 116) of randomly acquired fractures with seemingly normal distribution and we believe that we have thus adhered to most of the quality criteria set by Audigé et al. [27]. We believe that the normative "gold standard" that we have attempted to establish is fairly close to the "truth", based as it is on multiple classification rounds followed by analytical discussions. By comparison, the classification presented in the study of the epidemiology of proximal humeral fractures [16], was carried out by only one person and no intra-observer variations were tested.

Conclusions

The classification of humerus fractures in the Swedish Fracture Register is as accurate as in previous studies. We also believe that we offer a new way of interpreting the low kappa values of fracture classification by attempting to analyse the borderline problems that exist with any classification.

Abbreviations

AO: Arbeitsgemeinschaft für osteosynthesefragen; CT: Computed tomography; Eq5D: Euroqol 5 dimensions; ICD-10: International Classification of Diseases Tenth Revision; OTA: Orthopaedic Trauma Association; PROM: Patient Reported Outcome Measures; SFR: Swedish Fracture Register; SMFA: Short Musculoskeletal Function Assessment

Acknowledgements

The authors wish to thank Linda Akrami for statistical support. The authors also wish to thank all the orthopaedic surgeons at the department for entering detailed data on busy working days.

Funding

Not applicable

Authors' contributions

DW analysed and interpreted data and wrote the manuscript together with SS and CE, SS collected and analysed data and wrote the manuscript together with DW and CE, MS and MM were part of the consensus group, classified fractures and revised the manuscript, CE was part of the consensus group, classified fractures, analysed and interpreted data and wrote the manuscript together with DW and SS. All authors read and approved the final manuscript.

Competing interests
The authors declare that they have no competing interests.

Consent for publication
Not applicable

References

1. Siebenrock KA, Gerber C. The reproducibility of classification of fractures of the proximal end of the humerus. J Bone Joint Surg Am. 1993;75:1751–5.
2. Sjödén GO, Movin T, Güntner P, Aspelin P, Ahrengart L, Ersmark H, et al. Poor reproducibility of classification of proximal humeral fractures. Additional CT of minor value. Acta Orthop Scand. 1997;68:239–42.
3. Wennergren D, Ekholm C, Sandelin A, Möller M. The Swedish fracture register: 103,000 fractures registered. BMC Musculoskelet Disord. 2015;16:338.
4. Müller M, Koch P, Nazarian S, Schatzker J. The comprehensive classification of fractures of long bones. Berlin, Heidelberg, New York: Springer-Verlag; 1990.
5. Neer CS 2nd. Displaced proximal humeral fractures. I. Classification and evaluation. J Bone Joint Surg Am. 1970;52:1077–89.
6. Wennergren D, Ekholm C, Sundfeldt M, Karlsson J, Bhandari M, Möller M. High reliability in classification of tibia fractures in the Swedish fracture register. Injury. 2016;47:478–82.
7. Juto H, Möller M, Wennergren D, Edin K, Apelqvist I, Morberg P. Substantial accuracy of fracture classification in the Swedish Fracture Register: Evaluation of AO/OTA-classification in 152 ankle fractures. Injury. 2016. doi:10.1016/j.injury.2016.05.028. [Epub ahead of print].
8. Bergdahl C, Ekholm C, Wennergren D, Nilsson F, Möller M. Epidemiology and patho-anatomical pattern of 2,011 humeral fractures: data from the Swedish fracture register. BMC Musculoskelet Disord. 2016;17:159.
9. Zadeh LA. Fuzzy sets. Inf Control. 1965;8:338–53.
10. Shrader MW, Sanchez-Sotelo J, Sperling JW, Rowland CM, Cofield RH. Understanding proximal humerus fractures: image analysis, classification, and treatment. J Shoulder Elb Surg. 2005;14:497–505.
11. Sjödén GO, Movin T, Aspelin P, Güntner P, Shalabi A. 3D-radiographic analysis does not improve the Neer and AO classifications of proximal humeral fractures. Acta Orthop Scand. 1999;70:325–8.
12. Foroohar A, Tosti R, Richmond JM, Gaughan JP, Ilyas AM. Classification and treatment of proximal humerus fractures: inter-observer reliability and agreement across imaging modalities and experience. J Orthop Surg Res. 2011;6:38.
13. Bernstein J, Adler LM, Blank JE, Dalsey RM, Williams GR, Iannotti JP. Evaluation of the Neer system of classification of proximal humeral fractures with computerized tomographic scans and plain radiographs. J Bone Joint Surg Am. 1996;78:1371–5.
14. Sidor ML, Zuckerman JD, Lyon T, Koval K, Cuomo F, Schoenberg N. The Neer classification system for proximal humeral fractures. An assessment of interobserver reliability and intraobserver reproducibility. J Bone Joint Surg Am. 1993;75:1745–50.
15. Landis JR, Koch GG. The measurement of observer agreement for categorical data. Biometrics. 1977;33:159–74.
16. Court-Brown CM, Garg A, McQueen M. The epidemiology of proximal humeral fractures. Acta Orthop Scand. 2001;72:365–71.
17. Hertel R, Hempfing A, Stiehler M, Leunig M. Predictors of humeral head ischemia after intracapsular fracture of the proximal humerus. J Shoulder Elb Surg. 2004;13:427–33.
18. Sukthankar AV, Leonello DT, Hertel RW, Ding GS, Sandow MJ. A comprehensive classification of proximal humeral fractures: HGLS system. J Shoulder Elb Surg. 2013;22:e1–6.
19. Bruinsma WE, Guitton TG, Warner JP, Ring D. Interobserver reliability of classification and characterization of proximal humeral fractures. J Bone Joint Surg Am. 2013;95:1600–4.
20. Brorson S, Bagger J, Sylvest A, Hróbjartsson A. Low agreement among 24 doctors using the Neer-classification; only moderate agreement on displacement, even between specialists. Int Orthop. 2002;26:271–3.
21. Brunner A, Honigmann P, Treumann T, Babst R. The impact of stereo-visualisation of three-dimensional CT datasets on the inter- and intraobserver reliability of the AO/OTA and Neer classifications in the assessment of fractures of the proximal humerus. J Bone Joint Surg Br. 2009;91:766–71.
22. Yacoubian SV, Nevins RT, Sallis JG, Potter HG, Lorich DG. Impact of MRI on treatment plan and fracture classification of tibial plateau fractures. J Orthop Trauma. 2002;16:632–7.
23. Nguyen HT, Kreinovich V. How to fully represent expert information about imprecise properties in a computer system: random sets, fuzzy sets, and beyond: an overview. Int J Gen Syst. 2014;43:586–609.
24. Unal Y, Polat K, Kocer HE. Pairwise FCM based feature weighting for improved classification of vertebral column disorders. Comput Biol Med. 2014;46:61–70.
25. Herrera PJ, Dorado J, Riberio A. A novel approach for weed type classification based on shape descriptors and a fuzzy decision-making method. Sensors (Basel). 2014;14:15304–24.
26. Brorson S, Olsen BS, Frich LH, Jensen SL, Sørensen AK, Krogsgaard M, et al. Surgeons agree more on treatment recommendations than on classification of proximal humeral fractures. BMC Musculoskelet Disord. 2012;13:114.
27. Audige L, Bhandari M, Kellam J. How reliable are reliability studies of fracture classifications? A systematic review of their methodologies. Acta Orthop Scand. 2004;75:184–94.

7

Incidence of distal radius fracture surgery in Finns aged 50 years or more between 1998 and 2016 – too many patients are yet operated on?

Teemu P. Hevonkorpi[1,3*], Antti P. Launonen[1], Tuomas T. Huttunen[2], Pekka Kannus[3,4], Seppo Niemi[4] and Ville M. Mattila[1,3,5]

Abstract

Background: Although optimal treatment of distal radius fractures is controversial, surgery has gained popularity. The purpose of this study was to evaluate recent trends in the surgical treatment of distal radius fractures in Finns aged 50 years or more.

Methods: A nationwide hospital discharge register-based study was conducted among all patients 50 years of age or older who had a surgically treated distal radius fracture in Finland between 1998 and 2016. The number and rate of different surgical procedures were calculated per 100,000 person-years.

Results: Altogether 21,965 surgically treated distal radius fractures were identified. During the study period the rate of percutaneous pinning and external fixation diminished while the rate of plate fixation significantly increased. The rate of operative treatment increased continually from 1998 to 2008 whereupon the peak of the incidence was achieved. After 2008, the rate of operative treatment of distal radius fracture remained quite constant, ranging between 61.1 and 67.8 per 100,000 person-years.

Conclusions: Plate fixation has almost completely replaced both external fixation and percutaneous pinning in the surgical treatment of distal radius fractures in Finland. Despite growing evidence for less invasive treatment options in elderly patients, operative treatment of distal radius fracture is still rather popular today.

Keywords: Distal radius, Epidemiology, Surgical treatment, Volar plating, Forearm fractures

Background

Distal radius fracture (DRF) is the most common fall-related fracture [1, 2]. Its incidence peaks in children less than 15 years of age and in adults after the age of 50 [2]. Women have a greater risk of sustaining a distal radius fracture than men. In a Swedish population-based study, the incidence of DRF was 390 per 100,000 person-years in women and 120 per 100,000 person-years in men, giving a female to male ratio of 3.3:1 [3]. The overall incidence of DRFs in adults varies between 100 to 300 per 100,000 person-years [2–4]. Concerning secular trends, recent studies from Sweden, the Netherlands and Austria show that the incidence of DRFs has stabilized [5–8].

Even though non-operative treatment is still the most common treatment option for distal radius fractures, many investigators have reported about increase in the surgical activity [7, 9, 10]. In a Medicare patient cohort in the U.S.A., Chung and co-workers observed a trend of a decreasing rate of non-operative treatment. Coincidental with the change, the rate of open reduction and internal fixation increased and the rate of percutaneous approaches decreased [10]. These changes have been later confirmed by national studies in Finland (from 1998 to 2008) and Sweden (from 2004 to 2010) [7, 9]. To the best of our

* Correspondence: hevonkorpi.teemu.p@student.uta.fi
[1]Department of Orthopedics and Trauma Surgery, Tampere University Hospital, Tampere, Finland
[3]School of Medicine, University of Tampere, Tampere, Finland

knowledge, no national level epidemiological data on operative treatment of DRFs has been reported thereafter.

The trend towards open reduction and internal fixation (ORIF), mainly by volar locked plating, occurred internationally despite a lack of strong evidence to support its use. Recent high quality studies have shown that volar locked plating does not yield superior results over other surgical techniques after one-year follow-up [11–18]. In some studies, volar locked plating has been found to have advantages in comparison to external fixation and percutaneous pinning in the early rehabilitation period [13, 15, 17]. Long term results show, however, no difference between the methods [16, 18]. In addition, in the older age groups, non-surgical treatment seems to result in as good functional outcome as surgical treatment, however, with a lower rate of complications [11, 19].

The purpose of this study was to investigate recent trends in the incidence of DRF surgery in Finns aged 50 years or more and to assess to what extent these trends reflect current best evidence. We also examined the incidences of various types of surgical treatments performed for DRFs in patients aged 50 years or more.

Methods

To study the changes in the rates of different surgical techniques of the distal radius fractures over time we studied all persons 50 years of age and older in Finland between the 1st of January 1998 and 31st of December 2016. The distal radius fracture surgery data was obtained from the Finnish National Hospital Discharge Register (NHDR), which is an electronic hospital data registry containing variables such as personal identification number, sex, domicile, external cause of injury, diagnoses, and all surgical procedures performed during the hospital stay. The NHDR is mandatory for all hospitals in Finland including all private and public hospitals. The NHDR has been widely used in epidemiological research and the quality of the register is reportedly excellent [20, 21]. As a register-based blinded analysis, the study did not have identifiable individual participants and thus neither informed consent nor ethics approval was needed.

All Finnish adults aged 50 or older who underwent a surgical procedure for a distal radius fracture (ICD-10 code S52.5 or 52.6) were included. To analyse the rates of different surgical techniques the procedures were categorised into three groups according to the Nomesco (Nordic Medico-Statistical Committee) procedural classification: percutaneous pinning (procedural codes NCJ64 and NDJ64), external fixation (procedural codes NCJ70 and NDJ70), and plate fixation (NCJ62 and NDJ62). The NHDR does not include laterality of the fracture and thus in this study we included only the first distal radius fracture operation of each patient.

The main outcome variable was the number of patients who had a certain surgical procedure (pinning, external fixation or plate fixation) for a distal radius fracture. To calculate the population-based rates of surgical treatment, the annual population statistics were obtained from the Official Statistics of Finland [22], a statutory, computer-based population register of the country. In 1998, there were 5.15 million inhabitants in Finland of which 1.67 million (32,4%) were aged 50 years or more. The population structure in Finland has changed towards older so that in 2016 there were 5.50 million inhabitants of which 2.25 million (40,9%) were at least 50 years old. As the distal radius fractures (per 100,000 person-years) were based on the entire 50-year-old or older population of Finland between 1998 and 2016, no statistical probability estimation methods (intrinsically needed in cohort-based estimations) were used. This was in full accordance with our previous nationwide studies [9, 23].

Results

A total of 21,965 DRFs in patients aged 50 years or more were treated surgically in Finland between 1998 and 2016. There were 3,916 (17.8 %) men and 18,049 (82.2 %) women. Open reduction with plate fixation was the most common technique in the operative treatment of distal radius fractures (*n*=12,108, 55.1%), followed by external fixation (*n*=8,020, 36.5%) and percutaneous pinning (*n*=1,837, 8.4%) (Fig. 1).

A marked change in the type of surgical fixation occurred during the study period as external fixation was replaced by open reduction and plate fixation as the most common procedure. After a moderate increase in the early 2000s there was a nearly six-fold increase in the incidence of plate fixation between 2004 and 2008, after which the rate of increase started to slow down. The incidence of operative treatment in women altered between 58.3 to 112.4 per 100,000 person-years being considerably higher than in men (13.6 to 28.5) during the study period. In men the rate of plating increased quite similarly in all age groups (Fig. 2) whereas in older women a striking increase in plating occurred after 2004 (Fig. 3). The peak of the incidence of ORIF occurred in 2013. Between 2013-2014 the incidence of plate fixations declined from 59.1 to 52.7 per 100,000 person-years. The decline was observed in women of all age groups, whereas in men the decline was observed only in patients aged 50 to 59. After 2014, the incidence of ORIF has increased moderately but continually, yet remaining below the peak incidence of 2013. Coincidental with the overall increase in the rate of plate fixation, a decrease in the rate of the two other surgical techniques, mainly external fixation, was observed.

The overall activity of operative treatment of DRFs reached its peak in 2008 (73.3 per 100.000 person-years).

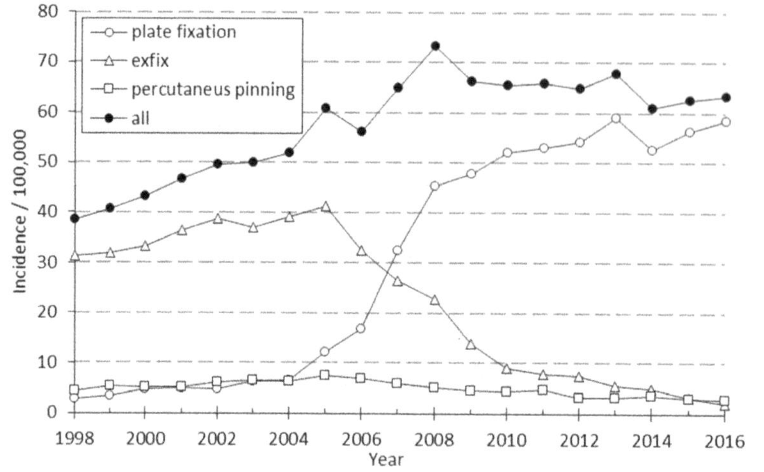

Fig. 1 The incidence of surgical techniques used in the treatment of DRF in 50-year-old or older Finns between 1998 and 2016

After that the incidence of external fixation has diminished year by year (from 22.9 in 2008 to 2.1 in 2016), thus stabilizing the increase in the use of ORIF. Between 2009 and 2016 the overall incidence of operative treatment of DRFs has remained rather stable, varying between 61.1 and 67.8 (Fig. 4).

Discussion

The main finding of the present study was that despite emerging evidence supporting non-operative treatment methods of distal radius fractures in elderly patients, the operative activity of this common injury has remained notably high in older adults.

The increase in operative activity seemed to arise primarily from the increased activity of ORIF and simultaneous decrease in percutaneous fixation and especially external fixation. The change occurred quickly and without clear support of scientific evidence [11, 19]. Interestingly, the increase in surgical activity seemed to result mainly from the increased rate of surgical treatment of older women. In men the changes were more moderate. Incidence ratio of surgical treatment between women and men varied from 3.2:1 to 4.6:1 during the study period. Assuming that incidence ratio of the DRF has remained in approximately 3.3:1 in Northern Countries [3], women are operated to a slightly greater extent.

It has been previously reported that there has been a significant increase in operative activity, especially in volar locked plating, in the treatment of distal radius fracture [5, 7, 9, 10]. However, in our study we noticed the rate of operative treatment to stabilize after 2008. Nevertheless, despite the stabilization of the overall incidence of operative treatment, the number of DRF operations in older men and women has remained notably high. Even though volar locked plate fixation may result in better anatomical reduction compared to percutaneous techniques or non-operative treatment, we may anticipate that anatomical restoration does

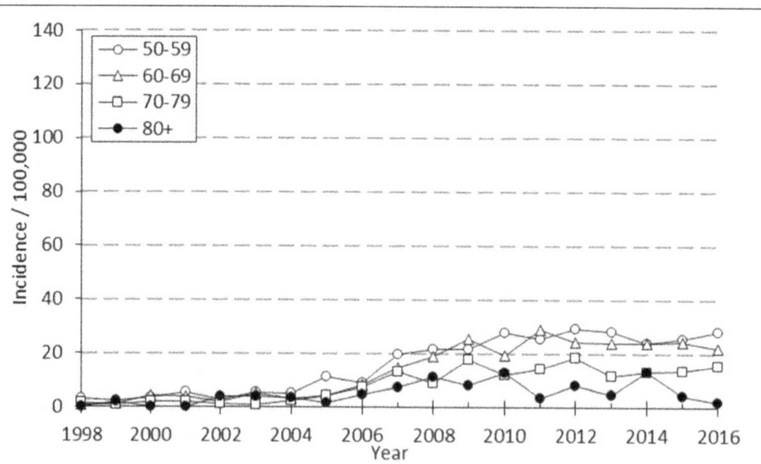

Fig. 2 The annual incidence of plate fixation by age in 50-year-old or older Finnish men between 1998 and 2016

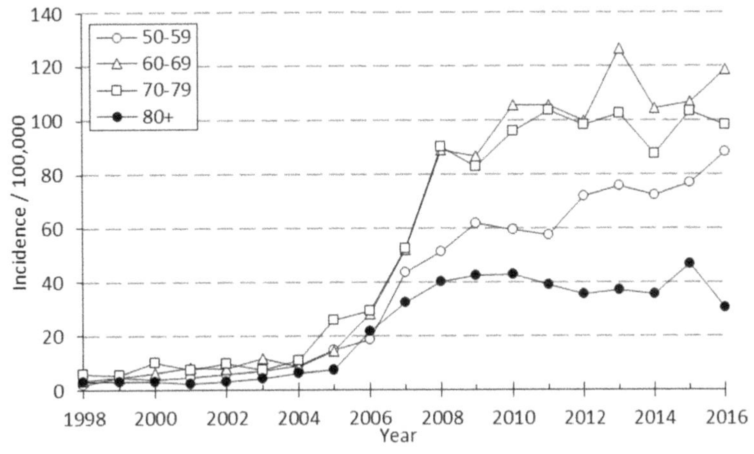

Fig. 3 The annual incidence of plate fixation by age in 50-year-old or older Finnish women between 1998 and 2016

not automatically yield good functional outcome in elderly people [15, 17].

In a previous study, Koval and co-workers reported of a decreasing trend of percutaneous techniques in the treatment of distal radius fractures among younger orthopaedic surgeons in the United States [24]. In a selected Medicare patient cohort, Chung et. al. observed a decreasing trend of closed treatment and an increase in the surgical management of distal radius fractures. They also noted a trend towards ORIF [10]. Similar findings have been reported from Finland, Sweden and the Netherlands [5, 7, 9]. In this study, we also noticed this significant increase in incidence of operative treatment of DRFs (from 38.5 per 100,000 person-years in 1998 to 63.4 per 100,000 person-years in 2016). At the same time, it seems that the total incidence of distal radius fracture has stabilized or even decreased, according to studies by de Putter et al., Dimai et al. and Wilcke and colleagues [5, 7, 8]. Put together, these findings suggest that nowadays orthopaedic surgeons lean towards surgery in the treatment of distal radius fractures. This is of interest since there is no high-quality scientific evidence that warrants increased surgical activity in the treatment of elderly people's distal radius factures [11, 19]. In fact, there is one randomized controlled trial supporting non-operative treatment of the distal radius fracture in the older age groups [11].

Unfortunately, the NHDR does not include laterality of the fracture and thus in this study we included only the first distal radius fracture operation of each patient. It is possible that same patient has had a contralateral distal radius fracture later on which has also been treated operatively. However, we consider that cases like this are infrequent and are unlikely to affect the results and conclusions of our study. In addition, nationwide incidence of distal radius fractures in Finland is not known since only patients treated operatively or hospitalised due to distal radius fracture are included in the NHDR.

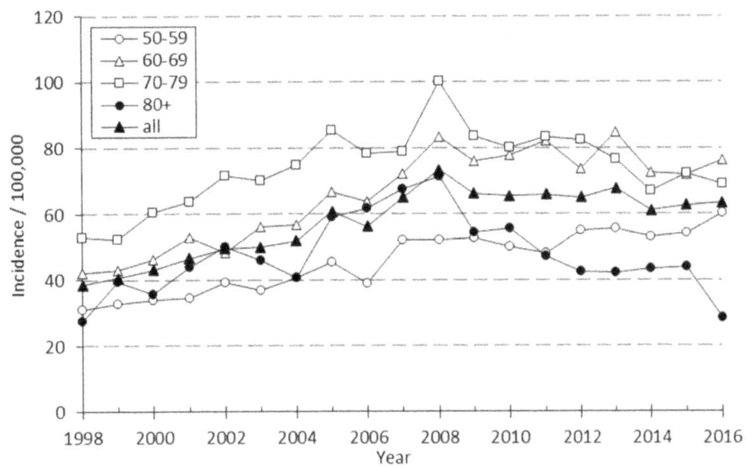

Fig. 4 The annual incidence of surgical treatment of DRF by age in 50-year-old or older Finns between 1998 and 2016

However, a previously published population-based study from Sweden showed that the incidence of distal radius fractures has not changed markedly during recent years [7]. Thus, we propose that the more pronounced incidence changes observed in the present study are unlikely to be explained by variations in DRF incidence alone. Smaller fluctuations in DRF surgery incidence, such as the 2008 peak or the decline after 2013, may well be related to the number of DRFs sustained by the population.

Conclusions

In Finland plate fixation has almost completely replaced both external fixation and percutaneous pinning in the surgical treatment of distal radius fractures. The observed change, which has occurred especially in the older age groups, is not in line with the best available evidence on optimal treatment of distal radius fractures. As various surgical treatment methods and conservative treatment produce rather similar functional results, we should be critical in the use of volar locked plate fixation in the treatment of older adults' DRFs. According to our results, current Finnish practice patterns in treating DRFs do not reflect the best available and most recent evidence. This should prompt a revision of the current Finnish Clinical Practice Guidelines on the treatment of DRFs.

Abbreviations

DRF: Distal radius fracture; ICD: International Classification of Diseases; NHDR: National Hospital Discharge Register; Nomesco: Nordic Medico-Statistical Committee; ORIF: Open reduction and internal fixation

Acknowledgements

Not applicable.

Funding

No external funding was received for the study.

Authors' contributions

TPH: main investigator, acquisition of the data, data analysis, interpretation of data, and writing of the manuscript. AL: design of the study, interpretation of data, and critical revision of the manuscript. TTH: design of the study, analysis of the data, interpretation of data, and critical revision of the manuscript. PK: design of the study, interpretation of data, and critical revision of the manuscript. SN: acquisition of the data, data analysis, and critical revision of the manuscript. VM: design of the study, acquisition of the data, interpretation of data, and critical revision of the manuscript. All authors have read and approved the final manuscript.

Consent for publication

Not applicable.

Competing interests

Teemu Hevonkorpi, Antti Launonen, Tuomas Huttunen, Pekka Kannus, Seppo Niemi and Ville Mattila declare that they have no conflicts of interest.

Author details

[1]Department of Orthopedics and Trauma Surgery, Tampere University Hospital, Tampere, Finland. [2]Department of Anesthesia, Tampere University Hospital, Tampere, Finland. [3]School of Medicine, University of Tampere, Tampere, Finland. [4]Injury & Osteoporosis Research Center, UKK Institute for Health Promotion Research, Tampere, Finland. [5]Department of Clinical Science, Intervention and Technology, Karolinska Institutet, Division of Orthopedics and Biotechnology, Karolinska Institutet and Department of Orthopedics at Karolinska University Hospital, Karolinska Institutet, Solna and Huddinge, Sweden.

References

1. Court-Brown CM, Clement ND, Duckworth AD, Biant LC, McQueen MM. The changing epidemiology of fall-related fractures in adults. Injury. 2017; https://doi.org/10.1016/j.injury.2017.02.021.
2. Court-Brown CM, Caesar B. Epidemiology of adult fractures: A review. Injury. 2006;37(8):691–7.
3. Brogren E, Petranek M, Atroshi I. Incidence and characteristics of distal radius fractures in a southern Swedish region. BMC Musculoskelet Disord. 2007;8:48.
4. Flinkkila T, Sirnio K, Hippi M, Hartonen S, Ruuhela R, Ohtonen P, Hyvonen P, Leppilahti J. Epidemiology and seasonal variation of distal radius fractures in Oulu. Finland. Osteoporos Int. 2011;22(8):2307–12.
5. de Putter CE, Selles RW, Polinder S, Hartholt KA, Looman CW, Panneman MJ, Verhaar JA, Hovius SE, van Beeck EF. Epidemiology and health-care utilisation of wrist fractures in older adults in The Netherlands, 1997-2009. Injury. 2013;44(4):421–6.
6. Mellstrand-Navarro C, Pettersson HJ, Tornqvist H, Ponzer S. The operative treatment of fractures of the distal radius is increasing: results from a nationwide Swedish study. Bone Joint J. 2014;96-B(7):963–9.
7. Wilcke MK, Hammarberg H, Adolphson PY. Epidemiology and changed surgical treatment methods for fractures of the distal radius: a registry analysis of 42,583 patients in Stockholm County, Sweden, 2004-2010. Acta Orthop. 2013;84(3):292–6.
8. Dimai HP, Svedbom A, Fahrleitner-Pammer A, Resch H, Muschitz C, Thaler H, Szivak M, Amrein K, Borgstrom F. Epidemiology of distal forearm fractures in Austria between 1989 and 2010. Osteoporos Int. 2014;25(9):2297–306.
9. Mattila VM, Huttunen TT, Sillanpaa P, Niemi S, Pihlajamaki H, Kannus P. Significant change in the surgical treatment of distal radius fractures: a nationwide study between 1998 and 2008 in Finland. J Trauma. 2011;71(4): 939–42. discussion 942-3
10. Chung KC, Shauver MJ, Birkmeyer JD. Trends in the United States in the treatment of distal radial fractures in the elderly. J Bone Joint Surg Am. 2009;91(8):1868–73.
11. Arora R, Lutz M, Deml C, Krappinger D, Haug L, Gabl M. A prospective randomized trial comparing nonoperative treatment with volar locking plate fixation for displaced and unstable distal radial fractures in patients sixty-five years of age and older. J Bone Joint Surg Am. 2011;93(23):2146–53.
12. Egol K, Walsh M, Tejwani N, McLaurin T, Wynn C, Paksima N. Bridging external fixation and supplementary Kirschner-wire fixation versus volar locked plating for unstable fractures of the distal radius: a randomised, prospective trial. J Bone Joint Surg Br. 2008;90(9):1214–21.
13. Jeudy J, Steiger V, Boyer P, Cronier P, Bizot P, Massin P. Treatment of complex fractures of the distal radius: a prospective randomised comparison of external fixation 'versus' locked volar plating. Injury. 2012;43(2):174–9.
14. Kreder HJ, Hanel DP, Agel J, McKee M, Schemitsch EH, Trumble TE, Stephen D. Indirect reduction and percutaneous fixation versus open reduction and internal fixation for displaced intra-articular fractures of the distal radius: a randomised, controlled trial. J Bone Joint Surg Br. 2005;87(6):829–36.
15. Wilcke MK, Abbaszadegan H, Adolphson PY. Wrist function recovers more rapidly after volar locked plating than after external fixation but the outcomes are similar after 1 year. Acta Orthop. 2011;82(1):76–81.
16. Gradl G, Gradl G, Wendt M, Mittlmeier T, Kundt G, Jupiter JB. Non-bridging external fixation employing multiplanar K-wires versus volar locked plating for dorsally displaced fractures of the distal radius. Arch Orthop Trauma Surg. 2013;133(5):595–602.

17. Karantana A, Downing ND, Forward DP, Hatton M, Taylor AM, Scammell BE, Moran CG, Davis TR. Surgical treatment of distal radial fractures with a volar locking plate versus conventional percutaneous methods: a randomized controlled trial. J Bone Joint Surg Am. 2013;95(19):1737–44.
18. Costa ML, Achten J, Parsons NR, Rangan A, Griffin D, Tubeuf S, Lamb SE, DRAFFT Study Group. Percutaneous fixation with Kirschner wires versus volar locking plate fixation in adults with dorsally displaced fracture of distal radius: randomised controlled trial. BMJ. 2014;349:g4807.
19. Lutz K, Yeoh KM, MacDermid JC, Symonette C, Grewal R. Complications associated with operative versus nonsurgical treatment of distal radius fractures in patients aged 65 years and older. J Hand Surg Am. 2014;39(7): 1280–6.
20. Huttunen TT, Kannus P, Pihlajamaki H, Mattila VM. Pertrochanteric fracture of the femur in the Finnish National Hospital Discharge Register: validity of procedural coding, external cause for injury and diagnosis. BMC Musculoskelet Disord. 2014;15:98–2474. 15-98
21. Sund R. Quality of the Finnish Hospital Discharge Register: a systematic review. Scand J Public Health. 2012;40(6):505–15.
22. Official Statistics of Finland (OSF). Official Statistics of Finland (OSF): Population structure [e-publication]. ISSN=1797-5395. Helsinki: Statistics Finland [referred: 3.9.2016]. Access method: http://pxnet2.stat.fi/PXWeb/pxweb/fi/StatFin/StatFin__vrm__vaerak/?tablelist=true&rxid=4890b256-f984-4cb7-b74f-bd55a47ab9c5.
23. Huttunen TT, Kannus P, Rolf C, Fellander-Tsai L, Mattila VM. Acute achilles tendon ruptures: incidence of injury and surgery in Sweden between 2001 and 2012. Am J Sports Med. 2014;42(10):2419–23.
24. Koval KJ, Harrast JJ, Anglen JO, Weinstein JN. Fractures of the distal part of the radius. The evolution of practice over time. Where's the evidence? J Bone Joint Surg Am. 2008;90(9):1855–61.

8

Impairment of early fracture healing by skeletal muscle trauma is restored by FK506

Brady J. Hurtgen[1], Beth E. P. Henderson[1], Catherine L. Ward[1], Stephen M. Goldman[1], Koyal Garg[1], Todd O. McKinley[2], Sarah M. Greising[1], Joseph C. Wenke[1] and Benjamin T. Corona[1*]

Abstract

Background: Heightened local inflammation due to muscle trauma or disease is associated with impaired bone regeneration.

Methods: We hypothesized that FK506, an FDA approved immunomodulatory compound with neurotrophic and osteogenic effects, will rescue the early phase of fracture healing which is impaired by concomitant muscle trauma in male (~4 months old) Lewis rats. FK506 (1 mg/kg; i.p.) or saline was administered systemically for 14 days after an endogenously healing tibia osteotomy was created and fixed with an intermedullary pin, and the overlying tibialis anterior (TA) muscle was either left uninjured or incurred volumetric muscle loss injury (6 mm full thickness biopsy from middle third of the muscle).

Results: The salient observations of this study were that 1) concomitant TA muscle trauma impaired recovery of tibia mechanical properties 28 days post-injury, 2) FK506 administration rescued the recovery of tibia mechanical properties in the presence of concomitant TA muscle trauma but did not augment mechanical recovery of an isolated osteotomy (no muscle trauma), 3) T lymphocytes and macrophage presence within the traumatized musculature were heightened by trauma and attenuated by FK506 3 days post-injury, and 4) T lymphocyte but not macrophage presence within the fracture callus were attenuated by FK506 at 14 days post-injury. FK506 did not improve TA muscle isometric torque production

Conclusion: Collectively, these findings support the administration of FK506 to ameliorate healing of fractures with severe muscle trauma comorbidity. The results suggest one potential mechanism of action is a reduction in local T lymphocytes within the injured musculoskeletal tissue, though other mechanisms to include direct osteogenic effects of FK506 require further investigation.

Keywords: Adaptive immune response, Composite injury, Inflammation, Immunomodulation, Musculoskeletal, Open fracture, Orthopaedic trauma, Skeletal muscle injury, Volumetric muscle loss, Tacrolimus

Background

Approximately 5 – 50% of open fractures present either delayed or non-union depending on injury severity and location, and patient characteristics [1, 2]. The concomitant loss of surrounding muscle tissue has been associated with poor healing outcomes in open fracture patients [2, 3] and experimentally confirmed in animal models [4, 5]. There are likely multiple mechanisms by which severe trauma to the surrounding musculature may impair fracture healing, to include impaired revascularization, loss of muscle-derived stem cells that support bone regeneration, and alteration of the local milieu of muscle-derived growth factors and myokines [6, 7]. However, heightened and prolonged immune responses are inherent to trauma [8] and are a principle mediator of musculoskeletal healing. It is therefore plausible that

* Correspondence: benjamin.t.corona.civ@mail.mil; corona.benjamin.t@gmail.com
[1]Extremity Trauma and Regenerative Medicine Task Area, US Army Institute of Surgical Research, 3698 Chambers Pass, BHT1, Fort Sam Houston, TX 78234, USA

severe muscle trauma compounds the local immune response and thereby impairs fracture healing.

We recently described the recruitment of $CD4^+$ (helper) and $CD8^+$ (cytotoxic) T lymphocytes to both damaged muscle and fracture callus following complex musculoskeletal injury [4]. The recruitment of T lymphocytes was amplified through 28 days post-injury in comparison to a simple fracture and was associated with impaired healing [4]. $CD4^+$and $CD8^+$ T lymphocytes are key components of the adaptive immune system and have been shown to regulate musculoskeletal tissue degeneration and repair [9, 10]. However, depletion studies also implicate lymphocytes as deleterious to fracture repair [11]. For instance, $CD4^+$ T cells can negatively influence the receptor activator of NF-kB-ligand/receptor activator of NF-kB/osteoprotegerin (RANKL/RANK/OPG) osteoclastogenesis pathway by activating stromal cells via cytokines and CD40-CD40L interactions and by activating bone destructing osteoclasts through the production of cytokines (RANKL and IL-17) [12]. $CD8^+$ T cells may also negatively influence fracture healing [13], however exact mechanisms are not well defined. Altogether, the activation, polarization, differentiation, and magnitude of specific T cell functions are influenced by the complexity of injury and may be both beneficial and detrimental for musculoskeletal regeneration.

Therapeutically targeting T lymphocytes is an attractive strategy to restore fracture healing following severe musculoskeletal trauma. A viable tool is FK506 (Tacrolimus) because it both directly and indirectly inhibits T cell mediated immune responses [14]. Tacrolimus is an FDA approved macrolide that inhibits IL-2 dependent T cell activation by inhibiting enzymatic activity of calcineurin and subsequent translocation of transcription factor nuclear factor of activated T cells (NFAT) [14]. FK506 is also effective in reducing gene expression of pro-inflammatory, but not anti-inflammatory cytokines [14] and therefore potentially promotes T helper 2 (Th2) versus T helper 1 (Th1) responses. Moreover, FK506 has been shown to directly mediate osteogenic differentiation of mesenchymal stem cells in vitro [15], and therefore may augment challenged fracture healing in vivo [16]. FK506 also has neurotrophic properties that may improve functional recovery of the traumatized musculature [17]. That being said, the treatment of simple fractures or rhBMP-2 treated segmental defects with systemic administration of FK506 did not augment fracture healing [16, 18]. However, it remains plausible that fracture healing impaired by compounding inflammation secondary to concomitant muscle trauma (i.e., open fracture) [4] may be rescued by FK506.

In the current study, we primarily tested the hypothesis that systemic FK506 administration improves the recovery of mechanical strength of fractured tibia when accompanied by comorbid muscle trauma using an established rat model of open fracture [4]. As a putative mechanism, the effect of FK506 administration on the innate and adaptive immune responses in the injured bone and muscle were evaluated.

Methods

Animals

All protocols and animal care guidelines were approved (A14-033) by the Institutional Animal Care and Use Committee at the United States Army Institute of Surgical Research. All components were conducted in compliance with the Animal Welfare Act, the Implementing Animal Welfare Regulations and in accordance with the principles of the Guide for the Care and Use of Laboratory Animals. Inbred male Lewis rats (350-400 g; ~4 months of age) were purchased from Harlan Laboratories and housed in a specific pathogen-free animal facility. All rats received a pre-surgical (~30 min prior) administration of buprenorphine-SR (1.2 mg/kg; s.c.) for pain management and a post-surgical x-ray was taken to ensure proper fracture fixation. All animals were euthanized while heavily sedated, by injection of Fatal Plus (sodium pentobarbital, 150 mg/kg; intracardiac).

Experimental design

Volumetric muscle loss (VML) injury has previously been shown to impair endogenous healing of rat tibia non-segmental osteotomy (OST) [4] and BMP-2 mediated healing of a segmental defect (SD) in the rat tibia [19] and femur [5]. The current work was designed to determine if the immunomodulatory compound, FK506, restores the early phase of recovery of tibia mechanical properties during endogenous bone regeneration of impaired fracture healing.

Male Lewis rats underwent surgical creation of an endogenously healing tibia osteotomy (OST) with or without concomitant ipsilateral tibialis anterior (TA) muscle VML injury (OST + VML). Briefly, the OST was performed approximately 5 mm proximal to the tibia-fibula junction and stabilized with a 1.25 mm Kirschner pin inserted in the medullary cavity from the tibial plateau [4]. VML injury was surgically created in the middle third of the adjacent TA muscle using a punch biopsy (6 mm), as we have reported previously [20, 21]. X-rays were acquired with 3 days post-injury to ensure adequate tibia stabilization. Injured rats were allotted randomly to systemic saline or FK506 treatment groups. FK506 (1 mg/kg; Sigma-Aldrich) was administered in sterile saline by daily injection (i.p.) beginning immediately after surgery and for 14 days post-injury, during the primary period post-injury when the musculoskeletal immune response is exacerbated in this model [4]. This dosage of FK506 has previously been shown to induce a therapeutic concentration of FK506 systemically [18].

Rats were followed out to 28 days post-injury, at which time musculoskeletal physiological and mechanical assessments were performed (n = 6-8/group; Statistical power (1-ß) was approximately 0.7). Previous reports using this and similar models have indicated that at this time post-injury fracture healing is not fully resolved, permitting observations of an impaired rate of healing by concomitant VML injury [4, 22, 23]. To determine if FK506 attenuated the cellular immune response in OST + VML, muscles samples were harvested at 3 days post-injury for flow cytometric analysis (n = 4/group). Additionally, tibiae were collected at 3 and 14 days post-injury, in a follow-on analysis for quantitative immunohistological analyses (n = 3/group; Fig. 1).

Bone mechanical testing

Three-point bending was performed on a set of rat tibiae at 28 days post-injury, using methods previously described [4]. Load-deflection curves were used to obtain maximum load and stiffness.

Muscle functional assessment

In vivo functional testing of TA muscles was performed at 28 days post-injury using methodology previously described [20, 21, 24]. Briefly, TA muscle in vivo physiological properties were measured in anesthetized rats (isoflurane 1.5 – 2.0%) using a dual-mode muscle lever system (Aurora Scientific, Inc., Mod. 305b). Subcutaneous needle electrodes were inserted in the posterior compartment of the lower limb on each side of the common peroneal nerve. Optimal voltage (2 – 5 V) was set with a series of tetanic contractions (5 – 10 contractions; 150 Hz, 0.1 ms pulse width, 400 ms train). Then, a skin incision was made at the antero-lateral aspect of the ankle and the distal tendons of the extensor digitorum longus and extensor hallicus longus muscles was isolated and severed above the retinaculum [20]. TA muscle maximal isometric tetanic torque was measured (150 Hz) with the ankle at a right angle.

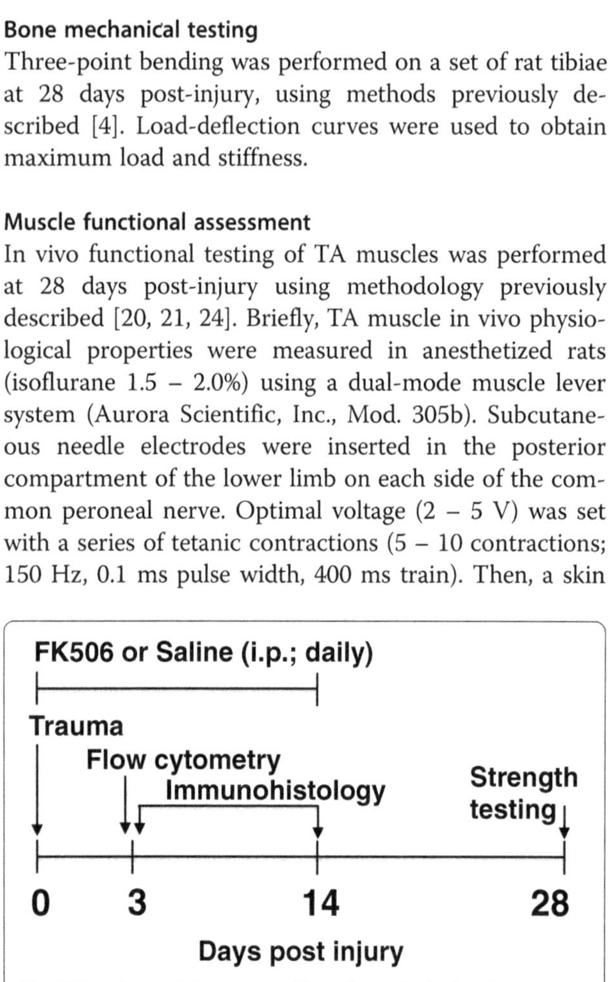

Fig. 1 Experimental time course. The schematic depicts the therapeutic regimen (FK506 or saline) and experimental assays carried out over the course of 28 days post OST + VML. Trauma consisting of OST + VML was generated at day 0. FK506 or saline control was administered daily by the intraperitoneal route from day 0 to day 14 following injury. At 3 days post-injury, flow cytometry and immunohistochemical analysis of damaged muscle and adjacent fracture region was carried out, immunohistochemical analysis was also analyzed at 14 days post-injury. At 28 days post-trauma strength testing assays of bone and muscle were carried out

Cellular isolation from muscle tissue

Cells were isolated from the middle third of the TA muscle that encompassed the muscle defect by enzymatic digestion as previously described [4]. Briefly, the defect was surgically isolated and the mass was determined. Tissue was incubated with collagenase type II and dispase for 90 min at 37 °C. Cells were further released by gentle mechanical disruption and filtered through a 70 μm cell strainer. Erythrocytes were lysed with ammonium-chloride-potassium lysing buffer and cells were filtered through a 40 μm cell strainer washed, and resuspended in PBS containing 0.5% FBS and 0.1% sodium azide. Viable cells were quantified using trypan blue exclusion and a hemocytometer.

Quantification of cellular infiltrates in muscle defect by flow cytometry

Muscle-derived cells were labeled with fluorochrome-conjugated antibodies and analyzed by flow cytometry as previously described [4]. Cells were incubated with anti-CD32 antibody to block Fc receptors and labeled with either cocktail monoclonal antibodies to identify macrophages or T lymphocytes. The macrophage (MØ) cell cocktail included anti-CD45 (clone OX-1), anti-CD11b (WT.5), anti-CD68 (ED1), anti-CD86 (24F), and anti-CD163 (ED2). The T lymphocyte cell cocktail consisted of anti-CD45, anti-CD3 (IF4), anti-CD4 (OX-35), and anti-CD8α (OX-8). Labeled cells were fixed with 1% paraformaldehyde and enumerated by fluorescence-activated cells sorting using a MACSQuant flow cytometer (Miltenyi Biotec). Data were analyzed using MACSQuantify software (Miltenyi Biotec). Gating strategies to identify cellular populations included the following: $CD45^+$ hematopoietic cells, $CD45^+CD11b^+CD68^+$ MØ, $CD45^+CD11b^+CD68^+CD86^+$ M1-like MØ, $CD45^+CD11b^+CD68^+CD163^+$ M2-like MØ, $CD45^+CD3^+CD4^+$ T helper and $CD45^+CD3^+CD8\alpha^+$ T cytotoxic lymphocytes. Cell numbers of each gated population were determined by multiplying the percentage of cells by the total number of viable cells recovered from the respective defect. All cell numbers were normalized per gram of excised muscle tissue.

Histology

Tibiae were fixed in 10% neutral buffered formalin and decalcified in a formic acid bone decalcifier (Immunocal, Decal Chemical Corp, Tallman NY) using similar methodology as previously described [4]. Samples were processed in paraffin and embedded in a longitudinal orientation. Tibiae were cut in 8 μm sections and deparafinized. Immunohistochemical (CD4, BioRad: MCA55GA, 1:100; CD8a, BD Pharmingen: 550,298, 1:100; CD68, BioRad: MCA341R, 1:200) staining was performed using standard methodology.

Bright field images were acquired with a Zeiss Axio Scan.Z1 and stitched into a large composite image. Composite images were saved separately as a 24-bit, 96 dpi color images. All images were analyzed in MetaMorph (Molecular Devices LLC., Sunnyvale CA). For display purposes only, images were produced in Keynote by down-converting, without introducing any changes in brightness or contrast. With each inflammatory marker (CD4, CD8, and CD68) the region of the callus between the bone and on the anterior aspect of the tibia was selected for analysis, care was taken to not select mineralized bone or skeletal muscle fibers (Additional file 1). The image was color thresholded (hue, saturation, and intensity) to identify individual inflammatory markers (by saturation threshold). The percentage of area covered was determined off of the area of the total selected region and were analyzed using binary images. Analyses were conducted by an investigator blinded to treatment group; in the event that multiple serial sections from a single tibia stained for the same inflammatory marker the percent area from each section was averaged and used for analysis (n = 3 rats/group/time/marker). Tibiae sections used as negative controls were used to verify analysis of inflammatory markers.

Statistics

Dependent variables were analyzed using one- or two-way ANOVA or Student's t-test. In the event of a significant ANOVA, Fisher's post-hoc testing was performed. Statistical significance was achieved at alpha of 0.05. Statistical testing was performed using Prism 6 for Mac OSX (Graphpad Inc). Data is presented as box (25 to 75 percentile with median line) and whisker (minimum and maximum response) plots.

Results

Systemic FK506 administration improves healing of fracture with concomitant VML injury but not recovery of muscle strength

Previously, the immunomodulatory drug FK506 did not improve healing of a simple femur OST without concomitant muscle trauma [18]. Herein, FK506 delivery also failed to improve healing of an isolated tibia OST, evidenced by similar mechanical properties of injured OST-only tibiae from saline or FK506-treated rats 28 days post-injury (Fig. 2a & b). However, often fracture occurs with a concomitant loss of surrounding musculature (e.g., Gustilo-Anderson type II and III open fracture), which can impair bone regeneration [4]. In a model of this clinical scenario, VML injury significantly reduced (OST + VML-saline) tibia mechanical strength (−41%; p = 0.028) and stiffness (−54%; p = 0.039) compared to OST-only groups 28 days post-injury, with 5 of 6 observations in the OST + VML-saline group having

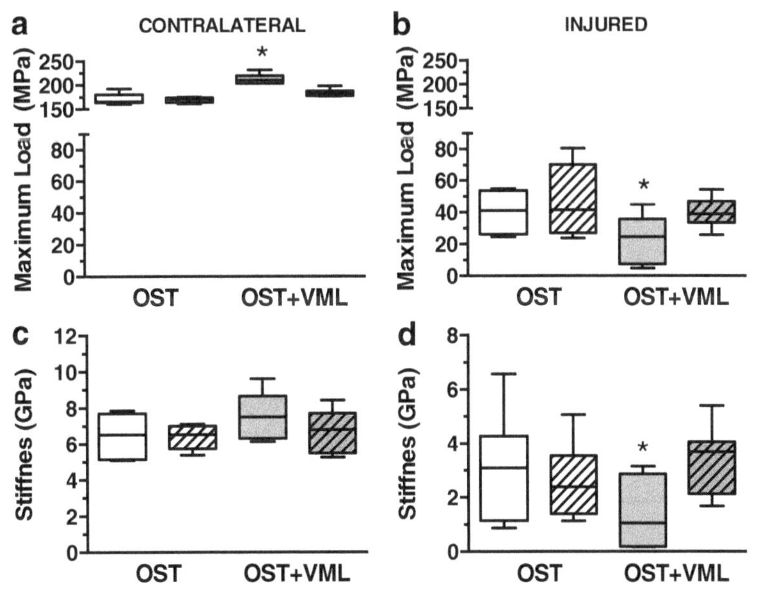

Fig. 2 Mechanical testing of bone following FK506 treatment of OST + VML injury. Three-point bending mechanical testing of (**a** & **c**) contralateral and (**b** & **d**) injured tibiae was performed at 28 days post-injury. * ≠ OST-saline & OST + VML-FK506; $p < 0.05$. Group responses are presented as box (25 to 75 percentile with median line) and whisker (minimum and maximum response) plots; n = 6-8/group

mechanical property values lesser than the median response of OST-saline (Fig. 2). Coinciding with diminished mechanical strength in the injured limb, the contralateral tibia mechanical strength was significantly increased in OST + VML treated with saline, compared to all other groups ($p < 0.001$). Notably, FK506 restored tibia mechanical properties in OST + VML rats to OST-only levels (Fig. 2b).

The effect of FK506 administration on in vivo isometric TA muscle strength was also assessed 28 days post-injury (Fig. 3). In OST-only groups, TA muscle strength was similar between saline and FK506-treated rats ($p = 0.112$). The surgical creation of VML injury (OST + VML-saline) resulted in a 33% decrease in neural-evoked isometric torque compared to OST-saline ($p < 0.001$), and FK506 administration did not ameliorate TA muscle strength deficits (OST + VML-saline vs. –FK506: $p = 0.492$).

Systemic FK506 administration modulates the immune response within VML injured muscle

VML injury induces a heightened and prolonged local pro-inflammatory immune response within the traumatized musculature that associates with impaired fracture healing [4]. To investigate the effect of systemic FK506 administration on the immune response to VML injury, first flow cytometric quantification of TA muscle infiltrating $CD45^+CD3^+CD4^+$ (T helper) and $CD45^+CD3^+CD8^+$ (T cytotoxic) lymphocytes was performed 3 days post-injury (Fig. 4a). In OST + VML groups, FK506 significantly reduced the number of $CD45^+CD3^+CD4^+$ cells by 51% ($p = 0.037$). $CD45^+CD3^+CD8^+$ cells were not significantly reduced by FK506 treatment (–43%; $p = 0.087$; Fig. 4b - d).

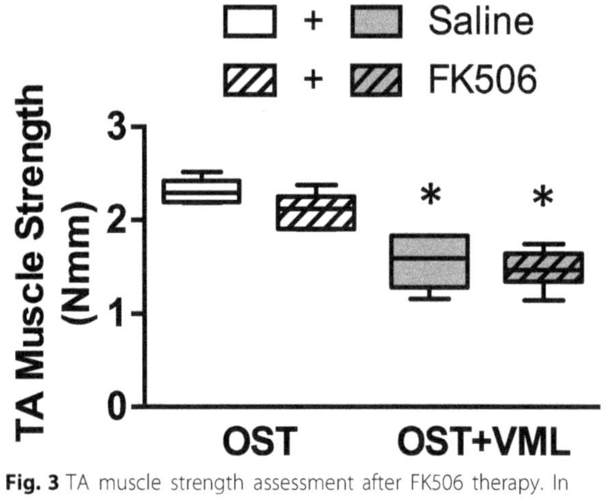

Fig. 3 TA muscle strength assessment after FK506 therapy. In vivo peak isometric tetanic torque was assessed at 28 days post-injury. *each OST + VML group < respective OST group, $p < 0.05$. Group responses are presented as box (25 to 75 percentile with median line) and whisker (minimum and maximum response) plots; n = 6-8/group

The effect of FK506 therapy on macrophage populations recruited to damaged muscle at 3 days post-injury was also investigated. Again, using flow cytometry we quantified muscle infiltrating $CD45^+$ (hematopoietic), $CD45^+CD11b^+CD68^+$ (MØ), $CD45^+CD11b^+CD68^+CD86^+$ (M1-like MØ), and $CD45^+CD11b^+CD68^+CD163^+$ (M2-like MØ) cells (Fig. 5a). FK506 reduced $CD45^+$ hematopoietic cells by 24% ($p = 0.008$) and $CD68^+$ macrophages by 22% ($p = 0.013$), but had no significant effect on M1 and M2 polarization or recruitment in comparison to saline treated animals (Fig. 5b - e).

Fracture site infiltration of T lymphocytes but not macrophages is attenuated by systemic FK506

As a potential link between heightened muscle inflammation and impaired fracture healing, it has been observed that conditions of heightened local and systemic inflammation correspondingly protract fracture site inflammation and disrupt bone regeneration [4, 25]. To further establish this relationship, the presence of $CD4^+$ and $CD8^+$ T cells and $CD68^+$ macrophages was quantified within the fracture callus at 3 and 14 days post-injury in saline or FK506-treated rats with OST + VML injury (Fig. 6). No differences in macrophage or lymphocyte markers were observed between groups during the early phase of repair at 3 days post-injury. At 14 days post-injury, the fractional area of $CD68^+$ expression was elevated in saline and FK506-treated rats compared to 3 days post-injury, but again no difference in macrophage marker presence was observed. The fractional area of both $CD4^+$ and $CD8^+$ expression was significantly elevated compared to 3 days post-injury in OST + VML treated with saline, which was significantly attenuated in FK506 treated rats (OST + VML-saline vs. -FK506: $CD4^+$ $p = 0.008$; $CD8^+$ $p = 0.001$).

Discussion

The primary finding of this study is that the FDA approved immunomodulatory drug, FK506 (Tacrolimus), improves the early recovery of tibia mechanical properties following osteotomy with concomitant severe muscle trauma (i.e., VML injury). Notably in this endogenously healing fracture model [4] and others that require rhBMP-2 treatment to recover [5, 19], VML injury impairs fracture healing and therefore the improvement in mechanical strength mediated by FK506 delivery reflects a restoration of the rate of endogenous fracture healing. These findings support the exploration of immunomodulatory therapies for augmentation of impaired fracture healing secondary to a loss of surrounding muscle tissue (e.g., type II and IIIa tibia open fracture).

In polytrauma and myopathy, heightened inflammation has been coupled with either poor fracture healing or poor bone health [25–29]. In each of these conditions,

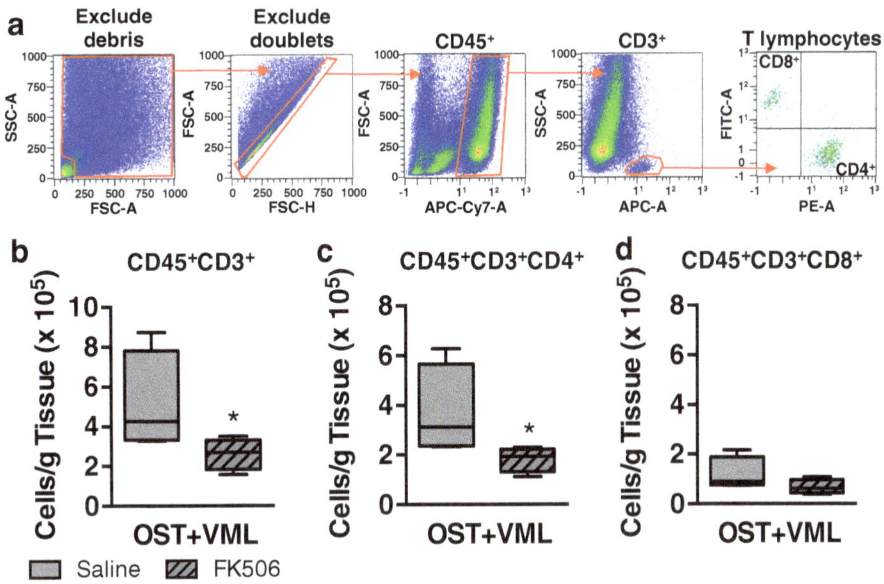

Fig. 4 Flow cytometric analysis of T lymphocytes infiltrating skeletal muscle after OST + VML treated with FK506. TA muscles were isolated from OST + VML groups treated with saline or FK506 at 3 days post-injury to evaluate immune cell infiltration by flow cytometry. The middle third region of the TA muscle was collected, digested, and cellular content was isolated. **a** Events were gated (red polygons) to eliminate debris and doublets, and cells were then gated for $CD45^+CD3^+$ T lymphocytes, $CD45^+CD3^+CD8^-CD4^+$ T helper lymphocytes, and $CD45^+CD3^+CD4^-CD8^+$ cytotoxic T lymphocytes. **b-d** Data for each cell population are normalized per gram of muscle tissue and presented as box (25 to 75 percentile with median line) and whisker (minimum and maximum response) plots; $n = 4$/group. $^*p < 0.05$

immunomodulation (i.e., macrophage or complement inhibition) has effectively improved bone healing [25, 30]. Similarly, under conditions of exacerbated inflammation, such as implantation of xenogeneic demineralized bone grafts in the abdominal musculature [31] or genetically modified xenogeneic muscle implants into femur segmental defect [16], FK506 has improved bone formation. However, previous work has shown that FK506 does not improve endogenous or rhBMP-2 mediated fracture healing without extensive muscle trauma [16, 18], which is likely because fractures without large muscle trauma do not result in excessive

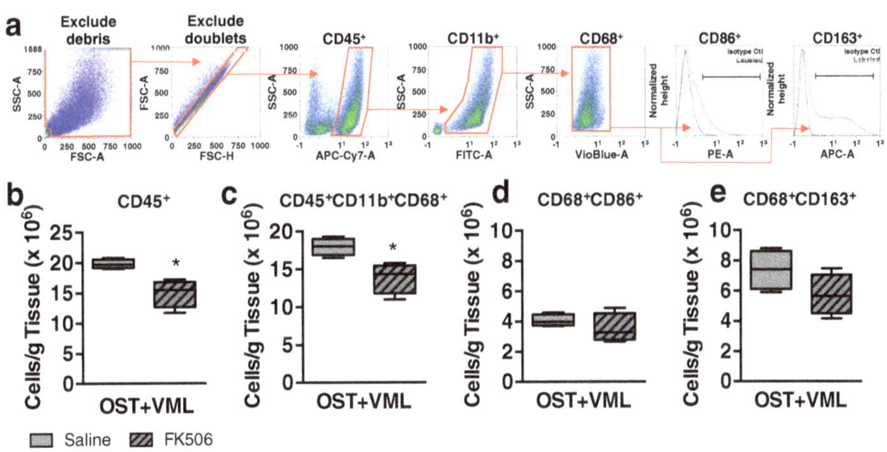

Fig. 5 Flow cytometric analysis of macrophages infiltrating skeletal muscle after OST + VML treated with FK506. TA muscles were isolated from OST + VML groups treated with saline or FK506 at 3 days post-injury to evaluate immune cell infiltration by flow cytometry. The middle third region of the TA muscle was collected, digested, and cellular content isolated. **a** Events were gated (*red polygons*) to eliminate debris and doublets, and cells were then gated for $CD45^+$ hematopoietic cells, $CD45^+CD11b^+CD68^+$ macrophages, $CD45^+CD11b^+CD68^+CD86^+$ M1-like macrophages (*black bar*), and $CD45^+CD11b^+CD68^+CD163^+$ M2-like macrophages (*black bar*); **b-e** Data for each cell population are normalized per gram of muscle tissue and presented as *box* (25 to 75 percentile with median line) and whisker (minimum and maximum response) plots; $n = 4$/group. $^*p < 0.05$

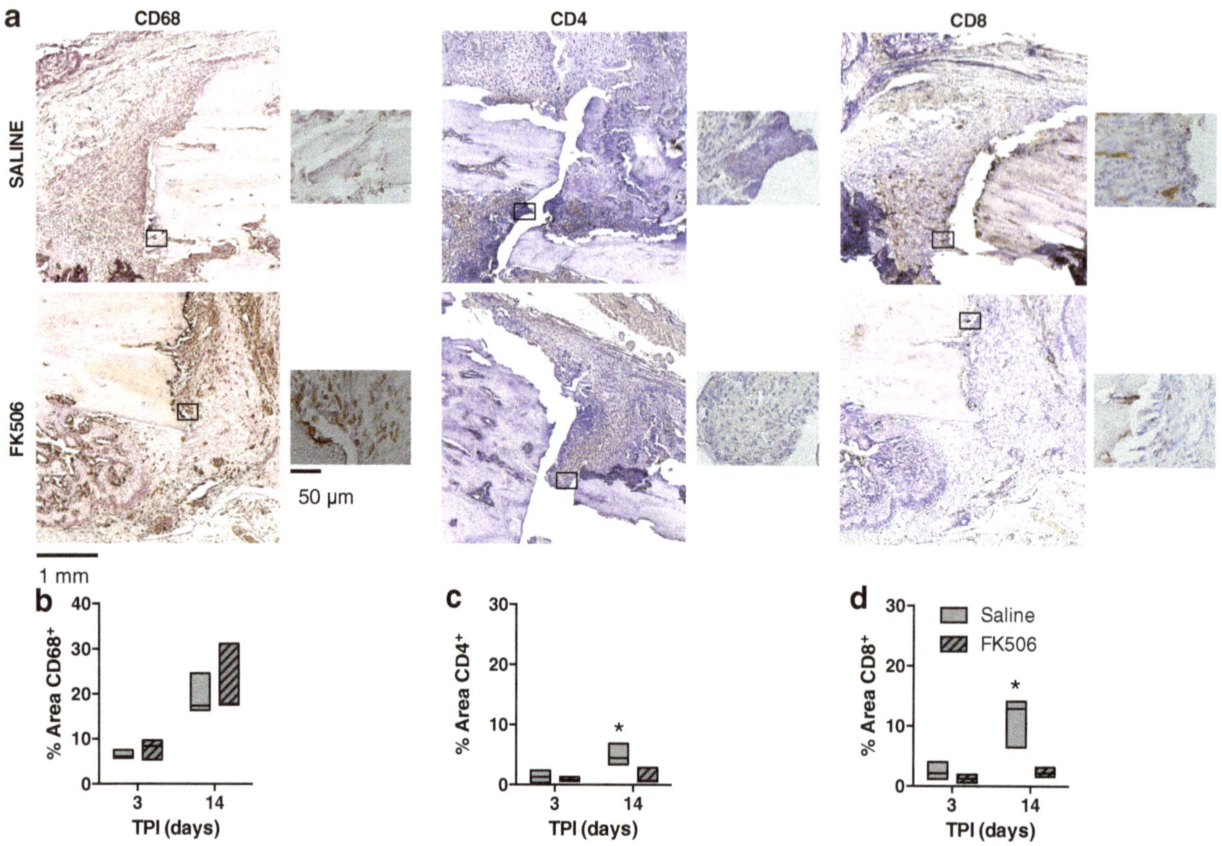

Fig. 6 Evaluation of immune cells infiltrating fracture callus of OST + VML treated with FK506 using immunohistological staining. Injured tibiae were collected at 3 and 14 days post-injury from OST + VML injured groups that received saline or FK506 treatment. Tissue was sectioned and immunohistochemical analysis was carried out to detect CD68$^+$ macrophages, CD4$^+$ T cells, and CD8$^+$ cytotoxic T cells, using horseradish peroxidase for detection. **a** Representative images from the fracture callus site for each treatment group at the 14 day time point is presented, with magnified inserts presented adjacent to image and identified by a box in the primary image. Scale bars = 1 mm and 50 µm, respectively. **b-d** The relative area of the fracture callus populated by CD68$^+$, CD4$^+$, and CD8$^+$ cells were quantified. Group responses are presented as floating box plots (minimum to maximum with median line); $n = 3$/group. * saline >3 day saline & 14 day FK506; $p < 0.05$. TPI, time post-injury

local immune responses [4]. The current findings agree with Voggenreiter et al. [18], as FK506 did not enhance healing of an osteotomy without VML injury, but go on to demonstrate that FK506 re-establishes the early recovery of mechanical properties in the presence of concomitant VML injury, which elicits exacerbated inflammation. In association with improved tibia mechanical properties, FK506 administration reduced the acute infiltration of T cells and macrophages in VML-injured musculature and T cells in the fractured bone within the first 2 weeks post-injury. These data therefore support further testing of the broad working hypotheses that: 1) VML injury prompts a heightened local immune response that disrupts fracture healing and 2) that an immunomodulatory therapy (e.g., FK506) normalizes the musculoskeletal immune response, and thereby rescues fracture healing.

While FK506 ameliorated the recovery of tibia mechanical properties, treatment did not improve neuromuscular strength after VML injury. Muscle strength deficits after VML injuries have been primarily attributed to the traumatic loss of contractile tissue [32, 33]. However, strength deficits are at least partially compounded by acute intramuscular nerve damage and it is suspected that the heightened immune response to VML injury causes secondary muscle damage. Given the well-known neurotrophic effects of FK506 [17, 34], it was therefore anticipated that FK506 administration would improve functional recovery of the remaining muscle mass. The systemic dose (1 mg/kg) used in this study was adequate to attenuate macrophage and lymphocyte infiltration within VML injured muscle, however, this dose has conflicting results regarding peripheral nerve regeneration [35, 36]. Collectively, these findings indicate that while attenuation of the heightened local immune response caused by VML injury may be beneficial to fracture healing, continued efforts are required to improve skeletal muscle regeneration and recovery of strength.

Improvement of fracture healing by FK506 was consistently associated with attenuated T lymphocyte infiltration within the traumatized muscle and bone. Given that T lymphocytes have been shown to drive the development and function of osteoclasts through the production of the pro-inflammatory cytokine IL-17 and RANKL [37], FK506 mediated attenuation of this degenerative interaction may explain the improved fracture healing. The restorative effects of FK506 on fracture healing may also occur through modulation of multiple types of immune cells. Several reports suggest FK506 modulates innate immune cells to generate reduced responses to innate stimuli [38–40]. For example, dendritic cells and macrophages pretreated with FK506 were shown to produce lower amounts of pro-inflammatory cytokines after exposure to lipopolysaccharide, a pathogen associated molecular pattern (PAMP) [38, 39]. PAMPs and damage-associated molecular patterns (DAMPs) both signal through Toll-like receptor (TLR) pathways that are damped in TLR-ligand stimulated peripheral blood mononuclear cells isolated from patients who received FK506 [40]. FK506 also affects the regulatory T (Treg) cell population, which is known to dampen pro-inflammatory immune responses [41]. It is clear that the entire T cell population is not detrimental to fracture repair but instead individual T cell subsets uniquely regulate or impair the fracture repair process [13, 42–46]. Given the myriad of cellular targets upon which FK506 may interact and general IL-2-mediated suppression of T lymphocytes by FK506, further study is required to assess whether such a broad therapeutic effect is necessary to restore fracture healing after severe musculoskeletal trauma.

We were surprised by the differential response of macrophages in the bone and muscle tissue. A previous report of *mdx* mouse pathology demonstrated a coordinated macrophage response between diseased muscle and adjacent fracture bone that corresponded with impaired fracture healing [25]. However, FK506 reduced $CD45^+$ cells, which were primarily (>90%) comprised of $CD68^+$ macrophages, in the muscle 3 days post-injury while cell numbers of this population were unchanged in the fracture site at 3 or 14 days post-injury. It is possible that the reduction of macrophages in the muscle could lead to overall reduced pro-inflammatory cytokine/chemokine levels that impact downstream wound healing events in muscle and bone. Alternatively, the activation levels of macrophages at the fracture may be reduced to allow for improved wound healing despite the cell numbers being unaltered by FK506. Further investigation is required to conclusively determine the impact of the macrophage response on fracture healing following complex musculoskeletal trauma.

It has been established that local musculature provides vascular, paracrine, mechanical, and cellular support to adjacent bone [6, 7]. The partial loss of surrounding skeletal muscle in similar rodent open fracture models indicate that associated impairment of fracture healing is not necessarily driven by deficient revascularization of the fracture [22, 23], highlighting a potential deficiency in the activity of myokines [47–49] and muscle derived stem cells [50, 51] in the support of fracture healing under these conditions. Interesting interplay between immune responses and IGF-1 signaling [52] and muscle stem cells [53] support the idea that that while controlled inflammation is beneficial to muscle-bone communication, exacerbated inflammation following severe soft tissue trauma may restrict muscle derived support of osseous regeneration and thus contribute to impaired fracture healing.

FK506 may also directly influence osteoblast and osteoclast activity [54–58] and thereby improve fracture healing. Notably, FK506 has also been shown to promote osteogenic differentiation of mesenchymal stem cells via BMP receptor signaling in vitro [15], highlighting the potential utility of this compound as an osteoinductive agent. In vivo FK506 had no effect on the quantity but improved the quality of bone formation in xenogeneic muscle graft-treated femur defect in athymic rats, potentially reflecting direct osteoblast/clast augmentation [25]. In relation to fracture healing, it is interesting that in animal models with a competent immune system, FK506 does not appear to augment endogenous or rhBMP-2 mediated bone regeneration when comorbid muscle trauma is not explicitly introduced, see Fig. 2 and [16, 18]. These findings suggest that in vivo the direct osteogenic effects of FK506 are more influential under conditions of heightened inflammation. Suffice to say that while impaired bone regeneration following open fracture can be driven by the dysregulated immune response provoked by VML injury [4], rescued fracture healing by FK506 may not be strictly related to immunomodulation.

There remain numerous questions regarding the use of FK506 or other immunomodulatory compounds for open fracture that are not addressed in this work. Notably, it is unclear whether FK506 is effective if delivered in a delayed manner, which is the likely clinical scenario. Relatedly, it is unclear if FK506 can be delivered either locally or systemically at an effective dose for musculoskeletal healing without potentiating infection. While these salient limitations are important to clinical translation, this initial study highlights the utility of FK506 in improving regeneration following complex musculoskeletal trauma.

Conclusions

In summary, the present study offers initial evidence that reduction of the dysregulated immune response triggered by complex musculoskeletal injury with FK506, an

FDA-approved drug (Tacrolimus), may play a role in rescuing impaired fractured healing; however, direct osteoinductive activity of the compound may also influence early fracture healing. In agreement with previous lymphocyte depletion studies [11], herein the data associate heightened T cell but not macrophage recruitment to the fracture site with impaired recovery of mechanical properties early during the fracture healing process. The current study also suggests that a mere attenuation of T cell infiltration within injured bone and adjacent muscle associates with improved bone healing. The results of this study highlights the potential of immunomodulatory drugs to treat orthopaedic musculoskeletal trauma and supports previous findings that the net T cell response to complex musculoskeletal injury is dysfunctional for efficient fracture healing.

Abbreviations

DAMPs: Damage-associated molecular patterns; NFAT: Nuclear factor of activated T cells; OPG: Osteoprotegrin; OST: Osteotomy; PAMP: Pathogen associated molecular pattern; RANK: Receptor activator of NF-kB; RANKL: Receptor activator of NF-kB-ligand; SD: Segmental defect; TA: Tibialis anterior; Th1: T helper 1; Th2: T helper 2; TLR: Toll-like receptor; Treg: Regulatory T cell; VML: Volumetric muscle loss

Funding

This work was supported by the United States Army Medical Research and Materiel Command, Combat Casualty Care Research Program (F_005_2015_USAISR; BTC), as well as the Orthopaedic Trauma Association (BTC & TOM).

Authors' contributions

All authors (BJH, BEPH, CLW, SMG, KG, TOM, SMG, JCW, and BTC) gave final approval of the manuscript to be published and agreed to be accountable for all aspects of the work. All authors were involved in data analysis and synthesis. BJH, CLW, BEPH, SMG, KG, SMG, and BTC performed all surgical procedures and data collection. BJH, SMG, TOM, and BTC drafted the original manuscript and all authors edited and/or approved the final draft of the manuscript.

Competing interests

The authors declare that they have no competing interests.

Consent for publication

Not applicable.

Declarations

The opinions or assertions contained herein are the private views of the authors and are not to be construed as official or as reflecting the views of the Department of the Army or the Department of Defense.

Author details

[1]Extremity Trauma and Regenerative Medicine Task Area, US Army Institute of Surgical Research, 3698 Chambers Pass, BHT1, Fort Sam Houston, TX 78234, USA. [2]Department of Orthopaedic Surgery, Indiana University School of Medicine, Indianapolis, IN, USA.

References

1. Mills LA, Simpson AH. The relative incidence of fracture non-union in the Scottish population (5.17 million): a 5-year epidemiological study. BMJ Open. 2013;3
2. Papakostidis C, Kanakaris NK, Pretel J, Faour O, Morell DJ, Giannoudis PV. Prevalence of complications of open tibial shaft fractures stratified as per the Gustilo-Anderson classification. Injury. 2011;42:1408–15.
3. Karladani AH, Granhed H, Karrholm J, Styf J. The influence of fracture etiology and type on fracture healing: a review of 104 consecutive tibial shaft fractures. Arch Orthop Trauma Surg. 2001;121:325–8.
4. Hurtgen BJ, Ward CL, Garg K, Pollot BE, Goldman SM, Mc Kinley TO, et al. Severe muscle trauma triggers heightened and prolonged local musculoskeletal inflammation and impairs adjacent tibia fracture healing. J Musculoskelet Neuronal Interact. 2016;16:122–34.
5. Willett NJ, Li MT, Uhrig BA, Boerckel JD, Huebsch N, Lundgren TL, et al. Attenuated human bone morphogenetic protein-2-mediated bone regeneration in a rat model of composite bone and muscle injury. Tissue Eng Part C Methods. 2013;19:316–25.
6. Bonewald LF, Kiel DP, Clemens TL, Esser K, Orwoll ES, O'Keefe RJ, et al. Forum on bone and skeletal muscle interactions: summary of the proceedings of an ASBMR workshop. J Bone Miner Res. 2013;28:1857–65.
7. Davis KM, Griffin KS, Chu TG, Wenke JC, Corona BT, McKinley TO, et al. Muscle-bone interactions during fracture healing. J Musculoskelet Neuronal Interact. 2015;15:1–9.
8. Evans KN, Forsberg JA, Potter BK, Hawksworth JS, Brown TS, Andersen R, et al. Inflammatory cytokine and chemokine expression is associated with heterotopic ossification in high-energy penetrating war injuries. J Orthop Trauma. 2012;26:e204–13.
9. Tidball JG, Villalta SA. Regulatory interactions between muscle and the immune system during muscle regeneration. Am J Physiol Regul Integr Comp Physiol. 2010;298:R1173–87.
10. Walsh MC, Kim N, Kadono Y, Rho J, Lee SY, Lorenzo J, et al. Osteoimmunology: interplay between the immune system and bone metabolism. Annu Rev Immunol. 2006;24:33–63.
11. Toben D, Schroeder I, El Khassawna T, Mehta M, Hoffmann JE, Frisch JT, et al. Fracture healing is accelerated in the absence of the adaptive immune system. J Bone Miner Res. 2011;26:113–24.
12. Jones D, Glimcher LH, Aliprantis AO. Osteoimmunology at the nexus of arthritis, osteoporosis, cancer, and infection. J Clin Invest. 2011;121:2534–42.
13. Reinke S, Geissler S, Taylor WR, Schmidt-Bleek K, Juelke K, Schwachmeyer V, et al. Terminally differentiated CD8(+) T cells negatively affect bone regeneration in humans. Sci Transl Med. 2013;5:177ra136.
14. Thomson AW, Bonham CA, Zeevi A. Mode of action of tacrolimus (FK506): molecular and cellular mechanisms. Ther Drug Monit. 1995;17:584–91.
15. Kugimiya F, Yano F, Ohba S, Igawa K, Nakamura K, Kawaguchi H, et al. Mechanism of osteogenic induction by FK506 via BMP/Smad pathways. Biochem Biophys Res Commun. 2005;338:872–9.
16. Liu F, Ferreira E, Porter RM, Glatt V, Schinhan M, Shen Z, et al. Rapid and reliable healing of critical size bone defects with genetically modified sheep muscle. Eur Cell Mater. 2015;30:118–30. discussion 130-111
17. Gold BG. FK506 and the role of immunophilins in nerve regeneration. Mol Neurobiol. 1997;15:285–306.
18. Voggenreiter G, Siozos P, Hunkemoller E, Heute S, Schwarz M, Obertacke U. Immunosuppression with FK506 has no influence on fracture healing in the rat. Bone. 2005;37:227–33.
19. Pollot BE, Goldman SM, Wenke JC, Corona BT. Decellularized extracellular matrix repair of volumetric muscle loss injury impairs adjacent bone healing in a rat model of complex musculoskeletal trauma. J Trauma Acute Care Surg. 2016;
20. Corona BT, Garg K, Ward CL, McDaniel JS, Walters TJ, Rathbone CR. Autologous minced muscle grafts: a tissue engineering therapy for the volumetric loss of skeletal muscle. Am J Physiol Cell Physiol. 2013;305:C761–75.
21. Garg K, Ward CL, Hurtgen BJ, Wilken JM, Stinner DJ, Wenke JC, et al. Volumetric muscle loss: persistent functional deficits beyond frank loss of tissue. J Orthop Res. 2015;33:40–6.
22. Utvag SE, Grundnes O, Rindal DB, Reikeras O. Influence of extensive muscle injury on fracture healing in rat tibia. J Orthop Trauma. 2003;17:430–5.
23. Utvag SE, Iversen KB, Grundnes O, Reikeras O. Poor muscle coverage delays fracture healing in rats. Acta Orthop Scand. 2002;73:471–4.

24. Garg K, Ward CL, Rathbone CR, Corona BT. Transplantation of devitalized muscle scaffolds is insufficient for appreciable de novo muscle fiber regeneration after volumetric muscle loss injury. Cell Tissue Res. 2014;358:857–73.
25. Abou-Khalil R, Yang F, Mortreux M, Lieu S, Yu YY, Wurmser M, et al. Delayed bone regeneration is linked to chronic inflammation in murine muscular dystrophy. J Bone Miner Res. 2014;29:304–15.
26. Recknagel S, Bindl R, Kurz J, Wehner T, Ehrnthaller C, Knoferl MW, et al. Experimental blunt chest trauma impairs fracture healing in rats. J Orthop Res. 2011;29:734–9.
27. Bhandari M, Tornetta P 3rd, Sprague S, Najibi S, Petrisor B, Griffith L, et al. Predictors of reoperation following operative management of fractures of the tibial shaft. J Orthop Trauma. 2003;17:353–61.
28. Novotny SA, Warren GL, Lin AS, Guldberg RE, Baltgalvis KA, Lowe DA. Prednisolone treatment and restricted physical activity further compromise bone of mdx mice. J Musculoskelet Neuronal Interact. 2012;12:16–23.
29. Mojumdar K, Liang F, Giordano C, Lemaire C, Danialou G, Okazaki T, et al. Inflammatory monocytes promote progression of Duchenne muscular dystrophy and can be therapeutically targeted via CCR2. EMBO Mol Med. 2014;6:1476–92.
30. Recknagel S, Bindl R, Kurz J, Wehner T, Schoengraf P, Ehrnthaller C, et al. C5aR-antagonist significantly reduces the deleterious effect of a blunt chest trauma on fracture healing. J Orthop Res. 2012;30:581–6.
31. Voggenreiter G, Assenmacher S, Kreuzfelder E, Wolf M, Kim MR, Nast-Kolb D, et al. Immunosuppression with FK506 increases bone induction in demineralized isogeneic and xenogeneic bone matrix in the rat. J Bone Miner Res. 2000;15:1825–34.
32. Ward CL, Ji L, Corona BT. An autologous muscle tissue expansion approach for the treatment of volumetric muscle loss. BioResearch Open Access. 2015;4
33. Corona BT, Wenke JC, Ward CL. Pathophysiology of volumetric muscle loss injury. Cells Tissues Organs.
34. Sawada S, Suzuki G, Kawase Y, Takaku F. Novel immunosuppressive agent, FK506. In vitro effects on the cloned T cell activation. J Immunol. 1987;139: 1797–803.
35. Udina E, Ceballos D, Verdu E, Gold BG, Navarro X. Bimodal dose-dependence of FK506 on the rate of axonal regeneration in mouse peripheral nerve. Muscle Nerve. 2002;26:348–55.
36. Wang MS, Zeleny-Pooley M, Gold BG. Comparative dose-dependence study of FK506 and cyclosporin A on the rate of axonal regeneration in the rat sciatic nerve. J Pharmacol Exp Ther. 1997;282:1084–93.
37. Singh A, Mehdi AA, Srivastava RN, Verma NS. Immunoregulation of bone remodelling. Int J Crit Illn Inj Sci. 2012;2:75–81.
38. Szabo G, Gavala C, Mandrekar P. Tacrolimus and cyclosporine A inhibit allostimulatory capacity and cytokine production of human myeloid dendritic cells. J Investig Med. 2001;49:442–9.
39. Jennings C, Kusler B, Jones PP. Calcineurin inactivation leads to decreased responsiveness to LPS in macrophages and dendritic cells and protects against LPS-induced toxicity in vivo. Innate Immun. 2009;15:109–20.
40. Howell J, Sawhney R, Testro A, Skinner N, Gow P, Angus P, et al. Cyclosporine and tacrolimus have inhibitory effects on toll-like receptor signaling after liver transplantation. Liver Transpl. 2013;19:1099–107.
41. Burrell BE, Nakayama Y, Xu J, Brinkman CC, Bromberg JS. Regulatory T cell induction, migration, and function in transplantation. J Immunol. 2012;189: 4705–11.
42. Buchwald ZS, Aurora R. Osteoclasts and CD8 T cells form a negative feedback loop that contributes to homeostasis of both the skeletal and immune systems. Clin Dev Immunol. 2013;2013:429373.
43. Colburn NT, Zaal KJ, Wang F, Tuan RS. A role for gamma/delta T cells in a mouse model of fracture healing. Arthritis Rheum. 2009;60:1694–703.
44. Croes M, Oner FC, van Neerven D, Sabir E, Kruyt MC, Blokhuis TJ, et al. Proinflammatory T cells and IL-17 stimulate osteoblast differentiation. Bone. 2016;84:262–70.
45. Lei H, Schmidt-Bleek K, Dienelt A, Reinke P, Volk HD. Regulatory T cell-mediated anti-inflammatory effects promote successful tissue repair in both indirect and direct manners. Front Pharmacol. 2015;6:184.
46. Ono T, Okamoto K, Nakashima T, Nitta T, Hori S, Iwakura Y, et al. IL-17-producing gammadelta T cells enhance bone regeneration. Nat Commun. 2016;7:10928.
47. Hamrick MW. A role for myokines in muscle-bone interactions. Exerc Sport Sci Rev. 2011;39:43–7.
48. Hamrick MW, Arounleut P, Kellum E, Cain M, Immel D, Liang LF. Recombinant myostatin (GDF-8) propeptide enhances the repair and regeneration of both muscle and bone in a model of deep penetrant musculoskeletal injury. J Trauma. 2010;69:579–83.
49. Hamrick MW, McNeil PL, Patterson SL. Role of muscle-derived growth factors in bone formation. J Musculoskelet Neuronal Interact. 2010;10:64–70.
50. Abou-Khalil R, Yang F, Lieu S, Julien A, Perry J, Pereira C, et al. Role of muscle stem cells during skeletal regeneration. Stem Cells. 2015;
51. Liu R, Birke O, Morse A, Peacock L, Mikulec K, Little DG, et al. Myogenic progenitors contribute to open but not closed fracture repair. BMC Musculoskelet Disord. 2011;12:288.
52. O'Connor JC, McCusker RH, Strle K, Johnson RW, Dantzer R, Kelley KW. Regulation of IGF-I function by proinflammatory cytokines: at the interface of immunology and endocrinology. Cell Immunol. 2008;252:91–110.
53. Zhang L, Wang XH, Wang H, Du J, Mitch WE. Satellite cell dysfunction and impaired IGF-1 signaling cause CKD-induced muscle atrophy. J Am Soc Nephrol. 2010;21:419–27.
54. Tang L, Ebara S, Kawasaki S, Wakabayashi S, Nikaido T, Takaoka K. FK506 enhanced osteoblastic differentiation in mesenchymal cells. Cell Biol Int. 2002;26:75–84.
55. Miyazaki M, Fujikawa Y, Takita C, Tsumura H. Tacrolimus and cyclosporine A inhibit human osteoclast formation via targeting the calcineurin-dependent NFAT pathway and an activation pathway for c-Jun or MITF in rheumatoid arthritis. Clin Rheumatol. 2007;26:231–9.
56. Igarashi K, Hirotani H, Woo JT, Stern PH. Cyclosporine A and FK506 induce osteoclast apoptosis in mouse bone marrow cell cultures. Bone. 2004;35:47–56.
57. Hirotani H, Tuohy NA, Woo JT, Stern PH, Clipstone NA. The calcineurin/nuclear factor of activated T cells signaling pathway regulates osteoclastogenesis in RAW264.7 cells. J Biol Chem. 2004;279:13984–92.
58. Dai W, Dong J, Fang T, Uemura T. Stimulation of osteogenic activity in mesenchymal stem cells by FK506. J Biomed Mater Res A. 2008;86:235–43.

9

Correlation analysis between the magnetic resonance imaging characteristics of osteoporotic vertebral compression fractures and the efficacy of percutaneous vertebroplasty

Wei Xu[1†], Silian Wang[2†], Chao Chen[1], Yifan Li[1], Yunhan Ji[3], Xiaodong Zhu[1] and Zhikun Li[1*]

Abstract

Background: To explore the relationship between the magnetic resonance imaging (MRI) characteristics of osteoporotic vertebral compression fractures (OVCFs) and the efficacy of percutaneous vertebroplasty (PVP).

Methods: A prospective study was conducted to analyze the clinical and imaging data of 93 patients with OVCFs treated via PVP. A visual analogue scale (VAS), the Oswestry Disability Index (ODI), and the Medical Outcomes Study(MOS) 36-Item short-form health survey (SF-36) were completed before surgery as well as 1 day and 1, 6, and 12 months after surgery. In addition, postoperative complications were recorded. According to the degree and ranges of bone marrow edema on MRI, the patients were divided into three groups: the mild (group A), moderate (group B), and severe (group C) bone marrow edema groups. Pain and dysfunction scores were compared across the three groups of patients before surgery as well as 1 day and 1, 6, and 12 months after surgery.

Results: The VAS, ODI, and SF-36 scores showed significant differences ($P < 0.05$) before and after surgery among the three groups. The ODI and SF-36 scores were significantly different ($P < 0.05$) at 1 day and 1 month after surgery among the three groups. Groups A and B showed significantly better pain relief than group C. Group B experienced better pain relief than group A. These results indicate that PVP was associated with better pain relief effects among patients with a greater extent of bone marrow edema. The edema ranges of the vertebral fractures were negatively correlated with the postoperative VAS and ODI scores 1 month after surgery, whereas the ranges were positively correlated with postoperative SF-36 scores 1 month after surgery.

Conclusions: PVP is an effective treatment for OVCFs. Better outcomes were observed among patients with severe or moderate bone marrow edema rather than those with mild bone marrow edema. A greater degree of pain relief after PVP was correlated with faster recovery of the postoperative function. However, this correlation gradually became weak over time and disappeared 6 months after surgery. Therefore, PVP should be an option for early stage OVCFs, especially among patients with bone marrow edema signs on MRI.

* Correspondence: scoliosis_lizk@126.com
[†]Equal contributors
[1]Department of Orthopedics, Tongren Hospital, Shanghai Jiao Tong University School of Medicine, 1111 XianXia Road, Shanghai 200336, People's Republic of China
Full list of author information is available at the end of the article

Background

Population aging contributes to the annual increase in the proportion of elderly people in China. To date, 88 million people are aged 65 years or over, which accounts for 7% of the total population and indicates a considerable number of elderly people. Osteoporosis is a common disease among the aged population, and it has increasingly drawn public attention due to concerns regarding population aging. Characterized by reduced bone mass, decreased bone strength, and bone microstructure degeneration, osteoporosis is a systemic disease that can cause increased bone fragility and risk of fracture [1]. The most serious consequence caused by osteoporosis is osteoporotic vertebral compression fracture (OVCF), which results in significant morbidity and decreased quality of life. The clinical manifestations of OVCFs are numerous, and the most serious symptom is severe pain [2–4]. Severe pain caused by OVCFs might not respond to conservative therapies including bed rest, the use of analgesics, and supportive devices; moreover, this pain can lead to many complications [5–7].

Percutaneous vertebroplasty (PVP) has become the gold standard to treat acute and chronic OVCFs, and it can effectively relieve the refractory pain in the middle or lower back caused by vertebral fractures [8–10]. However, a variety of factors can affect the degree of pain relief and functional recovery in individuals [11–13].

Pain relief in patients with OVCFs after PVP is associated with the duration of disease, bone density, the amount of injected bone cement, and the severity of vertebral compression. Magnetic resonance imaging (MRI) can sensitively detect the bone marrow edema caused by vertebral compression fractures, which can indicate acute or subacute fractures [14–16] and is considered as the best indication for PVP, However, the relationship between bone marrow edema and PVP was not further explained. In clinical practice, bone marrow edema signs on MRI among patients with vertebral compression fractures is a useful predictor for postoperative pain relief and functional recovery. The purpose of this study was to investigate the correlation between the MRI characteristics of OVCFs and the efficacy of PVP, the hypothesis of study is that the degree of edema predicts degree of success of injection.

Methods

Patient selection and grouping

In this study, we included patients with OVCFs who underwent PVP at Shanghai Tongren Hospital since January 2013. These patients signed an informed consent document before surgery. The Shanghai Tongren Hospital Ethics Committee reviewed and approved this study in January 2013 (project number: 20130111). The inclusion criteria were as follows: the diagnostic criteria for OVCFs were met; single-segment vertebral body compression fracture was confirmed; and preoperative MRI of the vertebral bodies was performed.

Compression fractures were diagnosed based on X-ray, Computed Tomography(CT), and MRI images. The diagnostic criterion for osteoporosis was a T-score of <– 2.5 in the dual-energy X-ray absorptiometry (DXA) of the lumbar spine and hip. All patients presented with pain in the lower back corresponding to the fracture site with or without anterior-thoracic or abdominal radiating pain. No symptoms of spinal cord or nerve root compression were reported. Surgical contraindications, including infection, hemorrhagic disease, and severe vertebral compression fractures, were ruled out.

MRI of the affected vertebral body was performed before surgery to identify the fracture site and distinguish new fractures from old fractures. A 1.5 T MRI scanner was used for this study. The fractures with bone marrow edema signals (i.e., low T1-weighted signals and high T2-weighted signals) were classified as newly onset fractures(usually within 2 weeks after the fracture). According to the degree and ranges of bone marrow edema on the MRI sagittal view, the patients were divided into group A (mild edema ranging from 1% to 24%), group B (moderate edema ranging from 25% to 74%), and group C (severe edema ranging from 75% to 100%), Fig. 1. Experienced radiologists completed the MRI evaluations. Percent = the area of bone marrow edema/ the area of the entire vertebral body*100%.

Methods

Surgical procedure

Under general anesthesia, the patients assumed the prone position with two hands alongside their heads. The effected vertebral body was confirmed via physical examination, X-ray,CT and MRI. Usually, we estimate the position of the vertebral body by the bone marker. For example, the iliac crest is at the L4/5 level. Place the K wires in the estimated position and identify the fracture vertebra by comparison with X-ray intraoperative and X-ray,CT,MRI pre-operation. It is necessary to make full use of the bone markers in the X-ray for positioning, and sometimes it needs to use multiple kirschner wire. For example, if T12 fracture, according to T12 whether there are ribs, vertebral body compression, greater osteophyte and so on to confirm the vertebral body. If L4 fracture, according to the position of sacrum, vertebral body compression, greater osteophyte and so on to confirm the vertebral body. A digital subtraction angiography (DSA) machine was used to locate the affected vertebral body and the medial edges of the bilateral pedicles to determine the puncture approach and position angle of the puncture needle and to mark the body's surface. The operative field was disinfected and draped.

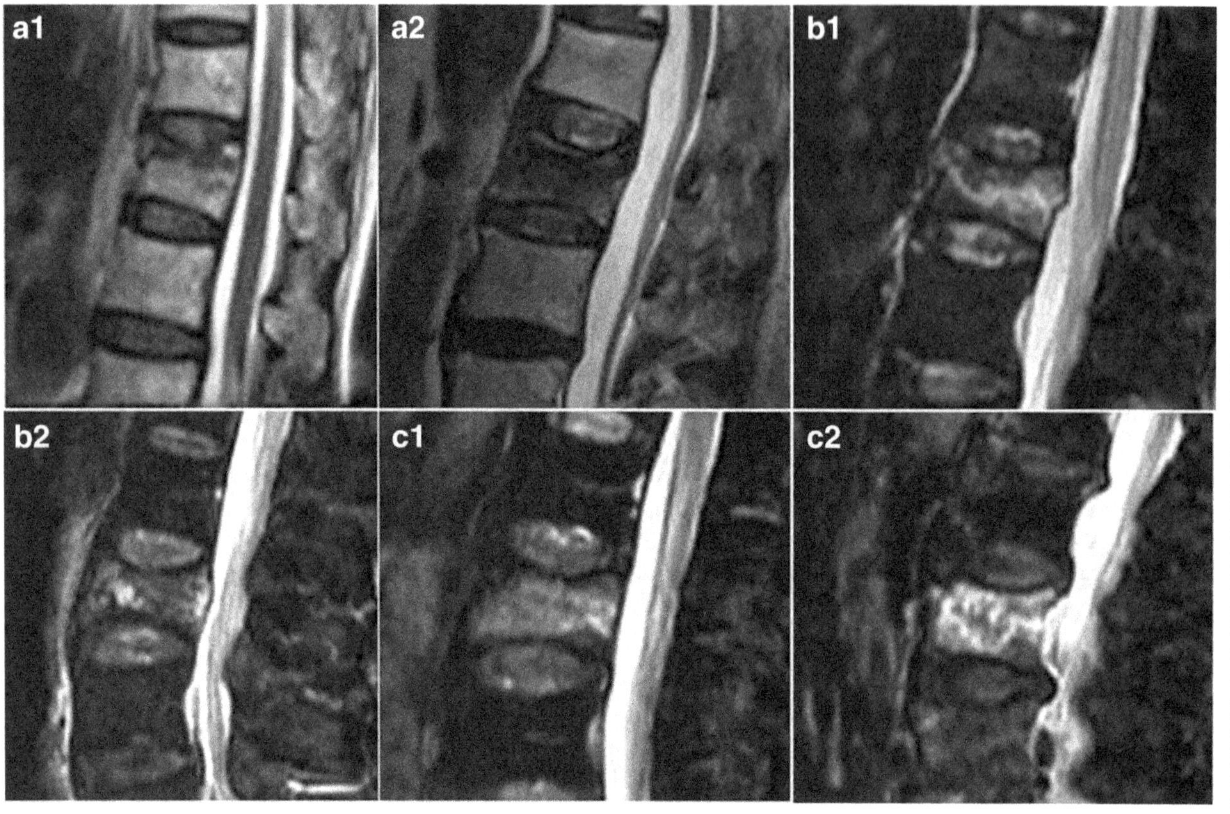

Fig. 1 According to the degree and ranges of bone marrow edema on the MRI sagittal view, the patients were divided into mild edema(a1、a2), moderate edema(b1、b2), and severe edema(c1、c2)

Under the fluoroscopic guidance of the DSA machine, the access needles (Stryker Inc., USA) were advanced into the anterior-middle 1/3 of the affected vertebral body along the sagittal plane. The position of the needle tip was confirmed via fluoroscopy (anteroposterior and lateral views). Standard bone cement, polymethyl methacrylate (stark, USA), was injected into the affected vertebral body until it was distributed to the posterior margin of the vertebral body or stop the injection when serious imaging complications are found. In other words, in intraoperative X-ray, a large amount of bone cement leaked outside the vertebral body. The amount of the injected bone cement was documented. The patient was required to use a waist supportive belt to help with ambulation for 2 weeks.

Clinical parameters

Patient age, gender, bone mineral density, amount of the injected bone cement, duration of disease, and degree of vertebral compression were documented. The degrees of vertebral compression fracture were defined as follows: A vertebral compression with less than 1/4 of the vertebral body height loss was recorded as 1; vertebral compression with 1/4 to 1/2 of the vertebral body height loss was recorded as 2; and vertebral compression with more than 1/2 of the vertebral body height loss was recorded as 3. Vertebral compression fractures of T1 through T10 were recorded as 1, T11 to L2 as 2, and L3 to L5 as 3.

Efficacy observations using a visual analogue scale (VAS), the Oswestry disability index (ODI), and the MOS item short-form health survey (SF-36) were completed before surgery as well as 1 day and 1, 6, and 12 months after surgery

a. A VAS was used to assess pain severity. The VAS (0–10) categories are as follows: 0, no pain; < 3, mildly tolerable pain; 4 to 6, moderate, reluctantly tolerable pain that affects sleep quality; and 7 to 10: severe or worst possible, an intolerable pain that affects appetite and sleep quality.
b. The ODI was used to evaluate the patient's daily activity and degree of dysfunction. The ODI questionnaire contains 10 items addressing pain intensity, lifting, ability to care for oneself, ability to walk, ability to sit, sex life (if able), ability to stand, social life, sleep quality, and ability to travel. Each item has six options, representing a 5-point scale. The total was calculated and then divided by 50 to obtain the ODI score. For practical application, the scores are multiplied by 100. Zero

represents no disability, and 100 denotes the maximum disability possible.

c. The SF-36 was used to evaluate the patient's physical and mental statuses. The SF-36 consists of eight scaled scores, including physical role functioning, social role functioning, physical functioning, mental health, emotional role functioning, vitality, bodily pain, and general health perceptions. Standard physical health and mental health scores are calculated based on the aforementioned eight sections.

Statistical analyses

The data are expressed as means±standard deviations. Statistical Product and Service Solutions(SPSS) 21.0 was used for statistical analysis. Paired t-tests were used to compare differences with regard to the VAS, ODI, and SF-36 scores within the three groups (i.e., comparisons before and after treatment in each group and comparisons between the groups). Independent-samples t-tests were used to compare the difference between groups. Spearman's rank correlation coefficient was used to analyze the correlation between the bone marrow edema signs of the fractured vertebral body and each efficacy parameter. $P < 0.05$ was considered as significant.

Results

General surgical data

As of August 2016, 93 patients were included in this study (Fig. 2), including 18 men and 75 women. The average age was 73.4 ± 10.3 years, ranging from 55 to 99 years. Their bone mineral density was − 2.9 ± 0.45. The amount of injected bone cement was 4.3 ± 0.8 mL. The duration of disease was 1.34 ± 0.561 days. Fifty-two and 44 of the 93 vertebral fractures were thoracic and lumbar vertebral fractures, respectively. The degree of vertebral compression fracture was 1.75 ± 0.747. The number of vertebral fracture segments was 1.96 ± 0.44. The aforementioned parameters did not significantly differ among the three groups ($P > 0.05$; Table 1).

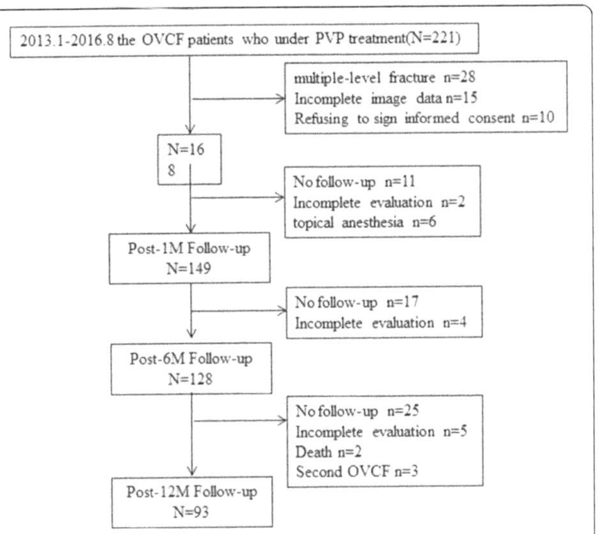

Fig. 2 Flow chart of follow-up

Observation of efficacy

The VAS, ODI, and SF-36 evaluations showed that postoperative pain was reduced significantly in groups A, B, and C ($P < 0.05$).

The VAS, ODI, and SF-36 scores did not significantly differ among the three groups ($P > 0.05$) before surgery. The VAS, ODI, and SF-36 scores significantly differed ($P < 0.05$) before and after surgery among the three groups. The ODI and SF-36 scores significantly differed ($P < 0.05$) 1 day and 1 month after surgery among the three groups. The VAS, ODI, and SF-36 scores did not significantly differ ($P > 0.05$) when comparing 1 month with 6 months and when comparing 6 months with 12 months after surgery. Significant pain relief was observed in groups A and B compared with group C. Group B achieved better pain relief than group A. These results indicate that patients with moderate or severe bone marrow edema can achieve better pain relief after PVP (Table 2).

Correlation analysis

The edema ranges of the vertebral fractures were negatively correlated with the postoperative VAS and ODI scores 1 month after surgery; however, the ranges were positively correlated with postoperative SF-36 scores 1 month after surgery. (Table 3).

Complications

The intraoperative leakage of bone cement into the anterior or posterior vertebral bodies of the three groups was noted in 5 and 1 patient(s), respectively. However, these patients were asymptomatic after surgery. After a 1-year follow-up period, no complaints (e.g., pain or progressive pain) were reported. No worsening dysfunction was evident in daily activity.

Discussion

In general, the pathogenesis of primary OVCFs of the spine can be divided into five phases [17, 18]: (1) the occurrence of fractures and vertebral ischemic changes; (2) vertebral bone marrow edemas that are present as high T2WI on MRI, although the lesion enhancement is not shown in the enhanced scan; (3) irregular enhancement at the compressive vertebral body can be noted during early stage of fracture healing due to increased blood supply during tissue repair; (4) the degree of enhancement at the compressive vertebral body gradually decreases during the late stage of fracture healing because the increased blood supply gradually becomes normal;

Table 1 Paired t-tests were used to compare differences with regard to the parameters within the three groups

Parameters	Group A($n = 30$)	Group B($n = 46$)	Group C($n = 11$)	P
Age(year)	73.9 ± 10.2	76.4 ± 10.8	71.2 ± 8.4	> 0.05
Gender(Female/Male)	21/9	20/6	19/7	> 0.05
BMD	−2.92 ± 0.46	−2.88 ± 0.42	− 2.96 ± 0.50	> 0.05
PMMA(ml)	4.2 ± 1.3	4.4 ± 1.5	3.8 ± 1.1	> 0.05
Time(day)	1.4 ± 0.563	1.31 ± 0.618	1.31 ± 0.549	> 0.05
Degree	1.70 ± 0.75	1.78 ± 0.758	1.76 ± 0.752	> 0.05
VB	1.93 ± 0.365	1.96 ± 0.469	2.0 ± 0.5	> 0.05

BMD bone mineral density, *PMMA*, the injection volume of PMMA in PVP operation, *Time* course of disease, *Degree* The degree of vertebral compression, *VB* Compression vertebral body

and (5) the compressive vertebral body is gradually replaced by adipose tissue during the chronic phase. Although the fractured vertebral body can be compressed into a "coin-like" tissue, the T1WI and T2WI signals gradually increased, especially the T1WI signal. If necrotic liquefaction is present in the fractured vertebral body, then the intensity of this vertebral body might not change during an enhanced scan. On the other hand, the mechanism of pain relief via PVP remains unclear and might involve the following aspects [14]. (1) Mechanical manipulation - The injection of bone cement can improve the biomechanical properties of the spine, fixate micro-fractures, and reduce the tiny migration of the fracture fragments, thereby reducing the stimulation to nociceptive nerve endings. Because trabecular spacing in the case of osteoporosis increases, bone cement can be filled into the entire vertebral body via increased trabecular spacing (i.e., vertebral augmentation that supports the vertebral body to effectively prevent vertebral collapse and compression fractures). (2) Thermal effect of the bone cement - The polymerization reaction of bone cement through which the peak temperature generated is between 52 and 93 °C can lead to necrosis of the surrounding tissue and the destruction of the nerve endings. Thus, pain subsides or is alleviated. (3) Chemical effects - Bone cement has its own cytotoxic effect that can kill the tumor tissue.

This study divided the patients into mild, moderate, and severe groups. Patient age, sex, bone mineral density, amount of injected bone cement, duration of disease, and degree of vertebral compression fracture before surgery did not significantly differ ($P > 0.05$). The results revealed significant differences in the VAS, ODI, SF-36 scores with regard to pain severity before and after surgery among patients with different bone marrow edema signs of vertebral fractures ($P < 0.05$), indicating that PVP is effective, regardless of the extent of bone marrow edema, Fig. 3. Moreover, these results indicate

Table 2 Paired t-tests were used to compare differences with regard to the VAS, ODI, and SF-36 scores within the three groups

Period		Group A($n = 30$)	Group B($n = 46$)	Group C($n = 17$)	P
Per	VAS	7.7 ± 1.3	8.4 ± 1.0	7.8 ± 1.3	> 0.05
	ODI	75.9 ± 5.1	83.1 ± 5.2	77.8 ± 4.4	> 0.05
	SF-36	24.5 ± 4.3	26.1 ± 3.5	25.2 ± 2.6	> 0.05
Post	VAS	4.0 ± 2.6	3.5 ± 2.0	3.0 ± 2.1	<0.05*
	ODI	33.4 ± 3.9	28.9 ± 3.3	23.3 ± 4.2	<0.05*
	SF-36	26.7 ± 4.3	30.2 ± 4.6	33.7 ± 5.2	<0.05*
Post-1 M	VAS	3.2 ± 1.5	3.0 ± 1.9	2.8 ± 1.5	>0.05
	ODI	26.1 ± 3.2	22.6 ± 3.0	19.5 ± 2.9	<0.05*
	SF-36	29.1 ± 3.5	35.1 ± 4.4	37.9 ± 4.8	<0.05*
Post-6 M	VAS	3.1 ± 1.5	3.0 ± 1.8	2.8 ± 1.6	>0.05
	ODI	22.2 ± 3.1	21.5 ± 2.9	21.8 ± 1.6	>0.05
	SF-36	35.3 ± 3.2	36.9 ± 3.9	35.1 ± 2.5	>0.05
Post-12 M	VAS	3.0 ± 1.2	2.9 ± 1.5	2.8 ± 1.5	>0.05
	ODI	21.2 ± 3.0	21.4 ± 2.6	21.9 ± 1.5	>0.05
	SF-36	34.3 ± 2.2	35.5 ± 3.7	35.4 ± 2.1	>0.05

Note: *P<0.05

Table 3 The spearman's relevance bewteen Vertebral marrow edema and VAS,ODI,SF-36

Evaluated Parameters		Correlation Coefficient	P
VAS	Per	−0.31	0.766
	Post	−0.522**	<0.001
	Post 1 M	0.001	0.991
	Post 6 M	0.121	0.246
	Post 12 M	0.15	0.884
ODI	Per	0.178	0.088
	Post	−0.808**	<0.001
	Post 1 M	−0.735*	<0.05
	Post 6 M	−0.135	0.196
	Post 12 M	0.112	0.283
SF-36	Per	0.086	0.414
	Post	0.802**	<0.001
	Post 1 M	0.688**	<0.05
	Post 6 M	0.002	0.987
	Post 12 M	0.071	0.500

Note:*P<0.05,**P<0.01

that patients with moderate or severe bone marrow edema can achieve better pain relief after PVP. Nevertheless, sharp decreases in the postoperative VAS and ODI scores and a rapid increase in the SF-36 score were observed in patients with larger ranges of bone marrow edema (group C). In patients with different degrees of bone marrow edema, the difference in efficacy was significant before and immediately after surgery; however, this difference gradually became smaller. On the 6th month after surgery, no difference in efficacy was observed among the three groups ($P < 0.05$). This result demonstrates that PVP is more effective in patients with larger ranges of bone marrow edema during the early stage (within 6 months) after surgery but has a similar effect 6 months after surgery (Fig. 4).

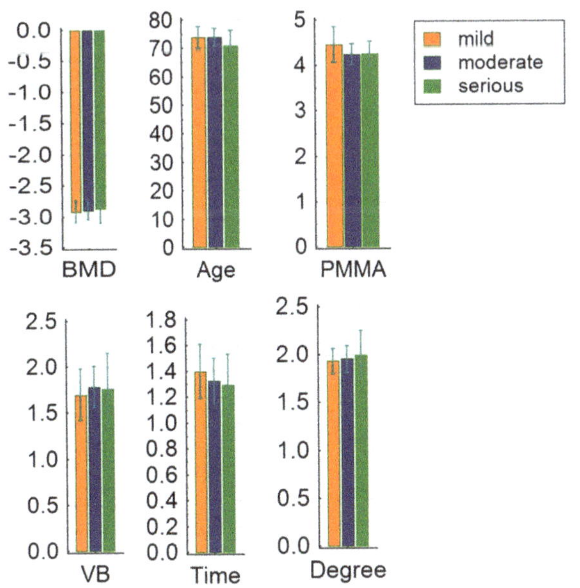

Fig. 3 Statistical graphs of various parameter in different groups

MRI is a routine examination before PVP among patients with OVCFs. In addition to its high resolution regarding soft tissue, the skeletal muscles, or the nervous system, MRI is sensitive to the presence, magnitude, and location of bone marrow edema of the vertebral compression fracture. The changes in bone marrow signal intensity can reflect the stages of OVCFs and the phases of bone healing [16, 19]. In general, OVCFs are present with low T1WI and high T2WI signals on MRI within 1 month after fractures and tend to become normal (i.e., isointense T1WI and T2WI) after 1 month; then, they return to normal bone marrow signals after complete healing or low T1WI and low T2WI signals due to tissue organization. Therefore, bone marrow edema in patients with OVCFs often indicates acute or subacute fractures, which can be effectively treated with PVP to alleviate pain symptoms. On the contrary, PVP is not suitable for the treatment of old vertebral compression fractures without bone marrow edema. Voormolen et al. [20] suggested that the extent of bone marrow edema on preoperative MRI is the only factor associated with pain relief. Thus, bone marrow edema is a useful sign for treatment selection [21]. Moreover, our results also suggest that PVP can alleviate pain symptoms in most patients with a small degree of bone marrow edema. Brown et al. [12] also reported that PVP effectively treats patients without abnormal signals on MRI; however, fluoroscopy revealed a correlation between findings from a physical examination and the compression segment in an imaging study. Nevertheless, we consider a small range of bone marrow edema as an unstable, deformed healing state in the compression body. The mechanism of pain in these patients differs from that in those with acute, subacute, and chronic fractures. The cause of pain might be due to the unstable state of spinal mechanics, the stimulation of Schmorl's nodes, or other changes in degeneration. Postoperative pain relief might be related to the correction of PVP with regard to the aforementioned factors. This interesting phenomenon should be verified in studies with larger sample sizes.

The advantages of this study are as follows. Because the degree of pain relief differs between local and general anesthesia [22], the latter was selected for all patients to avoid bias caused by different routes of anesthesia. The limitations of this study are listed below. (1) The follow-up visits were scheduled at 1, 6, and 12 months after surgery. The long follow-up intervals might affect the accurate evaluation of the changes in postoperative bone marrow edema and the clinical

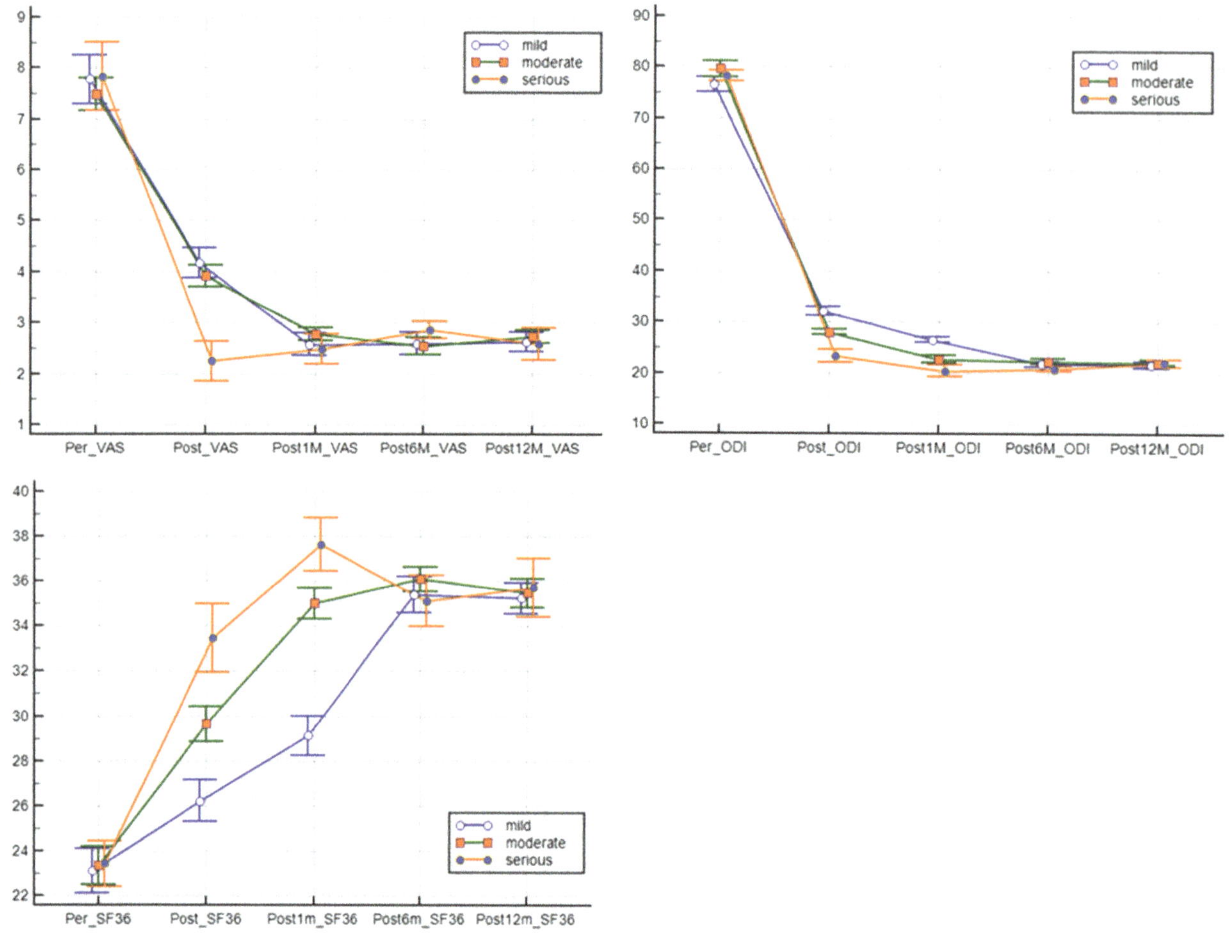

Fig. 4 Changes in VAS,ODI,SF-36 during different group follow-up

efficacy. The evaluation might only reflect the approximate trend of the changes. (2) This study is a single-center study with a small sample size.(3) The number of fracture vertebral body was not uniform (One, two, three vertebral bodies). Inconsistency of number will lead to bias from patients.

Conclusions

PVP is an effective treatment for OVCFs. The MRI characteristics of OVCFs are helpful in predicting their treatment outcomes. Better outcomes were observed among patients with severe or moderate bone marrow edema than among those with mild bone marrow edema. The greater degree of pain relief after PVP was correlated with the faster recovery of post-operative function. However, this correlation gradually became weak over time and disappeared 6 months after surgery. Therefore, PVP should be an option for early stage OVCFs, especially for patients with bone marrow edema signs on MRI.

Abbreviations

CT: Computed tomography; DSA: Digital subtraction angiography; DXA: Dual-energy X-ray absorptiometry; MOS: Medical outcomes study; MRI: Magnetic resonance imaging; ODI: Oswestry disability index; OVCFs: Osteoporotic vertebral compression fractures; PVP: Percutaneous vertebroplasty; SF-36: 36-Item short-form health survey; SPSS: Statistical product and service solutions; VAS: Visual analogue scale

Acknowledgements

Not applicable.

Funding

1. Health development planning commission of Changning qu in Shanghai.Award Number: 20164Y003 | Recipient: zhikun li, M.D.
2. Project supported by National Natural Science Foundation of China Award Number: 81501897 | Recipient: wei xu.
3. Scientific research funds of shanghai Tongren hospital Award Number: TRYJ201605 | Recipient: zhikun li, M.D.

Authors' contributions

LZK, XW conceived and designed the study. CC,WSL,JYH and LYF measure and record the data. LZK,XW and ZXD wrote the paper. ZXD reviewed manuscript and revised the manuscript critically for important intellectual content. All authors read and approved the manuscript.

Competing interests
The authors declare that they have no competing interests.

Author details
[1]Department of Orthopedics, Tongren Hospital, Shanghai Jiao Tong University School of Medicine, 1111 XianXia Road, Shanghai 200336, People's Republic of China. [2]Department of Radiology, Tongren Hospital, Shanghai Jiao Tong University School of Medicine, 1111 XianXia Road, Shanghai 200336, People's Republic of China. [3]Medical Services Section, Tongren Hospital, Shanghai Jiao Tong University School of Medicine, 1111 XianXia Road, Shanghai 200336, People's Republic of China.

References
1. Mattie R, Laimi K, Yu S, Saltychev M. Comparing percutaneous Vertebroplasty and conservative therapy for treating osteoporotic compression fractures in the thoracic and lumbar spine: a systematic review and meta-analysis. J Bone Joint Surg Am. 2016;98:1041–51.
2. Johnell O, Kanis JA. An estimate of the worldwide prevalence and disability associated with osteoporotic fractures. Osteoporos Int. 2006;17:1726–33.
3. Krueger A, Bliemel C, Zettl R, Ruchholtz S. Management of Pulmonary Cement Embolism after percutaneous Vertebroplasty and Kyphoplasty: a systematic review of the literature. Eur Spine J. 2009;18:1257–65.
4. Zoarski GH, Snow P, Olan WJ, Stallmeyer MJ, Dick BW, Hebel JR, De Deyne M. Percutaneous Vertebroplasty for osteoporotic compression fractures: quantitative prospective evaluation of long-term outcomes. J Vasc Interv Radiol. 2002;13:139–48.
5. Phillips FM. Minimally invasive treatments of osteoporotic vertebral compression fractures. Spine (Phila Pa 1976). 2003;28:S45–53.
6. G. Voggenreiter, 'Balloon Kyphoplasty Is Effective in deformity correction of osteoporotic vertebral compression fractures', Spine (Phila Pa 1976), 30 (2005), 2806–2812.
7. Yang EZ, Xu JG, Huang GZ, Xiao WZ, Liu XK, Zeng BF, Lian XF. Percutaneous Vertebroplasty versus conservative treatment in aged patients with acute osteoporotic vertebral compression fractures: a prospective randomized controlled clinical study. Spine (Phila Pa 1976). 2016;41:653–60.
8. Barr JD, Barr MS, Lemley TJ, McCann RM. Percutaneous Vertebroplasty for pain relief and spinal stabilization. Spine (Phila Pa 1976). 2000;25:923–8.
9. Diamond TH, Champion B, Clark WA. Management of Acute Osteoporotic Vertebral Fractures: a nonrandomized trial comparing percutaneous Vertebroplasty with conservative therapy. Am J Med. 2003;114:257–65.
10. Farrokhi MR, Alibai E, Maghami Z. Randomized controlled trial of percutaneous Vertebroplasty versus optimal medical Management for the Relief of pain and disability in acute osteoporotic vertebral compression fractures. J Neurosurg Spine. 2011;14:561–9.
11. Brown DB, Gilula LA, Sehgal M, Shimony JS. Treatment of chronic symptomatic vertebral compression fractures with percutaneous Vertebroplasty. AJR Am J Roentgenol. 2004;182:319–22.
12. Brown DB, Glaiberman CB, Gilula LA, Shimony JS. Correlation between Preprocedural Mri findings and clinical outcomes in the treatment of chronic symptomatic vertebral compression fractures with percutaneous Vertebroplasty. AJR Am J Roentgenol. 2005;184:1951–5.
13. M. Spalteholz, E. Strasser, T. Hantel, and R. H. Gahr, 'Prone Position in Balloon Kyphoplasty Leads to No Secondary Vertebral Compression Fractures in Osteoporotic Spine - a Mri Study', *GMS Interdiscip Plast Reconstr Surg DGPW*, 3 (2014), Doc17.
14. Do HM. Magnetic resonance imaging in the evaluation of patients for percutaneous Vertebroplasty. Top Magn Reson Imaging. 2000;11:235–44.
15. Modic MT, Steinberg PM, Ross JS, Masaryk TJ, Carter JR. Degenerative disk disease: assessment of changes in vertebral body marrow with Mr imaging. Radiology. 1988;166(1 Pt 1):193–9. https://doi.org/10.1148/radiology.166.1.3336678
16. Tang ZB, Lei Z, Yang HL, Chen KW. Value of bone scan imaging in determining painful vertebrae of osteoporotic vertebral compression fractures patients with contraindications to Mri. Orthop Surg. 2012;4:172–6.
17. Jin ZG, Shen SM, Gao JX, Wang XP, Liu HM, Lu WX, Shen K. Identification of fresh and old vertebral compression fractures by Mri. Fa Yi Xue Za Zhi. 2011;27:274–6.
18. Thawait SK, Kim J, Klufas RA, Morrison WB, Flanders AE, Carrino JA, Ohno-Machado L. Comparison of four prediction models to discriminate benign from malignant vertebral compression fractures according to Mri feature analysis. AJR Am J Roentgenol. 2013;200:493–502.
19. Park SY, Lee SH, Suh SW, Park JH, Kim TG. Usefulness of Mri in determining the appropriate level of cement augmentation for acute osteoporotic vertebral compression fractures. J Spinal Disord Tech. 2013;26:E80–5.
20. Voormolen MH, van Rooij WJ, Sluzewski M, van der Graaf Y, Lampmann LE, Lohle PN, Juttmann JR. Pain response in the first trimester after percutaneous Vertebroplasty in patients with osteoporotic vertebral compression fractures with or without bone marrow edema. AJNR Am J Neuroradiol. 2006;27:1579–85.
21. Mathis JM, Barr JD, Belkoff SM, Barr MS, Jensen ME, Deramond H. Percutaneous Vertebroplasty: a developing standard of Care for Vertebral Compression Fractures. AJNR Am J Neuroradiol. 2001;22:373–81.
22. Dahlstrand U, Sandblom G, Ljungdahl M, Wollert S, Gunnarsson U. TEP under general anesthesia is superior to Lichtenstein under local anesthesia in terms of pain 6 weeks after surgery: results from a randomized clinical trial. Surg Endosc. 2013;27(10):3632–8.

10

A novel cerclage wiring technique in intertrochanteric femoral fractures treated by intramedullary nails in young adults

You-Shui Gao*, Yan-Jie Guo, Xin-Gang Yu, Yang Chen, Chen Chen and Nan-Ji Lu

Abstract

Background: Intertrochanteric femoral fractures (IFFs) in young adults, generally due to severe trauma, are increasingly presented. Different from IFFs in the geriatric population, these fractures in young adults are always comminuted and substantially displaced. Natural traction induced by musculature following IFFs determines closed reduction on a fracture table is extremely difficult.

Methods: To achieve anatomical reduction before intramedullary nail (IMN) fixation, we made an extended or a mini petrotrochantetic incision to facilitate temporary reduction using a pointed clamp. Subsequently, a curved and cannulated wire-passer was employed to pass through a multistrand cable to surround displaced fragments and strengthen intertrochanteric fixation. Afterward, a standard procedure was conducted to nail the fracture.

Results: We used the surgical technique in 9 young patients with an age range of 28~ 48 years old. The fractures were categorized as AO/OTA 31-A2.2 (3 cases) and 31-A2.3 (6 cases). The injury-to-surgery interval was 2.5 days on average. Mean operation time was 55 min. All fractures achieved anatomical reduction and healed within 14 weeks postoperatively without cable breakage, implant irritation or deep infection.

Conclusions: In conclusion, the surrounding technique with cerclage wire in IFFs in young adults is an effective surgical technique with easily achieved anatomical reduction to facilitate operative maneuvers and fracture healing.

Keywords: Intertrochanteric femoral fractures, Cerclage augmentation, Intramedullary nail

Background

Intertrochanteric femoral fractures are frequent injuries in the elderly, mainly due to falling from a standing position [1]. Thankfully, these geriatric and osteoporotic femoral fractures can be fixed by intramedullary nails to facilitate an early leaving bed and support a desired functional recovery [2, 3]. In contrast, intertrochanteric femoral fractures in young adults are rarely seen and are mostly induced by high-energy injuries. Therefore, young intertrochanteric femoral fractures are comminuted and displaced at large. The muscular forces of the hip could deteriorate the fragment deformation, which makes anatomical reduction through closed maneuver quite difficult [4].

The story of subtrochanteric femoral fractures shows us that anatomical reduction through closed manipulation is of significant difficulty [4, 5]. To solve the problem, we can utilize techniques of assisted reduction and devices via a small lateral incision. Among these devices, various clamps and cerclage wire are frequently employed to achieve and maintain satisfactory reduction permanently or consistently [6–9].

In the current study, for comminuted and displaced intertrochanteric femoral fractures in young adults (Fig. 1), we made an extended or a mini lateral incision to palpate the displaced fragments. Afterward, a pointed reduction clamp was used to reposition the displaced fractures. Generally, the reduction could be easily maintained; however, loss of reduction could be encountered when reaming and with the entering of an intramedullary nail. Therefore, before making the starting point at the tip of the trochanter, we used a cerclage wire to assure the reduction for following manipulation of intramedullary nail fixation, while the displaced fragments

* Correspondence: gaoyoushui@sjtu.edu.cn
Department of Orthopaedic Surgery, Shanghai Jiao Tong University Affiliated Sixth People's Hospital, Shanghai 200233, China

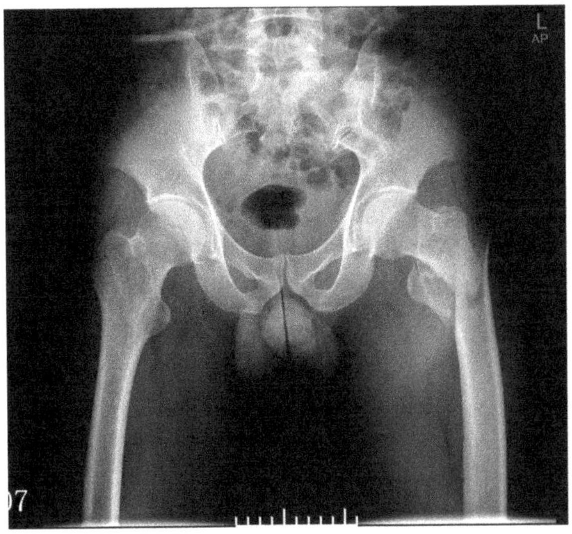

Fig. 1 A 38-year-old man who fell from height and had a comminuted intertrochanteric femoral fracture, which was graded as AO/OTA 31-A2.3

could be surrounded by the wire. The novelty of our surgical technique is reflected in two aspects. First, the circumferential level was above the lesser trochanter and close to the posterior cortex. The quality of bone structure (the calcar) here is the best. Therefore, the augmentation by cerclage could be effective and rigid. Second, the wire we used also surrounded the displaced greater trochanter, which became stable following tightening of the wire. Thus, in the young adults, early partial weight bearing was encouraged immediately postoperatively. We will describe the surgical technique in detail and present pilot clinical results. We believe the surgical technique is competent for irreducible intertrochanteric femoral fractures in young adults.

Methods

Surgical techniques

Under general anesthesia, the patient is placed supine on a fracture table. The injured lower limb is stabilized in a traction boot while the uninvolved limb is placed in abduction to facilitate intraoperative imaging. Closed reduction maneuvers should be attempted under fluoroscopic control, generally through axial traction and adduction and internal rotation of the involved limb. Occasionally, elevation of the distal limb is helpful to achieve satisfactory reduction. Attempts for closed reduction should be made no more than 3 times. In case of failure reduction, methods of open reduction can be used on the same fracture table.

The limb is then prepared and draped, and the axial traction should be relaxed. The proximal incision above the greater trochanter for routine entrance of an intramedullary nail is extended for 4~ 6 cm, or a separated lateral incision 3~ 5 cm long is made. Alternatively, a separated mini lateral incision is made. The fascia lata is incised, and the fibers of the vastus lateralis are split bluntly along the anterior edge of the proximal femur. The muscular forces always make the proximal fragment displaced to the position of adduction, internal rotation and anterior flexion (Fig. 2). In the lateral incision, the fracture site can be palpated. Gentle traction is applied to make the fractured main fragments to approximately the same level. In this scenario, a pointed reduction clamp is helpful to achieve temporary anatomical reduction (Fig. 3). The smooth medial edge of the femur (calcar) can be palpated intraoperatively; meanwhile, the quality of reduction should be confirmed under fluoroscopy. To avoid reduction loss, we use a cerclage wire to augment reduction. A wire passer is inserted from anteromedial femur (above the lesser trochanter) to posterolateral position. In the case of multiple greater-trochanter fragments (always displaced to the posterior), they can be surrounded by the wire as well (Fig. 4). We believe the advantages of cerclage wire-augmented reduction are clear: 1. a cerclage wire can surround more displaced fragments, which are commonly seen in young intertrochanteric fractures; 2. a cerclage wire can free the reduction clamp to facilitate following operation if necessary; 3. reaming and insertion of an intramedullary nail might cause loss of reduction, which can be effectively prevented by the wire augmentation; and 4. a cerclage wire is beneficial to prevent breakage of the lateral wall. The quality of reduction is reconfirmed under fluoroscopy.

Afterward, a standard procedure of intramedullary fixation is performed. In brief, following the starting point at the tip of the great trochanter is confirmed under fluoroscopy, and the proximal femur is reamed along the guide pin. In the current study, a proximal femoral nail antirotation (PFNA) (Synthes) was the fixation of choice, mainly based on the surgeons' preference. The nail is inserted to a proper depth, and a guide pin is drilled into the femoral head. It is important to obtain correct tip-to-apex distance (TAD, 5~ 10 mm) and anteversion angle (parallel to axial of the femoral neck). Afterwards, the screw blade is hammered into the femoral head and secured. Then the wire can be tightened to free the reduction clamp. We always find that the displaced fragments of the greater trochanter in posterior can achieve a better position on lateral view following clamp removal. Finally, the nail is stabilized with the static screw drilled. Usually, the end cap is used because hardware removal is preferable in young adults in China (Fig. 5).

Patients

Between July 2016 and June 2017, we consecutively treated 9 young adults with comminuted and displaced intertrochanteric femoral fractures. All of the patients

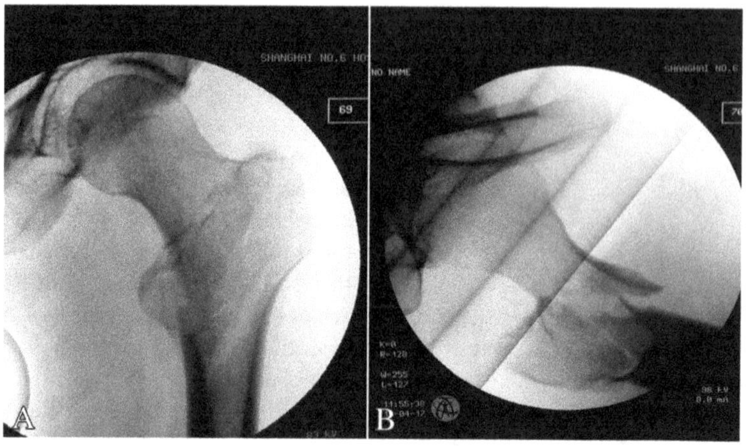

Fig. 2 Attempt for closed reduction on a traction table. **a** Under axial traction, internal rotation and elevation of the distal limb; anteroposterior imaging shows the closed reduction is acceptable. **b** Lateral imaging shows the reduction is unsatisfactory. Displacement of proximal fragment is significant determined by muscular forces

with such fractures underwent failure of closed reduction. Seven of the fractures were due to falling from height, and the other two were due to crash accidents. Eight patients were male, and one was female with an average age of 42.5 years (range, 28~ 48 years). According to AO/OTA classification, the fractures were categorized as 31-A2.2 in 3 cases and 31-A2.3 in 6 cases. The concomitant injuries included calcaneal fractures in 4 cases, wrist fractures in 2 and brain injuries in 2. The injury-to-surgery interval was 2.5 days (range, 2~ 5 days) on average.

Using the surgical techniques described above, we managed these intertrochanteric femoral fractures uneventfully. Calcaneal fractures in 3 and wrist fractures in 2 were treated surgically under the same anesthesia, following the surgical care of intertrochanteric femoral fractures. Other concomitant injuries were all treated conservatively. Mean operation time to manage intertrochanteric femoral fractures was 55 min (range, 45~ 70 min). Intraoperative blood loss was comparable to routine operations via closed reduction.

Postoperatively, anticoagulant drugs were prescribed to prevent deep vein thrombosis. We prefer to use low-molecular-weight heparin on hospitalization days and give patients Rivaroxaban or aspirin after discharge. Active exercises of the involved hip joint were initiated on the first postoperative day, while partial load bearing was determined on the patient's general condition and concomitant injuries. The study has been approved by the ethics committee of Shanghai Sixth People's Hospital.

Results

All patients achieved anatomical reduction and underwent routine follow-up until fracture healing. There was no early complication, such as infection, or late complication, such as delayed union, nonunion, implant

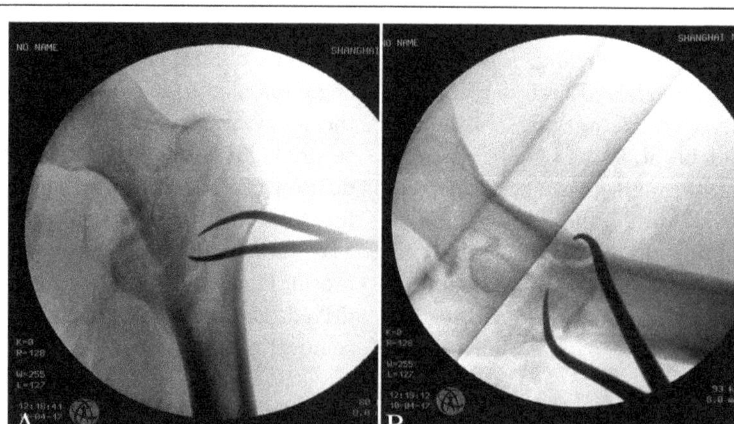

Fig. 3 Open reduction with the help of a clamp. **a** A pointed reduction clamp is used to achieve anatomical reduction through a lateral incision. **b** The lateral view shows previous displacement is no longer in existence

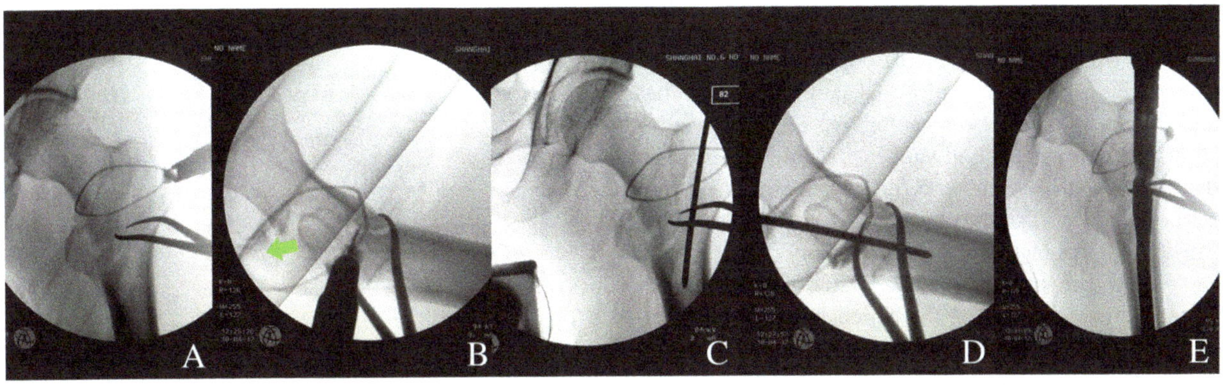

Fig. 4 Cerclage wiring and entrance of intramedullary nail. **a** A circumferential wire is used to augment anatomical reduction. The wire surrounds the medial calcar above the fractured lesser trochanter and the lateral wall. **b** The lateral imaging shows the displaced fragment of the greater trochanter is also encircled (green arrow). Following entry of a guide pin from the tip of the greater trochanter, anteroposterior (**c**) and lateral (**d**) imaging show the reduction is maintained. **e** A proximal femoral nail antirotation (PFNA) is inserted to an appropriate depth

breakage or cutoff. The fracture had obvious callus formation within 14 weeks. Afterward, patients were encouraged to perform full weight bearing. The patients returned to their previous position with a total treatment duration of 16 weeks on average (range, 14~ 20 weeks).

Discussion

Anatomical reduction is of critical importance in young intertrochanteric femoral fractures. Surgical maneuvers require satisfactory reduction achieved [10–14]. It is always highlighted to not ream an unreduced fracture [15]. Otherwise, intraoperative complications, including perforation and dehiscence of the femur, deterioration of fracture dislocation, and neurovascular damage, might be encountered. Anatomical reduction is also the prominent determinant of fracture healing and functional recovery.

To achieve satisfactory reduction, many assistant surgical techniques have been attempted for irreducible and unstable intertrochanteric fractures. In brief, a mini incision is always made as the pathway to palpate the displaced fracture. The lateral musculature can be bluntly detached to adapt the reduction devices. Previous studies recommended reduction clamp, pointed reduction clamp, bone hooks and bucking bar to obtain reduction [7, 16]. However, the reduction is not easy to be maintained during reaming and nail fixation. Alternatively, the surgeon has to be exposed under fluoroscopy radiation. Undoubtedly, loosening of reduction device before reaming or nail insertion could result in loss of reduction and delay of operation.

Cerclage wiring, a simple and historical surgical technique, has been used in fracture fixation solely or in combination with other implants, and gets its popularity in arthroplasty [17–28]. The concern with cerclage is the potential disruption to regional blood circulation, consequently delaying the fracture healing. The frustration

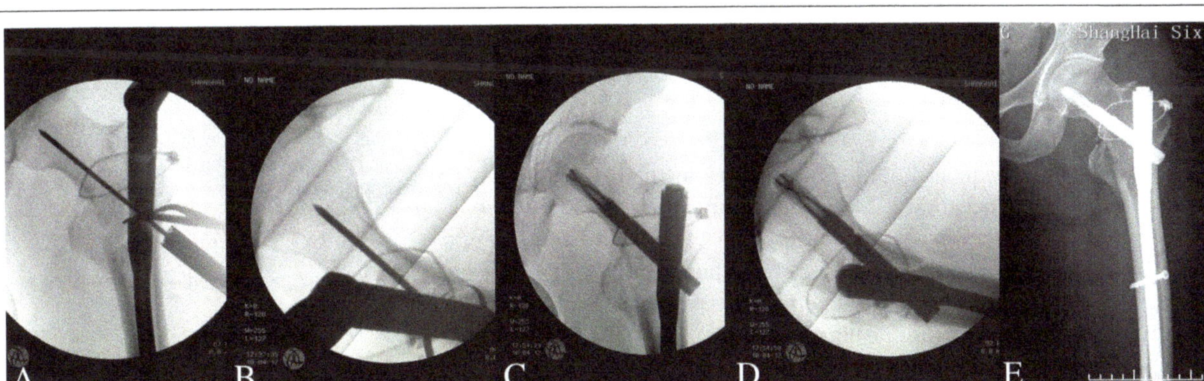

Fig. 5 Routine maneuvers of nail fixation. Anteroposterior (**a**) and lateral (**b**) imaging show the guide pin for the blade. The pin should be in parallel with the axis of the femoral neck in both planes with correct tip-to-apex distance. Anteroposterior (**c**) and lateral (**d**) view shows anatomical reduction and satisfactory fixation by PFN-A. The wire is tightened, and the displaced fragments of the greater trochanter get a better position. **e** Postoperatively, anteroposterior radiograph shows the perfect combination of the wire and the nail

might also include more operation time, cost and bleeding [29]. An animal study showed cable cerclage around the femoral cortex significantly decreased blood circulation in the area [30]. However, Apivatthakakul and colleagues found that percutaneous cerclage wiring resulted in minimal disruption of the blood supply of the femur through cadaveric injection study [31]. The experiment on cerclage-bone interface mechanics revealed cerclage provided a point contact fixation on the femoral shaft with blood-supply preserving principle [32]. Clinically, plenty of recent studies confirmed the beneficial effects of cerclage wiring in the care of peritrochanteric femoral fractures as well as in humeral shaft fractures and acetabular fractures. It seems that a cerclage wire facilitates fracture reduction and does not interrupt fracture healing.

To cerclage or not might become an ongoing debate. Nevertheless, the benefits and potential detriments of a wire should be noted for young surgeons. Closed reduction and intramedullary nail fixation has become the treatment of choice for unstable intertrochanteric femoral fractures [33]. To minimize detrimental effects, one can use temporary cerclage wiring technique alternatively. It should be highlighted that reduction was obtained with clamps and maintained with a wire in the current study. Wire should not act in a reduction role because the increased compression during tightening might induce iatrogenic fractures. The wire can also secure posterior fragments. The lateral wall of the trochanter is protected by a wire, which has been widely used in revision of hip arthroplasty.

The limitations of the current study should be noted as well. The number of treated cases is small due to the rarity of intertrochanteric fractures in young adults. Although all fractures healed in the follow-up, the implant is not removed to date, and long-term results have to be observed. In our early practice, we only maintained the reduction with a clamp and never used a wire temporarily or permanently. However, the clamp might become loosened when reaming. Although surgeons might prefer their familiar techniques, we believe cerclage wiring is simple and direct in the care of difficult intertrochanteric fractures.

Conclusions

Cerclage wiring is a beneficial surgical technique in the care of young intertrochanteric femoral fractures that are irreducible through closed maneuvers. The wire is helpful to maintain the reduced fractures, to facilitate reaming and nailing, to reduce intraoperative complications and not to hinder fracture healing.

Acknowledgements

We would like to thank all nurses, radiologists and medical students for their great contributions during intraoperative cooperation, postoperative care and following up. All data were collected at the Hip Fracture Ward of Emergency and Department of Orthopedic Surgery, Shanghai Jiao Tong University Affiliated Sixth People's Hospital.

Authors' contributions

YSG participated in study design, data collection and drafted the manuscript. YJG collected and analyzed the data, and searched the literatures. XGY collected and analyzed the data, discussed the results. YC participated in study design, critically read and revised the manuscript. CC participated in data collection, critically read and revised the manuscript. NJL participated in study design and critically revised the manuscript. All authors cared patients, read and approved the final manuscript.

Competing interests

The authors declare that they have no competing interests.

References

1. Koval KJ, Zuckerman JD. Hip fractures: II. Evaluation and treatment of intertrochanteric fractures. J Am Acad Orthop Surg. 1994;2(3):150–6.
2. Chughtai M, Khlopas A, Mont MA. Fixation methods in the management of hip fractures. Lancet. 2017;389(10078):1493–4.
3. Sabandam SN, Chandrasekharan J, Mounasamy V, Mauffrey C. Intertrochanteric fractures: a review of fixation methods. Eur J Orthop Surg Traumatol. 2016;26(4):339–53.
4. Kregor PJ, Obremskey WT, Kreder HJ, Swiontkowski MF. Evidence-based orthopaedic trauma working group. Unstable pertrochanteric femoral fractures. J Orthop Trauma. 2005;19(1):63–6.
5. Afsari A, Liporace F, Lindvall E, Infante A Jr, Sagi HC, Haidukewych GJ. Clamp-assisted reduction of high subtrochanteric fractures of the femur. J Bone Joint Surg Am. 2009;91(8):1913–8.
6. Codesido P, Mejia A, Riego J, Ojeda-Thies C. Cerclage wiring through a mini-open approach to assist reduction of subtrochanteric fractures treated with cephalomedullary fixation: surgical technique. J Orthop Trauma. 2017; 31(8):e263–8.
7. Ruecker AH, Rueger JM. Pertrochanteric fractures: tips and tricks in nail osteosynthesis. Eur J Trauma Emerg Surg. 2014;40(3):249–64.
8. Hoskins W, Bingham R, Joseph S, Liew D, Love D, Bucknill A, Oppy A, Griffin X. Subtrochanteric fracture: the effect of cerclage wire on fracture reduction and outcome. Injury. 2015;46(10):1992–5.
9. Kim JW, Park KC, Oh JK, Oh CW, Yoon YC, Chang HW. Percutaneous cerclage wiring followed by intramedullary nailing for subtrochanteric femoral fractures: a technical note with clinical results. Arch Orthop Trauma Surg. 2014;134(9):1227–35.
10. Babhulkar S. Unstable trochanteric fractures: issues and avoiding pitfalls. Injury. 2017;48(4):803–18.
11. Tsang ST, Aitken SA, Golay SK, Silverwood RK, Biant LC. When does hip fracture surgery fail? Injury. 2014;45(7):1059–65.
12. Ciufo DJ, Zaruta DA, Lipof JS, Judd KT, Gorczyca JT, Ketz JP. Risk factors associated with cephalomedullary nail cutout in the treatment of trochanteric hip fractures. J Orthop Trauma. 2017;31(11):583–8.
13. Palm H, Teixidor H. Proximal femoral fractures: can we improve further surgical treatment pathways? Injury. 2015;46(Suppl 5):S47–51.
14. Studer P, Suhm N, Wang Q, Rosenthal R, Saleh HA, Jakob M. Displaced trochanteric fragments lead to poor functional outcome in pertrochanteric fractures treated by cephalomedullary nails. Injury. 2015;46(12):2384–8.
15. Haidukewych GJ. Intertrochanteric fractures: ten tips to improve results. J Bone Joint Surg Am. 2009;91(3):712–9.
16. Ban I. Circumferential wires as a supplement to intramedullary nailing in unstable trochanteric hip fractures. Acta Orthop. 2013;84(2):227.
17. Angelini A, Battiato C. Past and present of the use of cerclage wires in orthopedics. Eur J Orthop Surg Traumatol. 2015;25(4):623–35.
18. Kulkarni SG, Babhulkar SS, Kulkarni SM, Kulkarni GS, Kulkarni MS, Patil R. Augmentation of intramedullary nailing in unstable intertrochanteric fractures using cerclage wire and lag screws: a comparative study. Injury. 2017;48(Suppl 2):S18–22.
19. Abdelkhalek M, Ali AM, Abdelwahab M. Cemented bipolar hemiarthroplasty with a cerclage cable technique for unstable intertrochanteric hip fractures in elderly patients. Eur J Orthop Surg Traumatol. 2013;23(4):443–8.
20. Angelini A, Battiato C. Combination of low-contact cerclage wiring and osteosynthesis in the treatment of femoral fractures. Eur J Orthop Surg Traumatol. 2016;26(4):397–406.
21. Apivatthakakul T, Phornphutkul C. Percutaneous cerclage wiring for reduction of periprosthetic and difficult femoral fractures. A technical note. Injury. 2012;43(6):966–71.

22. Ban I, Birkelund L, Palm H, Brix M, Troelsen A. Circumferential wires as a supplement to intramedullary nailing in unstable trochanteric hip fractures. 4 reoperations in 60 patients followed for 1 year. Acta Orthop. 2012;83(3):240–3.
23. Gavanier B, Houfani F, Dumoulin Q, Bernard E, Mangin M, Mainard D. Osteosynthesis of periprosthetic type a and B femoral fractures using an unlocked plate with integrated cerclage cable and trochanteric hook: a multicenter retrospective study of 45 patients with mean follow-up of 20 months. Injury. 2017;48(12):2827–32.
24. Gordon K, Winkler M, Hofstädter T, Dorn U, Augat P. Managing Vancouver B1 fractures by cerclage system compared to locking plate fixation – a biomechanical study. Injury. 2016;47(Suppl 2):S51–7.
25. Müller T, Topp T, Kühne CA, Gebhart G, Ruchholtz S, Zettl R. The benefit of wire cerclage stabilisation of the medial hinge in intramedullary nailing for the treatment of subtrochanteric femoral fractures: a biomechanical study. Int Orthop. 2011;35(8):1237–43.
26. Han KJ, Lee DH, Bang JY. Do cerclage cables delay the time to bone union in patients with an unstable humeral shaft fracture treated with intramedullary nails? Yonsei Med J. 2017;58(4):837–41.
27. Lin HH, Hung SH, Su YP, Chiu FY, Liu CL. Cerclage wiring in displaced associated anterior column and posterior hemi-transverse acetabular fractures. Injury. 2012;43(6):917–20.
28. Grimsrud C, Monzon RJ, Richman J, Ries MD. Cemented hip arthroplasty with a novel cerclage cable technique for unstable intertrochanteric hip fractures. J Arthroplast. 2005;20(3):337–43.
29. Cebesoy O, Subasi M, Isik M. Cerclage cable in fracture: frustration or necessity? Int Orthop. 2011;35(5):783–4.
30. Karakoyun O, Sahin E, Erol MF, Karıksız M, Küçükkaya M. Effect of cable cerclage on regional blood circulation in rabbits: a scintigraphic study. J Orthop Surg (Hong Kong). 2016;24(3):367–9.
31. Apivatthakakul T, Phaliphot J, Leuvitoonvechkit S. Percutaneous cerclage wiring, does it disrupt femoral blood supply? A cadaveric injection study. Injury. 2013;44(2):168–74.
32. Lenz M, Perren SM, Gueorguiev B, Richards RG, Krause F, Fernandez Dell'Oca A, Höntzsch D, Windolf M. Underneath the cerclage: an ex vivo study on the cerclage-bone interface mechanics. Arch Orthop Trauma Surg. 2012; 132(10):1467–72.
33. Evaniew N, Bhandari M. Cochrane in CORR®: intramedullary nails for extracapsular hip fractures in adults (review). Clin Orthop Relat Res. 2015; 473(3):767–74.

11

Associations between post-operative rehabilitation of hip fracture and outcomes: national database analysis

Bowen Su[1], Roger Newson[1], Harry Soljak[2] and Michael Soljak[3,1*]

Abstract

Background: Rehabilitation programmes are used to improve hip fracture outcomes. There is little published trial clinical trial or population-based data on the effects of the type or provider of rehabilitation treatments on hip fracture outcomes. We evaluated the associations of rehabilitation interventions with post-operative hip fracture outcomes.

Methods: Cross-sectional (2013–2015) analysis of data from the English National Hip Fracture Database (NHFD) from all 191 English hospitals treating hip fractures. Of 62,844 NHFD patients, we included 17,708 patients with rehabilitation treatment and 30-day mobility data, and 34,142 patients with rehabilitation treatment and discharge destination data. The intervention was early mobilisation rehabilitation treatments delivered by a physiotherapist (PT, physical therapist in North America) or other clinical staff as identifiable in NHFD. We used ordinal logistic and propensity scoring regression models to adjust for confounding variables including age, sex, pre-fracture mobility, operative delay, and cognitive function and peri-operative risk scores.

Results: In both the adjusted multivariate and propensity-weighted analyses, mobilisation on the day or the day following surgery is associated with better mobility function 30 days after discharge. However patients mobilised by a PT did not have better mobility compared to mobilisation by other professionals. Patients who received a PT assessment were not protected from poorer mobility 30 days after discharge, compared with those who did not receive an assessment. The discharge destination outcome is also better in mobilised than unmobilised patients, whether done by a PT or another health professional, and the difference persists, slightly attenuated, after propensity weighting.

Conclusions: In addition to the type of health professional initiating mobilisation, data on rehabilitation treatment activity and post-operative gait speed is needed to determine optimum rehabilitation dosage and functional outcome. After adjustment patients mobilised by non-PTs did as well as patients mobilised by PTs, suggesting that PTs' current roles in very early rehabilitation should be reconsidered, with a view to redeploying them to more specialised later rehabilitation activity.

Keywords: Hip fracture, Rehabilitation, Physical therapy, Clinical audit

* Correspondence: michael.soljak@ntu.edu.sg
[3]Centre for Population Health Sciences (CePHaS), Lee Kong Chian School of Medicine, Nanyang Technological University, Singapore 308232, Singapore
[1]Department of Primary Care & Public Health, School of Public Health, Imperial College London, W6 8RP, London, UK
Full list of author information is available at the end of the article

Background

Hip fractures in later life result in a high morbidity and mortality rate, with an often permanent decline in mobility, independence and quality of life [1]. Over a third of patients will have died 1 year after the fracture, compared with an expected annual mortality of about 10% in this age group [2]. One-year mortality after hip fracture has declined over the last decade in the United Kingdom (UK), [3] but the three-fold difference in one-year mortality between hip fracture patients and the general population has remained.

Although surgery is generally successful, few people recover fully, and there is a significant impact on their quality of life. Most survivors fail to regain former levels of mobility and activity, many become more dependent, and around 10% are unable to return to their previous residence [1, 4]. Many older people often already have loss of skeletal strength from osteoporosis, and sarcopenia, which is in itself a risk factor for falls and fractures [5]. In addition, people suffering a hip fracture frequently have other medical and physical problems, including impaired physical and cognitive function [6, 7]. There is also a significant psychological effect of hip fracture [8].

A variety of post-operative rehabilitation programmes are used to improve mobility, maximise physical function and prevent or reverse physical deconditioning. A 2009 Cochrane review of inpatient multi-disciplinary rehabilitation found a lack of evidence regarding what components of rehabilitation were essential for mobility recovery [9]. A 2010 Cochrane review of rehabilitation interventions for improving physical and psychosocial functioning included nine small heterogeneous trials involving 1400 participants [10]. It found conflicting results for specialist-nurse led care and educational and motivational interventions. A 2011 Cochrane review of interventions for improving mobility after hip fracture included 19 trials involving 1589 older adults, but these were mainly small, and often with methodological flaws [1]. Several recent studies in small populations evaluated the effectiveness of physiotherapy interventions in people with hip fracture [11–14]. However there has been little published rehabilitation research using large population-based datasets, [15] and rehabilitation data in the English National Hip Fracture Database Audit (NHFD) has not been extensively analysed previously. Furthermore, the results of randomised controlled trials are not necessarily replicated in "real world evidence" from unselected populations. The primary objectives of our evaluation were to use recent data from the [3] to:

- evaluate, after appropriate case-mix adjustment, the associations of rehabilitation (including physiotherapy) interventions with post-operative hip fracture mobility
- evaluate the associations of rehabilitation interventions with postoperative discharge destination and return to the same setting as pre-fracture.

The secondary objectives were:

- To assess the data quality of relevant NHFD variables
- To assess the appropriateness of current NHFD variables to audit rehabilitation interventions and to make recommendations for improvement

Methods

Data source

The NHFD is a clinically-led, web-based audit of hip fracture care and secondary prevention in England, Wales, Northern Ireland and the Channel Islands. All 253 eligible hospitals who treat hip fractures are registered with NHFD, and 98% participate by regularly uploading case records in a standard dataset format. All patients aged 60 and over with a hip fracture coded as S72.0, S72.1, S72.2 in ICD-10, including subtrochanteric fractures, are submitted, regardless of the fracture mechanism. The NHFD is approved by the NHS England Health Research Authority Confidentiality Advisory Group to collect patient data without consent under Section 251 exemption, so no ethical approval was required for this study. We carried out the same data quality checks used by NHFD on the 2013–15 data we received [16].

Exposure variables

To measure the effects of rehabilitation it would be most useful to have an activity type variable which described the type of rehabilitation delivered by specialist, mainly PT staff and the intensity e.g. number of sessions. As this is not part of the NHFD dataset we were forced to use proxies for rehabilitation activity or exposure. We used "mobilised on day of or day following surgery" as one measure of rehabilitation exposure. It is recognised that not all patients will be suitable for such mobilisation, and this field only seeks to capture how quickly individuals progress in initial physiotherapy. A patient would be described as 'mobilised' if they are able to sit or stand out of bed on the day of their return from operation, or on the following day. We used the variable "assessed by PT on day of or day after surgery" as another measure of rehabilitation exposure. Unfortunately these two variables are optional so some data is missing.

Predictor variables

We used demographic variables known to be associated with hip fracture outcomes, including age, sex, and delay from admission to operation. The Abbreviated Mental Test Score (AMTS), which is assessed pre-operatively, is a simple and robust 10 item screening tool for acute patients. In AMTS poor cognitive function = 0 and good cognitive function = 10. The American Society of Anaesthesiologists (ASA) score is a preoperative risk score based on the presence of co-morbidities at the time of surgery. An ASA score > 2 is associated with increased risk additional to that of classification of operation and duration of surgery.

Outcome variables

The first outcome variable was 30-day mobility score on a scale from 1 to 5, which counter-intuitively is higher for less mobile patients in NHFD. A new single mobility score has recently (2015) replaced all four measures previously used by the NHFD. In order to replace missing values of the single mobility score in older data, we used the translational matrix shown in Additional file 1: Table S1 in the online Supplementary Data file.

The second outcome variable was discharge destination from acute orthopaedic ward in combination with the location from which the patient was admitted. For the preoperative setting we used "admitted from". The method for combining the two variables is shown in Additional file 1: Table S2. Discharge destination models were fitted using the 30-day discharge destination combined with preoperative setting expressed on an integer scale from 1 to 4, with higher integers indicating better outcomes (1 = "Dead", 2 = "Worse", 3 = "Same", 4 = "Better").

Statistical analysis

Ordinal logistic regression models can be used where the outcome variable is nominal or ordinal i.e. with more than two levels [17, 18]. In mathematical notation:

$$L(\beta) = \_n\sum i = 1y1ig1(xi) + y2ig2(xi)$$
$$\text{-In}(1 + eg1(xi) + eg2(xi)).$$

We tested all the variables of interest in the NHFD dataset to check whether they were statistically associated with discharge destination (χ^2 tests and likelihood ratio tests). These variables were used to fit the ordinal logistic regression models. We used the *predict* command in Stata 14 to compute the ordinal-logistic odds ratio. We computed the c-statistic for a predictive score to measure the performance of the model.

Propensity score methods can be used for confounding control in non-experimental research [19]. We also carried out a propensity scoring or matching analysis, which is often used to obtain a better estimate of effect size in real-world examples. Propensity score models do not rely on modelling the outcome, but on a model of the treatment given the confounders [20, 21].

The mobility outcome was mobility at 30 days post-operatively. The Mobility models were fitted by using complete cases only. The treatment or exposure variable was mobilisation on the day of or day after surgery. Confounders were gender, age at discharge, hours elapsed between admission and surgery, pre-operation AMTS, ASA grade, and pre-fracture mobility score (1 to 5 or missing).

We defined a propensity score for mobilisation treatment with respect to confounders, using a logistic regression model, then defined weights to estimate the average treatment effect (ATE), [21] equal to the reciprocal of the fitted probability of mobilisation for the mobilised and non-mobilised patients respectively. More information on the propensity scores, weights and balance checks is provided in the online Additional file 1: Figures S3-S5. Having defined the propensity weights, we used Poisson regression models, with Huber variances, to regress the 30-day mobility score with respect to the binary treatment variable (mobilisation), with two mean mobility scores for mobilised and unmobilised patients, respectively. The first model was unadjusted/unweighted, and the second model was weighted using the ATE weights. For both models, we estimated the ATE using the Stata 14 add-on package *scenttest,* [22] which carries out a scenario *t*-test between the mobilised and unmobilised scenarios. We carried out balance checks for the propensity score using the Stata add-on package *somersd* [23].

Discharge destination models were fitted as for Mobility. We defined a propensity score for mobilisation treatment with respect to confounders, using a multinomial logistic regression model. For each patient, we defined three propensity scores, one per mobilisation group, as the fitted probability of the patient being in the mobilisation group. We then defined weights for estimation of the ATE [21]. Therefore we were directly standardising the sample to a hypothetical target population, with the same distribution of covariates as the sample, but with no association between treatment-propensity and treatment. The unadjusted Somers' *D* suggested that our ATE weights had balanced the propensity score. We then used Poisson regression models and the Stata packages as for the mobility outcome.

Results

Patient numbers are shown in the flowchart in Additional file 1: Figure S1. Of a total of 62,844 patients, there were 17,708 patients with non-missing values both for the treatment exposure and for 30-day mobility, and 34,142 patients with non-missing values both for the treatment variable and for the discharge-destination outcome, because as the latter did not require contacting patients but could be obtained from electronic health records (EHRs) it was easier to collect. Therefore, all analyses were subject to the caution of high missingness levels for the treatment exposure and the outcome.

Mobility

Most of the baseline characteristics of the complete cases in the Mobility model population after data translation are shown in Table 1. For further background, Additional file 1: Table S3 in the online Supplementary Data shows the mobility characteristics of the whole (both complete and incomplete cases) Mobility model outcome population before data translation. For comparison, Additional file 1: Table S4 shows the baseline characteristics of mobility variables before and after mobility data translation. Additional file 1: Table S5 shows all the baseline characteristics of Mobility Model population after data translation, for complete cases only.

Table 1 Key baseline characteristics of complete cases of the Mobility model population after data translation

Variables	Mobility model	
	Frequency	Percentage %
Age group		
60–69	1681	7.3
70–79	4384	19.0
80–89	10,471	45.5
> 90	6504	28.2
Total	23,040	100.0
Sex		
Male	6228	27.0
Female	16,812	73.0
Total	23,040	100.0
Pre Fracture Mobility		
Freely mobile without aids	7939	34.5
Mobile outdoors with one aid	4646	20.2
Mobile outdoors with two aids or frame	2619	11.4
Some indoor mobility but never goes out	7132	31.0
No functional mobility	391	1.7
Missing	313	1.4
Total	23,040	100.0
Mobility at 30 days		
Freely mobile without aids	452	2.0
Mobile outdoors with one aid	1746	7.6
Mobile outdoors with two aids or frame	3759	16.3
Some indoor mobility but never goes out	14,032	60.9
No functional mobility	3051	13.2
Missing	0	0.0
Total	23,040	100.0
Physiotherapy assessment		
No	399	1.7
Yes	22,546	97.9
Missing	95	0.4
Total	23,040	100.0
Mobilised on day of or day following surgery		
No	3332	14.5
Yes-physiotherapy	13,210	57.3
Yes-Other	661	2.9
Missing	5837	25.3
Total	23,040	100.0

X^2 tests (Additional file 1: Table S1) showed patients' pre-fracture mobility levels were most strongly associated with mobility 30 days after discharge, and AMTS, ASA grade and patients' age were also strongly associated with post fracture mobility. Gender and whether patients received PT assessment were weakly associated with post fracture mobility.

Table 2 shows the univariate and multivariate ordinal logistic regression analyses of the mobility model (as noted in the Methods a higher score indicates worse mobility). After adjustment, mobilisation on the day or the day following surgery is associated with a lower mobility score i.e. better mobility function 30 days after discharge. In the univariate analysis, mobilisation by a PT day or the day following surgery was more protective from a high score than mobilisation by other health professionals. However, in the adjusted/multivariate analysis, patients mobilised by a PT were not protected from poorer mobility compared to mobilisation by other professionals. Similarly, in both analyses, patients who received a PT assessment were not protected from poorer mobility 30 days after discharge, compared with those who did not receive an assessment.

We assessed discrimination of the ordinal logistic model in the same way as a traditional logistic model, using area under the receiver operating characteristic curve [24]. We fitted three different models but there was no difference in discrimination between them (area under the receiver operating characteristic curve = 0.755).

To further investigate associations of early mobilisation we then carried out a propensity-adjusted analysis comparing 30-day mobility between mobilised and unmobilised patients i.e. a two-category outcome (by grouping the PT and non-PT mobilisation). The Somers' *Ds* of the propensity score suggested that our ATE weights had balanced the propensity score between the treatment groups. We used the propensity weights to estimate the ATE, equal to the difference between the two scenario means, with PT and Other grouped together. The results in Additional file 1: Figure S2 show that the mobilisation-propensity score predicts mobilisation, with a Somers' D of 0.298. The ATE-adjusted scenario means are a little closer together than the unadjusted scenario means. The outcome is better (lower mobility score) in mobilised (=Yes) patients than in unmobilised patients (=No), whether the mobilisation is done by a PT or by somebody else, and the difference

Table 2 Univariate & multivariate ordinal logistic analysis for mobility (NB higher score = less mobile) 30 days after discharge model

	Univariate Analysis		Multivariate Analysis	
	ORs (95% CIs)	*P* value	ORs (95% CIs)	*P* value
Age 60–69	1		1	
70–79	1.067 (1.036–1.099)	< 0.001	1.139 (0.936–1.388)	0.196
80–89	0.857 (0.842–0.872)	< 0.001	1.628 (1.310–2.024)	< 0.001
> 90	1.513 (1.876–2.778)	< 0.001	2.269 (1.865–2.760)	< 0.001
Sex Male	1		1	
Female	1.018 (1.470–1.558)	0.54	0.931 (0.877–0.989)	0.02
Mobilised day of/after surgery No			1	
Yes-PT	0.438 (0.415–0.463)	< 0.001	0.541 (0.511 0.573)	< 0.001
Yes-Other	0.354 (0.304–0.413)	< 0.001	0.472 (0.403–0.553)	< 0.001
ASA grade Normal healthy individual	1		1	
Mild systemic disease that does not limit activity	2.627 (2.241–3.080)	< 0.001	1.601 (1.359–1.885)	< 0.001
Severe systemic disease that limits activity but is not incapacitating	6.987 (5.970–8.178)	< 0.001	2.453 (2.081–2.892)	< 0.001
Incapacitating systemic disease which is constantly life-threatening	12.096 (10.184–14.368)	< 0.001	3.078 (2.567–3.690)	< 0.001
Moribund - not expected to survive 24 h with or without surgery	36.562 (20.941–63.834)	< 0.001	7.057 (3.824–13.025)	< 0.001
Unknown	8.536 (6.734–10.820)	< 0.001	2.35 (1.828–3.021)	< 0.001
AMTS Score Poor cognitive function 0	1.263 (1.055–1.511)	0.084	1.179 (0.979–1.420)	0.084
1	1		1	
2	0.906 (0.723–1.136)	0.339	0.896 (0.710–1.132)	0.339
3	0.858 (0.683–1.077)	0.53	0.931 (0.736–1.178)	0.53
4	0.737 (0.589–0.923)	0.038	0.789 (0.626–0.995)	0.038
5	0.747 (0.600–0.929)	0.188	0.861 (0.687–1.079)	0.188
6	0.647 (0.522–0.802)	0.033	0.787 (0.631–0.982)	0.033
7	0.474 (0.388–0.580)	< 0.001	0.626 (0.509–0.771)	< 0.001
8	0.378 (0.313–0.456)	< 0.001	0.571 (0.470–0.693)	< 0.001
9	0.262 (0.219–0.314)	< 0.001	0.465 (0.386–0.560)	< 0.001
Good cognitive function 10	0.163 (0.137–0.193)	< 0.001	0.373 (0.312–0.446)	< 0.001
Not done	0.328 (0.266–0.405)	< 0.001	0.473 (0.382–0.587)	< 0.001
PT assessment No	1		1	
Yes	1.191 (0.996–1.424)	0.055	1.267 (1.056–1.520)	0.008
Pre Fracture Mobility Freely mobile no aids	1		1	
Mobile outdoors one aid	2.043 (1.901–2.197)	< 0.001	1.621 (1.503–1.749)	< 0.001
Mobile outdoors two aids or frame	2.813 (2.568–3.082)	< 0.001	1.956 (1.778–2.150)	< 0.001
Some indoor mobility never goes out	7.872 (7.315–8.472)	< 0.001	3.729 (3.442–4.039)	< 0.001
No functional mobility	53.419 (42.656 66.899)	< 0.001	27.849 (21.388–34.512)	< 0.001
Unknown	10.046 (7.929–12.727)	< 0.001	3.892 (3.051–4.964)	< 0.001
Delay (hours) to operation < 24	1		1	
24–48	0.304 (0.237–0.389)	< 0.001	0.999 (0.999–1.002)	0.95
48–70	0.336 (0.269–0.419)	< 0.001	0.999 (0.999–1.002)	0.95
> 70	0.338 (0.272–0.419)	< 0.001	1	

persists (slightly attenuated) after propensity weighting. The unadjusted results suggest that patients mobilised by a non-PT have a lower propensity score i.e. are better mobilised than patients mobilised by a PT, but the propensity-adjusted results suggest that this crude difference may easily be due to differences in the patients. This might happen if more vulnerable patients were allocated mostly to PTs and less vulnerable patients were allocated mostly to non-PTs. More detail about propensity scores and weights is provided in the online Additional file 1: Figure S3 is a forest plot of confounder categories vs Somers' D score which shows that ATE-weighted propensity scores for confounders are greatly reduced.

To further investigate the associations with who performs early mobilisation we then carried out a propensity-adjusted analysis comparing 30-day mobility score between mobilised (mobilised by PT or mobilised by other professionals) and unmobilised patients i.e. using three categories to separate the effects of PTs and other staff (Fig. 1). The results in Fig. 1 show that the mobilisation-propensity score predicts mobilisation, with a Somers' D of 0.298, as for the two-scenario analysis. The ATE-adjusted scenario means are a little closer together than the unadjusted scenario means, but not a lot. The outcome is better in mobilised patients than in unmobilised patients, whether the mobilisation is done by a PT or by somebody else. And the difference persists (slightly attenuated) after propensity weighting. However, it does not seem to make much difference whether the mobilisation is done by a PT or by somebody else, at least after propensity weighting.

Discharge destination

Additional file 1 Table S2 shows the baseline characteristics of the discharge destination model population. We again used propensity weights to estimate the ATEs, equal to the differences between the three scenario means (fully mobilised by PT, fully mobilised by others and fully non-mobilised) (Fig. 2). For this outcome a higher score indicates a better outcome. The mobilisation-propensity score predicts discharge destination, with a Somers' D of 0.332. Figure 2 shows that the ATE-adjusted scenario means are a little closer together than the unadjusted scenario means. The outcome is better in mobilised than unmobilised patients, whether done by a PT or by somebody else, and the difference persists (slightly attenuated) after propensity weighting. The results are quite similar to the 30 day Mobility model, suggesting that this is a reliable association.

Discussion

Summary

In summary, we investigated the associations of early mobilisation, as a proxy for rehabilitation, mainly delivered by PTs, with two outcome variables, both before and after adjustment for confounding variables. In both in the 30 day mobility and discharge destination outcome models, we confirmed that patients mobilised early had a better outcome than those not mobilised early, whether they were mobilised by PTs or by non-PTs. The unadjusted analyses suggest that patients mobilised by non-PTs were less immobile at 30 days, but after adjustment, patients mobilised by non-PTs did as well as patients mobilised by PTs. There are a number of possible explanations for this: there may be no actual difference, PTs could mobilise more vulnerable patients with a worse prognosis, or non-PTs such as nurses may deliver more rehabilitation sessions. However we also showed that 57% of patients are currently being mobilised early by a PT and only 3% by "Others", presumably nurses. If our findings are confirmed, PTs' roles in early rehabilitation should be reconsidered, with a view to redeploying them to more effective rehabilitation activity.

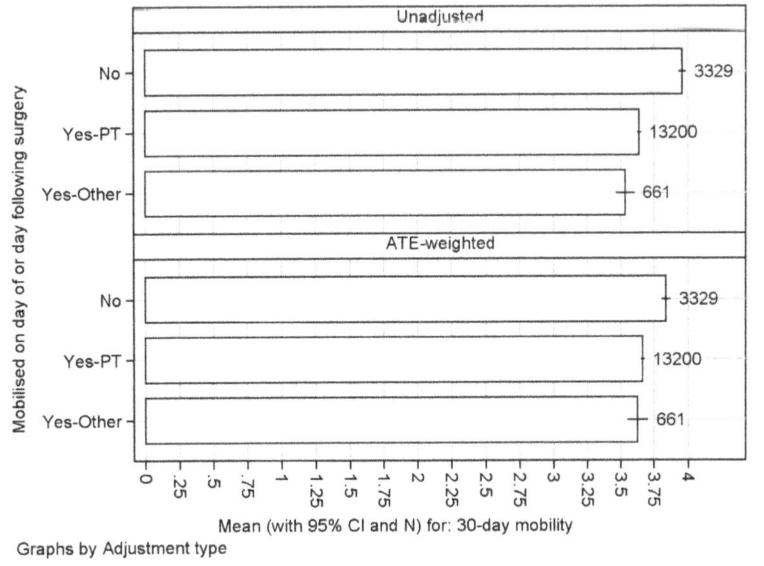

Fig. 1 Unadjusted and adjusted difference in average treatment effect (ATE) of no mobilisation (=no) or PT mobilisation (=yes-PT) or Other mobilisation (yes-Other) on day/day after surgery for 30-day mobility outcome (Numbers of scores are shown to right of each bar)

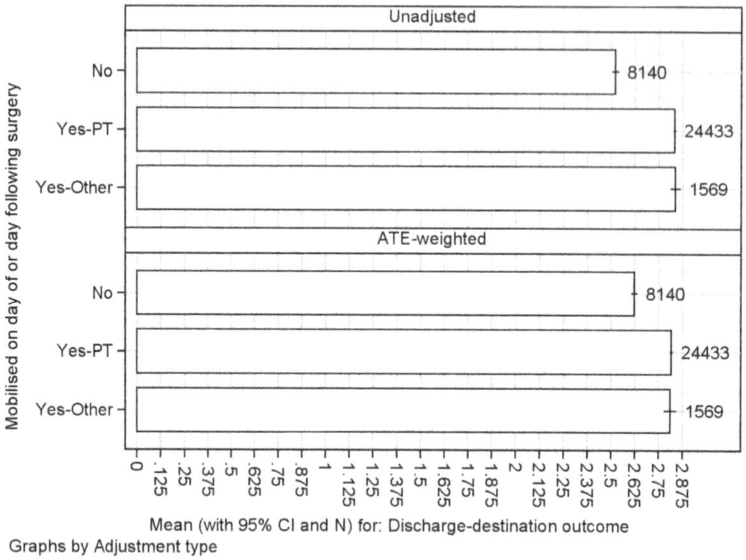

Fig. 2 Unadjusted and adjusted difference in average treatment effect (ATE) of mobilisation on day/day after surgery for discharge-destination outcome (Numbers of scores are shown to right of each bar)

There are few published cohort studies which have analysed rehabilitation exposures and outcomes, and in most instances they only measured effects of transfers to rehabilitation facilities. For example, in an Austrian cohort of 281 patients, [25] patients who were transferred to a nearby acute geriatric hospital for rehabilitation had significantly higher functional outcome scores. A study from the Scottish Hip Fracture Audit of 2708 patients aimed to determine whether place of residence is associated with a difference in access to comprehensive rehabilitation, rather than the effects of rehabilitation exposure [15]. It found that previously mobile care home patients were less likely to return to pre-admission levels of function at 120 days post fracture.

Strengths & limitations

We used two methods and two outcomes and obtained similar results from both, suggesting that our findings are robust. However, both the models could be applied to only the sub-population of patients with complete exposure and outcome data.

Unmeasured confounding is another limitation. Although we adjusted for five confounders, it is possible that other patient factors influenced outcomes. For example, a US study was assessed the relationship between self-reported disease burden and functional improvement during and after inpatient rehabilitation [26]. Compared with patients without chronic conditions, those who had a stroke had significantly worse self-care, transfer and locomotion ratings.

The biggest limitation in our analysis is that we were forced to use binary variables for early mobilisation or PT assessment as a proxy for rehabilitation, because there is inadequate data about the process of rehabilitation in the NHFD. There is likely to be great variation in the amount of early mobilisation rehabilitation, and there is little published data on the dose-response relationship. The hip fracture guideline from the UK's National Institute for Health & Care Excellence found only one, small randomised controlled trial with 60 patients of early versus delayed mobilisation, and three randomised studies with a total of 288 patients using three different types of PT programmes, which were not comparable and so could not be meta-analysed [27]. The American Academy of Orthopaedic Surgeons guidelines for the management of hip fractures in the elderly recommend intensive supervised occupational therapy and physiotherapy in hospital and home, [28] but the studies it quotes as evidence carried out extensive home rehabilitation programmes, [29] for example an intervention group received a median of 4.5 home visits, (PT median 3, minimum 0– maximum 7 visits; occupational therapist median 1.5, minimum 0–maximum 8 visits; and 11 patients were visited by a nurse) [30]. Real world rehabilitation may not have such a high dose.

Conclusions

In the real world the effectiveness of interventions which were efficacious in clinical trials may be sub-optimal. Given appropriate measurement, observational research using large databases such as our study can provide valuable evidence of clinical effectiveness. We found that early mobilisation is associated with better mobility function. NHFD data collection could be improved to capture dosage of rehabilitation activity by PTs and other healthcare professionals. This should not be done by manual data entry into NHFD, but by linkage of electronic data from hospital and community-based information systems. Unfortunately there is no national dataset for paramedical activity delivered to inpatients, which would allow this data to be linked with NHFD. NHFD should ask NHS Digital to produce such a dataset. In the interim, adding two variables in NHFD to capture a meaningful numerical rehabilitation outcome such as gait speed, and rehabilitation activity such as number of sessions, should be considered. The latter would help to determine the dose-response relationship of rehabilitation.

Future research and audit should aim to confirm our finding that, after adjustment, the results of early mobilisation by nurses seems to be similar to that achieved by PTs, although this could be a result of PTs treating patients with greater morbidity or frailty.

Additional file

Additional file 1: Table S1. Mobility variables translation matrix. **Table S2.** construction of admission/discharge destination outcome variable. **Figure S1.** Flowchart of mobility and discharge destination models. **Table S3** all baseline characteristics of mobility outcome population (both complete and incomplete cases) before data translation. **Table S4.** Frequency of mobility categories before and after data translation. **Table S5.** all baseline characteristics of Mobility Model population after data translation, complete cases only. **Table S6.** Strength of association between patient characteristics used in the Mobility models and mobility 30 days after discharge. **Figure S2** unadjusted and adjusted difference in average treatment effect (ATE) of no mobilisation (=no) or mobilisation (=yes) on day/day after surgery for 30-day mobility outcome. **Table S7** baseline characteristics of the discharge destination model. **Figure S3** chart of confounder categories vs Somers' D score for two category mobility outcome. **Figure S4.** Somers' D of propensity score and component covariates with respect to: mobilisation = No. **Figure S5.** Somers' D of propensity score and component covariates with respect to: mobilisation==No.

Acknowledgements/funding

This study was funded by a research grant from the UK Chartered Society of Physiotherapy (CSP). The funder was not involved in the design or conduct of the study. However we wish to acknowledge helpful comments received from an Expert Group coordinated by CSP, and from Prof Josip Car, Centre for Population Health Sciences (CePHaS), Lee Kong Chian School of Medicine, Nanyang Technological University, Singapore. We acknowledge the support of the National Hip Fracture Database, which is commissioned by the Healthcare Quality Improvement Partnership and managed by the Care Quality Improvement Department of the Royal College of Physicians, as part of the Falls and Fragility Fracture Audit Programme.

Authors' contributions

MS conceived the study and obtained funding and data. HS drafted the Background and Results sections. RN devised the statistical methods and carried out final analyses with BS. BS managed the data and carried out most of the analyses. RN performed the final statistical analyses. BS produced the draft tables and all authors contributed to subsequent drafts. MS edited and approved the final version. All authors read and approved the final manuscript.

Competing interests

The authors declare that they have no competing interests.

Author details

[1]Department of Primary Care & Public Health, School of Public Health, Imperial College London, W6 8RP, London, UK. [2]Department of Anaesthetics, St Peter's Hospital, Chertsey KT16 0PZ, UK. [3]Centre for Population Health Sciences (CePHaS), Lee Kong Chian School of Medicine, Nanyang Technological University, Singapore 308232, Singapore.

References

1. Handoll HHG, Sherrington C, Mak JCS. Interventions for improving mobility after hip fracture surgery in adults. Cochrane Database of Systematic Reviews. 2011;(3). https://doi.org/10.1002/14651858.CD001704.pub4.
2. Crotty M, Whitehead C, Miller M, Gray S. Patient and caregiver outcomes 12 months after home-based therapy for hip fracture: a randomized controlled trial. Arch Phys Med Rehabil. 2003;84(8):1237–9. 1233p
3. Boulton C, Bunning T, Burgon V, Cromwell D, Johansen A, Rai S, Stanley R, Tsang C, Wakeman R. National hip Fracture Database Annu Rep 2016. In: Falls and Fragility Fracture Audit Programme (FFFAP): Clinical Effectiveness and Evaluation Unit (CEEU), Royal College of Physicians; 2016.
4. Porell FW, Carter MW. Risk of mortality and nursing home institutionalization after injury. J Am Geriatr Soc. 2012;60(8):1498–503. 1496p
5. Landi F, Liperoti R, Russo A, Giovannini S, Tosato M, Capoluongo E, Bernabei R, Onder G. Sarcopenia as a risk factor for falls in elderly individuals: results from the ilSIRENTE study. Clin Nutr. 2012;31(5):652–8.
6. Leigheb F, Vanhaecht K, Sermeus W, Lodewijckx C, Deneckere S, Boonen S, Boto PA, Mendes RV, Panella M. The effect of care pathways for hip fractures: a systematic overview of secondary studies. Eur J Orthop Surg Traumatol. 2013;23(7):737–45.
7. Diamantopoulos AP, Hoff M, Hochberg M, Haugeberg G. Predictors of short- and long-term mortality in males and females with hip fracture - a prospective observational cohort study. PLoS One. 2013;8(10):e78169.
8. Zidén L, Wenestam C, Hansson-Scherman M. A life-breaking event: early experiences of the consequences of a hip fracture for elderly people. Clin Rehabil. 2008;22(9):801–11. 811p
9. Handoll HH, Cameron ID, Mak JC, Finnegan TP. Multidisciplinary rehabilitation for older people with hip fractures. Cochrane Database Syst Rev. 2009;4:CD007125.
10. Crotty M, Unroe K, Cameron Ian D, Miller M, Ramirez G, Couzner L. Rehabilitation interventions for improving physical and psychosocial functioning after hip fracture in older people. In: Cochrane Database of Systematic Reviews: John Wiley & Sons, ltd; 2010.
11. Ziden L. The break remains-elderly people's experiences of a hip fracture one year after discharge. Physiotherapy (United Kingdom). 2011;97:eS1377.
12. Peiten JB, Krug E, van Baardewijk LJ, van der Linden EHMJ, Haas R, Krijnen P, Schipper IB. Intensive rehabilitation in selected hip fracture patients may optimize care efficiency: a retrospective comparison study. J Rehabil Med. 2015;47(3):278–81.
13. Lahtinen A, Leppilahti J, Harmainen S, Sipila J, Antikainen R, Seppanen ML, Willig R, Vahanikkila H, Ristiniemi J, Rissanen P, et al. Geriatric and physically oriented rehabilitation improves the ability of independent living and physical rehabilitation reduces mortality: a randomised comparison of 538 patients. Clin Rehabil. 2015;29(9):892–906.
14. Ohoka T, Urabe Y, Shirakawa T. Therapeutic exercises for proximal femoral fracture of super-aged patients: effect of walking assistance using body weight-supported treadmill training (BWSTT). Physiotherapy. 2015;101:e1124–5.
15. Burleigh E, Smith R, Duncan K, Lennox I, Reid D. Does place of residence influence hospital rehabilitation and assessment of falls and osteoporosis risk following admission with hip fracture? Age Ageing. 2011;40(1):128–32.
16. Tsang C, Cromwell D. Statistical methods developed for the National hip Fracture Database Annu Rep, 2014. London: Royal College of Surgeons of England; 2014.
17. Hosmer JDW, Lemeshow S, Sturdivant RX. Logistic Regression Models for Multinomial and Ordinal Outcomes, Applied Logistic Regression: John Wiley & Sons, Inc.; 2013. p. 269–311.

18. Agresti A. Modelling ordered categorical data: recent advances and future challenges. Stat Med. 1999;18(17–18):2191–207.
19. Heinze G, Jüni P. An overview of the objectives of and the approaches to propensity score analyses. Eur Heart J. 2011;32(14):1704–8.
20. Garrido MM, Kelley AS, Paris J, Roza K, Meier DE, Morrison RS, Aldridge MD. Methods for constructing and assessing propensity scores. Health Serv Res. 2014;49(5):1701–20.
21. Guo L-L, Li L, Liu Y-W, Herr K. Evaluation of two observational pain assessment scales during the anaesthesia recovery period in Chinese surgical older adults. J Clin Nurs. 2015;24(1/2):212–21. 210p
22. Newson R: SCENTTEST: Stata module to compute scenario arithmetic means and their difference. Downloaded from https://econpapers.repec.org/software/bocbocode/s457904.htm on 15 January 2016.
23. Newson R: SOMERSD: Stata module to calculate Kendall's tau-a, Somers' D and median differences. Downloaded from https://ideas.repec.org/c/boc/bocode/s336401.html on 15 January 2016.
24. Zou KH, O'Malley AJ, Mauri L. Receiver-operating characteristic analysis for evaluating diagnostic tests and predictive models. Circulation. 2007;115(5):654–7.
25. Kammerlander C, Gosch M, Kammerlander-Knauer U, Luger TJ, Blauth M, Roth T. Long-term functional outcome in geriatric hip fracture patients. Arch Orthop Trauma Surg. 2011;131(10):1435–44.
26. Mathew RO, Hsu W-H, Young Y. Effect of comorbidity on functional recovery after hip fracture in the elderly. Am J Phys Med Rehabils. 2013;92(8):686–96.
27. National Institute for Health and Clinical Excellence: Clinical guideline: the management of hip fracture in adults. In. Edited by Excellence NIfHaC, vol. CG124. London; 2011, updated 2014.
28. American Academy of Orthopaedic Surgeons. Management of Hip Fractures in the Elderly. Illinois: American Academy of Orthopaedic Surgeons; 2017.
29. Crotty M, Whitehead CH, Gray S, Finucane PM. Early discharge and home rehabilitation after hip fracture achieves functional improvements: a randomized controlled trial. Clin Rehabil. 2002;16(4):406–13.
30. Ziden L, Kreuter M, Frandin K. Long-term effects of home rehabilitation after hip fracture - 1-year follow-up of functioning, balance confidence, and health-related quality of life in elderly people. Disabil Rehabil. 2010;32(1):18–32.

12

Anteromedial fractures of the ulnar coronoid process: correlation between surgical outcomes and radiographic findings

Alvin Chao-Yu Chen*, Chun-Jui Weng, Ying-Chao Chou and Chun-Ying Cheng

Abstract

Background: This study aimed to report the radiographic findings and surgical outcomes of anteromedial facet (AMF) fracture of the ulnar coronoid process and to suggest an optimal approach.

Methods: In this retrospective study, 20 consecutive patients with unilateral AMF fracture of coronoid process were surgically treated and divided into two groups without (group A) and with (group B) additional proximal ulnar fractures in equal case number. Time from injury to surgery averaged 4.38 ± 2.56 weeks. Mayo Elbow Performance Score (MEPS) and Shortened Disability of the Arm and Shoulder and Hand (quickDASH) score were used for functional evaluation. Cohen kappa coefficient (kappa) analysis was used to determine interobserver reliability on a radiographic reading.

Results: All cases had a mean follow-up of 2.3 years. MEPS at 2 years averaged 87.75 ± 12.51; quickDASH, 7.05 ± 6.19. A significantly higher MEPS was found in subtype 3 than in subtype 2 ($p = 0.036$) and in group B than in group A ($p = 0.020$). Significantly lower quickDASH cores were found in group B than in group A ($p = 0.011$). Kappa analysis showed moderate agreement in the O'Driscoll classification (kappa = 0.56) and substantial agreement in categorization of the additional proximal ulnar fractures (kappa = 0.76).

Conclusions: Additional proximal ulnar lesions were considered an integral part of varus posteromedial rotatory instability and required further categorization in the management of AMF fractures. Significantly better functional outcomes were achieved when those lesions were fully addressed.

Keywords: Elbow, Instability, Coronoid fracture, Anteromedial facet, Lateral collateral ligament, Varus instability

Background

Traditionally, the severity of coronoid fractures and their correlation with elbow stability were classified by fracture fragment size [1]. Previous studies have shown that the coronoid process consists of an anterior projection and an anteromedial facet (AMF). While the anterior projection was an anterior buttress of the elbow joint with > 25% involvement leading to gross instability [2–4], the AMF served as medial extension of the proximal ulna and was prone to fracture in resisting varus rotatory force [5, 6]. A more extensive classification system was proposed based on both fracture size and location to help analyze trauma mechanisms and predict associated injuries. However, coronoid fractures of the AMF, unlike those in terrible triad injuries, commonly show a diverse presentation [7]. Anatomically, fractures of the AMF may consist of simple avulsion of the sublime tubercle, a medial cortex split, and coronoid tip fracture with a tiny or large anterior fragment. The use of a strategic surgical approach is critical. The purpose of this study is to report the surgical outcomes of a consecutive case series and suggest an optimal surgical approach through a retrospective analysis of the surgical and radiographic findings of AMF fracture dislocation.

* Correspondence: alvinchen@cgmh.org.tw
Department of Orthopaedic Surgery, Bone and Joint Research Center, Chang Gung Memorial Hospital-Linkou & University College of Medicine, 5th, Fu-Shin St., Kweishan District, Taoyuan 333, Taiwan, Republic of China

Methods

Between 2007 and 2014, 20 patients with a displaced AMF fracture of the ulnar coronoid process and elbow subluxation were diagnosed with VPMRI by one orthopedic surgeon and one radiologist and referred for definite management. Chang Gung Institutional Review Board approval (IRB 201701326B0) was obtained for a retrospective review of all 20 patients' records and radiographs. The report of patients' data was in compliance with the Helsinki Declaration. Written consent to participate in the study was obtained from all the patients. Among them, 17 were primary injuries, while three were revision cases that had failed previous open reduction and internal fixation surgery. All patients underwent surgical fixation by the same surgeon, including five women and 15 men with an average age of 43.65 ± 12.17 years (range, 26–67 years). Twelve were in the left elbow; the other eight were in the right elbow. Three patients had concomitant ulnar neuropathy. The mean time interval from injury to surgery was 4.38 ± 2.56 weeks (range, 0–10). Based on radiographic findings, all 20 patients were divided into two groups. Patients without additional proximal ulnar lesions was in group A and served as a control; patients with additional proximal ulnar lesions, group B.

Radiographic assessment

Preoperative plain X-ray and computed tomography (CT) images were retrospectively reviewed by two of the authors (one orthopedic trauma surgeon [WCJ] and one elbow surgeon [ACC]). Based on the O'Driscoll classification for AMF fracture, two were subtype 1, nine were subtype 2, and nine were subtype 3. Furthermore, additional fractures of the proximal ulna beyond the definition of the O'Driscoll classification were found in 10 cases (Fig. 1). A coronoid base fracture was found in one case of subtype 2 and three cases of subtype 3. An articular depression between the AMF and the coronoid base (Fig. 2a) was found in one case of subtype 2 and three cases of subtype 3. An olecranon fracture was found in three cases, one of each subtype (Fig. 2b). Accordingly, we divided the 20 cases into two radiographic groups: group A, 10 cases without additional fractures; and group B, 10 cases with additional fractures. The patients' demographic data are listed in Table 1.

Surgical strategy and technique

Two kinds of surgical approaches for treating AMF of the coronoid process were used according to the preoperative radiographic analysis. For the three cases of olecranon fracture, a posterior global approach was adopted; for the other 17 cases, a medial over-the-top approach was used. A lateral incision was added whenever exposure of the lateral collateral ligament (LCL) was necessary. The surgical strategy was based on the O'Driscoll classification as well as the presentation of additional fractures (Fig. 3). To treat olecranon fracture, dorsal plating was applied for length and alignment restoration in two cases and a revision Kirschner wire with tension band fixation was performed in one case. A hybrid of internal fixation was used for coronoid fracture depending on the fracture patterns (Fig. 4). For large

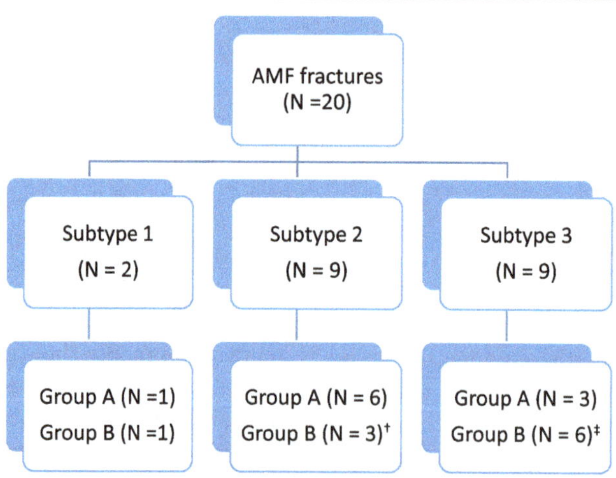

† 1 patient of coronoid base fracture; 1 patient coronoid articular depression fracture; 1 patient of coronoid base + coronoid articular depression + olecranon fracture

‡ 4 patients of coronoid base fractures; 1 patient of coronoid articular depression fracture; 1 patient of coronoid base + articular depression fracture

Fig. 1 Patient allocation according to fracture patterns

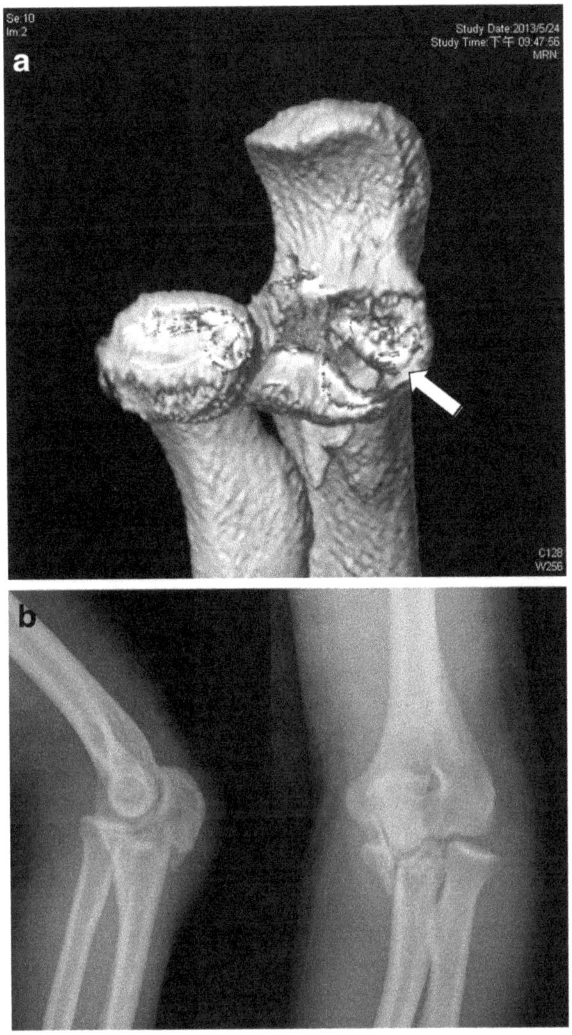

Fig. 2 Two cases of anteromedial facet fractures. **a** Three-dimensional computed tomography scans showing an articular depression fracture (white arrow) close to the base of the coronoid process. **b** Plain radiographs showing an olecranon fracture with a displaced anteromedial facet fracture of the coronoid process

Table 1 Demographic data of patients

Characteristics	Group A	Group B
Mean age (years)	47	40.3
Gender		
Women	3	2
Men	7	8
O'Driscoll's classification type 2 fracture		
Subtype 1	1	1
Subtype 2	7	3
Subtype 3	2	6
Time to surgery (weeks)	2.2	1.3

reducible fragments of the anterior coronoid without comminution, retrograde pinning followed by cannulated screw fixation from the dorsal proximal ulna was performed. Eighteen of our 20 cases (90%) showed an anteromedial rim split fracture accompanied by articular depression in four cases (20%) and was buttressed using a pre-contoured mini-plate (Synthes, Switzerland) or a Coronoid Plate (Acumed, OR, USA). The sublime tubercle avulsion fracture in nine cases (45%) was reduced and fixed with an interfragmental screw or suture anchor for securing the anterior band of the medial collateral ligament. After the fracture fixation, lateral elbow stability was checked under a mini-c-arm image intensifier. Three cases showed greater than grade II laxity and were treated with LCL repair using suture anchor fixation. In three cases (15%) of concomitant ulnar neuropathy with injury, surgical decompression and anterior transposition of the ulnar nerve was performed.

Postoperatively, the elbow was immobilized in a long arm splint at 90° of flexion and neutral rotation for 2 weeks; a gentle active motion was then initiated with a hinged brace for another 4 weeks. After that, the hinged brace was used only intermittently without range of motion limitations. Daily and occupational activities were allowed at 3 months after surgery.

Functional and radiographic assessment

Postoperatively, all patients attended regular outpatient clinic follow-up appointments at 2 weeks, 3 months, 6 months, 1 year, and 2 years. The Mayo Elbow Performance Score (MEPS) was used for functional survey and the Shortened Disability of the Arm and Shoulder and Hand (quickDASH) score was used for the subjective disability evaluation. The MEPS is a widely-used, physician-based elbow performance index for evaluating clinical outcomes of a variety of elbow disorders and showed validated reliability and accuracy for evaluating the treatment results of elbow fractures and dislocation [8]. Being a shortened version of the DASH Outcome Measure, the quickDASH uses 11 items (scored 1–5) instead of 30 items as in the DASH measurement to evaluate perceived physical function and symptoms in people with musculoskeletal disorders of the upper limb [9]. A radiographic examination was performed next to surgery day, and 3 months, 1 year, and 2 years after surgery.

Statistical analysis

Functional outcomes according to MEPS and quickDASH score were compared between different subtypes and between group A and B using an independent t-test. P values < 0.05 were considered statistically significant. Interobserver consistencies in radiographic diagnoses were analyzed between two observers using Cohen's kappa coefficient (kappa) analysis, in which a

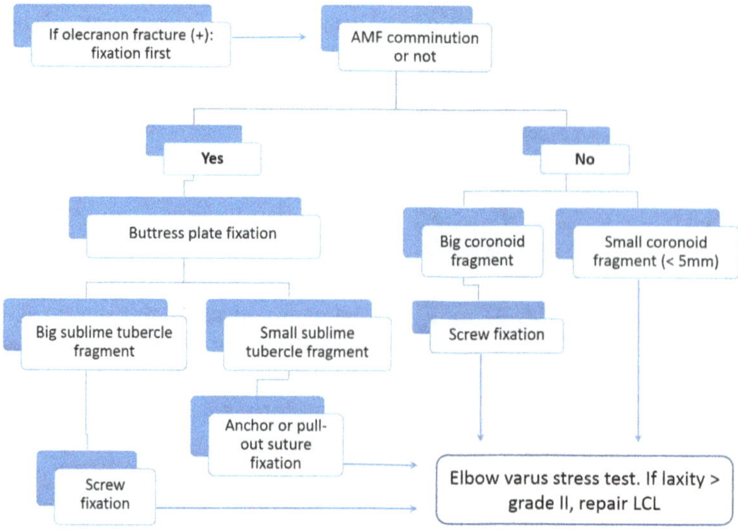

Fig. 3 Treatment algorithm. AMF, anteromedial facet; LCL, lateral collateral ligament

kappa of 0.41–0.60 meant moderate agreement and a kappa > 0.60 indicated substantial agreement.

Results

All patients underwent a clinical survey at an outpatient clinic with a mean follow-up of 2.3 years (range, 2–3.8 years). Radiographic union was defined by surgeon and radiologist consensus and was achieved in all cases at about 3 months after surgery. A functional survey was performed at 2 years with a mean MEPS of 87.75 ± 12.51 (range, 55–100) and quickDASH score of 7.05 ± 6.19 (range, 0–22). On MEPS grading, excellent results were achieved in 10 cases, while good results were achieved in eight. Fair and poor outcomes were achieved in one case each.

Comparisons of different subtypes and radiographic groups are detailed in Fig. 5. Better functional outcomes were found in subtype 3 than in subtype 2, with a significant difference in MEPS ($p = 0.036$) but not in quick-DASH scores ($p = 0.85$). The differences in functional scores between subtypes 1 and 2 and between subtypes 1 and 3 were insignificant. Functional outcomes were also compared between groups A and B. Significantly better outcomes were found in group B than in group A in both MEPS ($p = 0.020$) and quickDASH score ($p = 0.011$).

There were no immediate surgical complications such as neurovascular injury, wound problem, infection, or secondary displacement after fixation. Three cases of preoperative ulnar neuropathy were treated surgically with nerve transposition and achieved neurological recovery. No residual lateral instability was found after 3 months of follow-up. There were two cases of inferior outcomes: one received surgical fixation 1 week after acute trauma and had heterotopic ossification along the medical capsule postoperatively with a final range of motion of 5–80° and showed poor outcome on MEPS grading, while the other was a revision case that was treated with coronoid fixation at 3 weeks after the primary surgery. Partial resorption of the AMF fragment after revision surgery was found, and the final motion arc was 5–95° with residual instability.

Analysis of interobserver consistency on radiographic readings showed moderate agreement in the O'Driscoll classification (kappa = 0.56) and substantial agreement in the categorization of additional proximal ulnar fractures (kappa = 0.76). In cases of disagreement, reports of fracture classification and the categorization of additional fractures were empirically based on the surgeon's recommendations.

Discussion

The ulnar coronoid is a critical stabilizer in elbow trauma [10], and fractures involving > 25% of the coronoid height resulted in significant elbow instability [11]. O'Driscoll proposed a new classification of coronoid process fracture based on fracture size and location [5]. Reflecting the elbow injury mechanism, the O'Driscoll classification became popularly adopted as treatment guidance [12, 13]. Unlike the common fracture pattern of the anterior coronoid in terrible triad injuries, AMF fracture corresponding to O'Driscoll classification type 2 fracture shows a diverse presentation in fracture patterns and locations. Cases of type 2 fractures were further divided into three subtypes to cover different presentations of AMF fractures involving the coronoid tip, anteromedial cortex, sublime tubercle, or a combination thereof. Resulting from varus rotational injury force, AMF fractures could be associated with LCL insufficiency and lead to VPMRI [14].

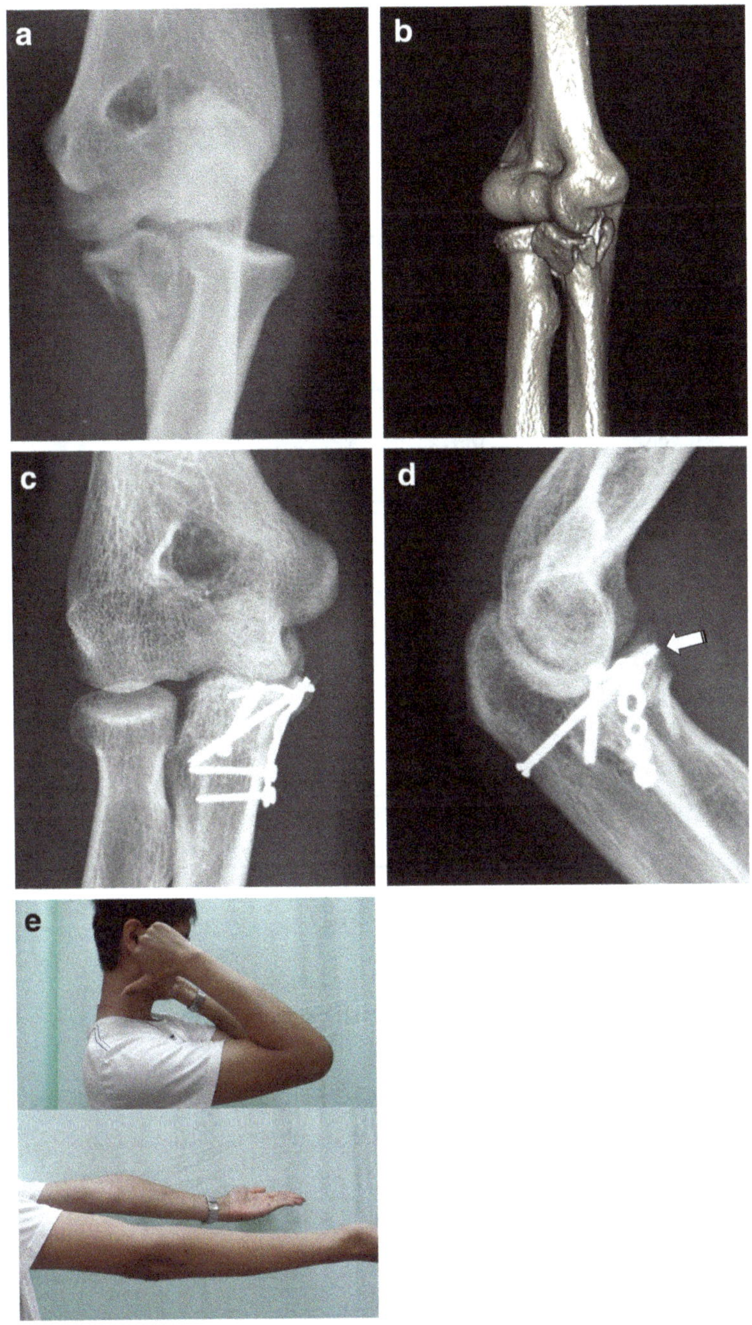

Fig. 4 Anteromedial facet fracture with varus instability. **a** Plain radiograph. **b** Three-dimensional computed tomography image showing a large coronoid fragment. **c** Postoperative anteroposterior radiograph. **d** Postoperative lateral radiograph; the white arrow shows retrograde screw fixation of a coronoid base fracture. **e** Patient photo at 10 weeks after surgery showing good range of motion

The surgical approach to VPMRI includes fracture fixation, ligament repair, or both, but treatment priority has yet to be determined. A recent comparison study consisting of 18 patients with O'Driscoll type 2 fractures proposed a strategic approach to fix big coronoid fragment with or without ligament repair but to leave the small fragment alone [15]. We believed all the bony constructs should be repaired as possible, and adopted the "fracture-fixation" strategy that meant we fixed all the coronoid and proximal ulnar fractures first. Small or comminuted coronoid fragments were buttressed with low-profile plates and augmented by anchor or transosseous suture. After restoration of bony constructs, we then verified stability and repaired the LCL whenever residual instability persisted. Since AMF is mechanically considered the primary constraint against varus rotatory force in the elbow joint [6], anatomical restoration with secure

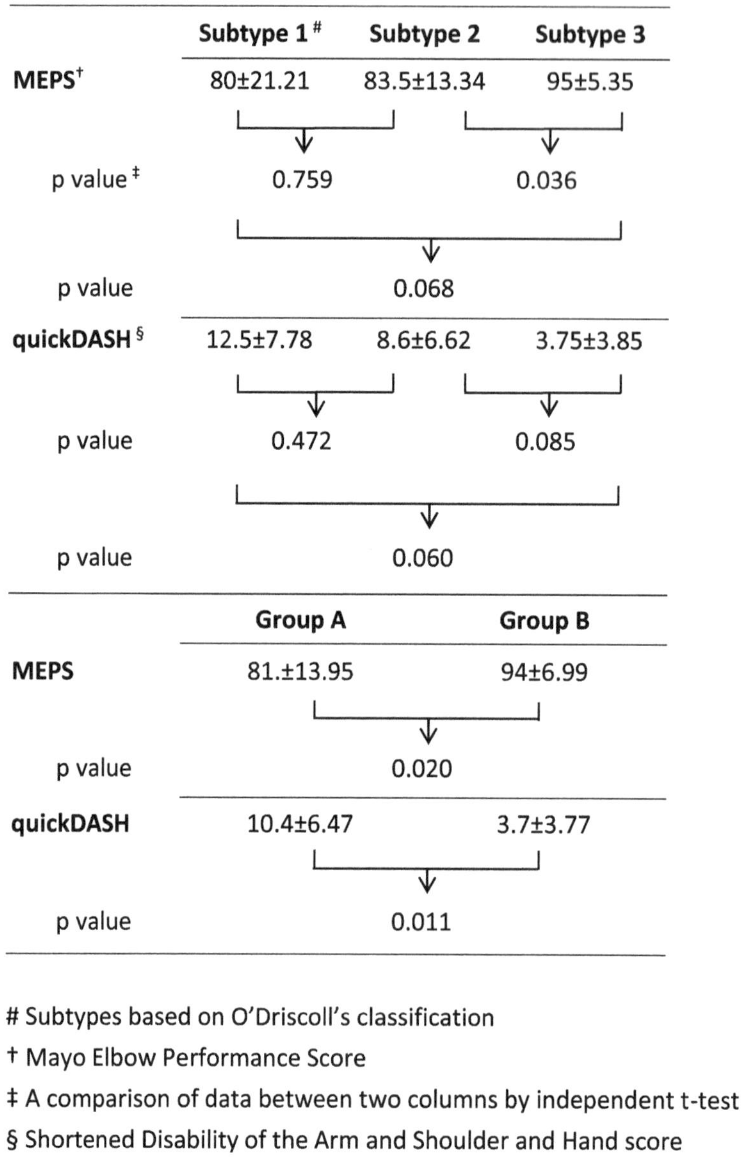

Fig 5 Comparison of functional assessment according to MEPS and DASH scores

fixation was recommended and critical in the treatment of AMF fractures with or without LCL insufficiency. Although a previous biomechanical study [16] and clinical report [17] documented that the direct management of LCL per se could improve the instability associated with AMF fractures, consensus is lacking regarding LCL injury severity. While surgical indications and LCL repair timing have yet to be established, LCL repair alone may not be beneficial whenever surgical reduction and secure fixation are achievable.

Despite the establishment of comprehensive classification systems and increased understanding of the pathophysiology, a definite treatment protocol and optimal surgical strategy have yet to be determined. In addition to the fracture patterns described in the O'Driscoll type 2 coronoid fracture, there could be various additional lesions over the proximal ulna. A recent study using CT images and a fracture mapping technique demonstrated considerable variability in coronoid fracture patterns and thus recommended that the present classification was insufficient for predicting coronoid fracture type [18]. Radiographs in half of our cases showed concomitant proximal ulnar fractures including olecranon, coronoid base, and coronoid articular depression fractures. All of those additional lesions were considered an integral part of VPMRI that needed to be fully addressed during surgical management. To our knowledge, the present study was the first to discuss the radiographic correlations of concomitant proximal ulnar injuries with AMF fractures and compared their treatment results. Significantly better functional outcome in cases of concomitant proximal ulnar lesions supported our surgical strategy and may encourage the surgeon to address all of the injured components in addition to AMF fractures. A more extended radiographic classification to include the proximal ulnar lesions is essentially important to categorize the injury patterns of AMF fractures. The use of a combined analysis of preoperative radiographic findings and injury mechanisms may enable surgeons to develop a meticulous surgical plan and thorough intervention of AMF fractures and the associated VPMRI.

This study had several limitations. First, it was a retrospective study from a consecutive series of 20 cases. Second, despite being a case-comparison study, the surgical approach and fixation modality was empirically determined through the planning and experience of a single surgeon. Third, there was a relatively small sample size in each group. Since we treated only referred cases from the primary trauma unit of our hospital and other institutes, a delay in definite treatment could have an adverse effect in either group. For future investigations, comparison studies with larger case numbers are necessary to further categorize associated injuries and clarify the critical role of the lateral elbow tissue in AMF fracture and VPMRI.

Conclusions

An innovative surgical strategy was proposed according to radiographic findings. With consideration of additional proximal ulnar lesions, AMF fractures could be further classified and thoroughly treated before proceeding to the intraoperative varus stress test to determine the indication for LCL repair. Significantly better functional outcomes were found when the associated proximal ulnar lesions were fully addressed during the surgical management of AMF fractures.

Abbreviations

AMF: Anteromedial facet; CT: Computed tomography; DASH: Shortened Disability of the Arm and Shoulder and Hand; LCL: Lateral collateral ligament; MEPS: Mayo Elbow Performance Score; VPMRI: Varus posteromedial rotatory instability

Authors' contributions

ACC formulated the outline, searched and retrieved the articles, and drafted the manuscript. CJW assisted in data collection and calculation. YCC and CYC assisted in the outline and drafting/revision of the manuscript. All authors read and approved the final manuscript.

Consent for publication

We have obtained written consent to publish from the participants.

Competing interests

The authors declare that they have no competing interests.

References

1. Regan W, Morrey BF. Fractures of the coronoid process of the ulna. J Bone Joint Surg Am. 1989;71:1348–54. PMID: 2793888
2. Matzon JL, Widmer BJ, Draganich LF, Mass DP, Phillips CS. Anatomy of the coronoid process. J Hand Surg Am. 2006;31:1272–8. https://doi.org/10.1016/j.jhsa.2006.05.010.
3. Ring D. Fractures of the coronoid process of the ulna. J Hand Surg Am. 2006;31:1679–89. PMID: 17145391
4. Beingessner DM, Dunning CE, Stacpoole RA, Johnson JA, King GJW. The effect of coronoid fractures on elbow kinematics and stability. Clin Biomech. 2007;22:183–90. https://doi.org/10.1016/j.clinbiomech.2006.09.007
5. O'Driscoll SW, Jupiter JB, Cohen MS, Ring D, McKee MD. Difficult elbow fractures: pearls and pitfalls. [review] [91 refs]. Instr Course Lect. 2003;52: 113–34. PMID: 12690844
6. Pollock JW, Brownhill J, Ferreira L, McDonald CP, Johnson J, King G. The effect of anteromedial facet fractures of the coronoid and lateral collateral ligament injury on elbow stability and kinematics. J Bone Joint Surg Am. 2009;91:1448–58. https://doi.org/10.2106/JBJS.H.00222.
7. Doornberg JN, Ring D. Coronoid fracture patterns. J Hand Surg Am. 2006;31: 45–52. https://doi.org/10.1016/j.jhsa.2005.08.014.
8. Cusick MC, Bonnaig NS, Azar FM, Mauck BM, Smith RA, Throckmorton TW. Accuracy and reliability of the Mayo elbow performance score. J Hand Surg Am. 2014;39:1146–50. https://doi.org/10.1016/j.jhsa.2014.01.041.
9. Mintken PE, Glynn P, Cleland JA. Psychometric properties of the shortened disabilities of the arm, shoulder, and hand questionnaire (QuickDASH) and numeric pain rating scale in patients with shoulder pain. J Shoulder Elb Surg. 2009;18:920–6. https://doi.org/10.1016/j.jse.2008.12.015.
10. Morrey BF. Complex instability of the elbow. Instr Course Lect. 1998;47:157–64. PMID: 9571413
11. Closkey RF, Goode JR, Kirschenbaum D, Cody RP. The role of the coronoid process in elbow stability. A biomechanical analysis of axial loading. J Bone Joint Surg Am. 2000;82:1749–53. PMID: 11130649
12. Sanchez-Sotelo J, O'Driscoll SW, Morrey BF. Medial oblique compression fracture of the coronoid process of the ulna. J Shoulder Elbow Surg. 2005; 14:60–4. https://doi.org/10.1016/j.jse.2004.04.012.
13. Steinmann SP. Coronoid process fracture. J Am Acad Orthop Surg. 2008;16: 519–29. PMID: 18768709
14. Ramirez MA, Stein JA, Murthi AM. Varus posteromedial instability. Hand Clin. 2015;31:557–63. https://doi.org/10.1016/j.hcl.2015.06.005.
15. Rhyou IH, Kim KC, Lee JH, Kim SY. Strategic approach to O'Driscoll type 2 anteromedial coronoid facet fracture. J Shoulder Elb Surg. 2014;23:924–32. https://doi.org/10.1016/j.jse.2014.02.016.
16. Pollock JW, Pichora J, Brownhill J, Ferreira LM, McDonald CP, Johnson JA, King GJ. The influence of type II coronoid fractures, collateral ligament injuries, and surgical repair on the kinematics and stability of the elbow: an in vitro biomechanical study. J Shoulder Elb Surg. 2009; 18:408–17. https://doi.org/10.1016/j.jse.2009.01.009.
17. Park SM, Lee JS, Jung JY, Kim JY, Song KS. How should anteromedial coronoid facet fracture be managed? A surgical strategy based on O'Driscoll classification and ligament injury. J Shoulder Elb Surg. 2015;24:74–82. https://doi.org/10.1016/j.jse.2014.07.010.
18. Mellema JJ, Doornberg JN, Dyer GSM, Ring D. Distribution of coronoid fracture lines by specific patterns of traumatic elbow instability. J Hand Surg Am. 2014;39:2041–6. https://doi.org/10.1016/j.jhsa.2014.06.123.

13

Epidemiology, treatment and mortality of trochanteric and subtrochanteric hip fractures: data from the Swedish fracture register

Leif Mattisson[1*], Alicja Bojan[2] and Anders Enocson[1,3]

Abstract

Background: Hip fractures are a major worldwide public health problem and includes two main types of fractures: the intracapsular (cervical) and the extracapsular (trochanteric and subtrochanteric) fractures. The aim of this study on patients with trochanteric and subtrochanteric hip fractures was to describe the epidemiology, treatment and outcome in terms of mortality within the context of a large register study.

Methods: A descriptive epidemiological register study including patients registered in the national Swedish Fracture Register from January 2014 to December 2016. Inclusion criteria were all primary surgically treated traumatic non-pathological trochanteric and subtrochanteric femoral fractures in patients aged 18 years and above. Individual patient data (age, gender, injury location, injury cause, fracture type, treatment and timing of surgery) were retrieved from the register database. Mortality data was obtained via linkage to the Swedish Death Register.

Results: A total of 10,548 consecutive patients were identified and included in the study. The mean (±SD) age for all patients was 82 ± 11 years and the majority of the patients were females (69%). Most of the fractures were caused by a fall at the same level (83%) at the patients' accommodation (75%). Fractures were classified using the AO/OTA classification as 31-A1 in 29%, as 31-A2 in 49% and as 31-A3 in 22% of the cases. The most commonly used implant was a short antegrade intramedullary nail (42%), followed by a plate with sliding hip screw (37%). With increasing fracture complexity, the proportion of intramedullary nails was increasing, and also the use of long versus short nails. The majority of the patients were operated within 36 h (90%). There was a higher mortality at 30 days and 1 year for males, and for all those who were delayed to surgery > 36 h.

Conclusion: Safety measures to prevent fall at elderly patient's accommodation might be a way to reduce the number of trochanteric and subtrochanteric hip fractures. Surgery as soon as possible without delay should be considered to reduce the mortality rate. The selection of surgical methods depends on the fracture complexity.

Keywords: Hip fracture, Trochanteric fracture, Surgical treatment, Epidemiology, Register study

* Correspondence: leif.mattisson@sll.se
[1]Department of Clinical Science and Education, Södersjukhuset, Karolinska Institutet. Department of Orthopaedics, Stockholm South General Hospital, 11883 Stockholm, Sweden
Full list of author information is available at the end of the article

Background

Hip fractures are a major public health problem and can lead to disability, reduced quality of life and increased mortality. Hip fractures in general are affecting around 1.5 million people per year worldwide, with the highest rates found in Scandinavia and the lowest in Africa [1, 2]. The number of hip fractures is likely to increase as the number of elderly people is increasing and worldwide it has been estimated that the number of hip fractures will rise to 2.6 million by 2025, and to 6.25 million in 2050 [1, 3]. The hip fractures are a heterogenous group with two main types of fractures: the intracapsular (cervical) and the extracapsular (trochanteric and subtrochanteric) fractures.

The absolute majority of the trochanteric and subtrochanteric hip fracture patients are fragile patients with a tendency to fall and an increased risk of major morbidity and mortality [4–7]. It is important to provide adequate management to these patients and the treatment of choice is normally surgical with internal fixation. The surgical options for these fractures commonly include plating with sliding hip screw or intramedullary nailing, with nailing today being the predominant procedure in many parts of the world [8, 9].

Although most of the authors in the literature recommend that hip fracture patients should be operated without delay to allow early mobilization and thereby reducing mortality and morbidity, the topic is still controversial and the effect of the time to surgery on mortality is debated [10–13].

The Swedish Fracture Register (SFR) is a nationwide register in which data on fracture epidemiology is reported. Previous publications from the register on specific fractures includes humeral and clavicle fractures [14, 15].

The aim of this study on patients with trochanteric and subtrochanteric hip fractures was to describe the epidemiology, treatment and outcome in terms of mortality within the context of a large register study.

Methods

The SFR started in 2011 and collects information on fractures in extremities, pelvis and spine. The database is national and the data is registered locally at the affiliated departments. Detailed data on fracture epidemiology and treatment is registered and all fractures are registered regardless of treatment type – surgical or non-surgical. To be included in the register the patients need to have a permanent Swedish personal identity number and only fractures that have occurred in Sweden are registered. At the start of this study in January 2014 the number of affiliated departments was 24, and end of the study in December 2016 the number of affiliated departments was 39. The total number of departments in Sweden that are treating fractures is estimated to 54. Data on patient mortality is obtained to the register via linkage to the national Swedish Death Register.

Inclusion criteria in this study were primary surgically treated traumatic non-pathological trochanteric and subtrochanteric femoral fractures in patients aged 18 years and above, occurring from January 2014 to December 2016.

Variables

Epidemiologic data (patient age and gender), injury data (injury location, cause and date), fracture data (fracture type, treatment and timing of surgery) and mortality data were retrieved from the register database.

Injury location was categorized as: at the patients' residence or accommodation, in a public place, in a street/road or in an unspecified place. The cause of injury was divided into: a fall at the same level, an unspecified fall, a fall from height, a traffic injury or any other cause. There is no strict guideline for classification of the energy level in the SFR, and it is up to the registering doctor to distinguish between high- and low-energy trauma mechanism. Fractures were classified according to the AO/OTA classification [16] and the ICD-10 code. Surgical implants were categorized as: a short or long antegrade intramedullary nail, a retrograde intramedullary nail, a plate with sliding hip screw, any other type of plate fixation, a hip arthroplasty or any other type of implant. The experience of the main surgeon was divided into: a specialist in orthopaedic surgery, an orthopaedic registrar or any other surgeon. Starting in early 2015, the time of the radiograph confirming the fracture and the time of the start of the operation was included in the register. From these variables, the time (in hours) from the radiograph to the start of the surgery was calculated.

Patient mortality was presented as 30-day and 1-year mortality.

Statistics

Because of the descriptive nature of the study, statistical testing of the variables was not performed. Variables are presented as proportions of all registered fractures, meaning the available number of inputs in the register excluding any missing values. For scale variables mean ± standard deviations (SD) are presented. The statistical software used was IBM SPSS Statistics, Version 23 for Windows (SPSS Inc., Chicago, USA).

Results

Patient and fracture epidemiology

A total of 10,548 entries fulfilling the inclusion criteria were identified in the register and included in the study. The majority of the patients were female (69.4%, n = 7317/10548) and the mean (±SD) age for all patients was 82.4 ± 10.5 years. The mean (±SD) age was higher for females (83.9 ± 9.1 years) compared to males (78.9 ± 12.3 years) (Fig. 1).

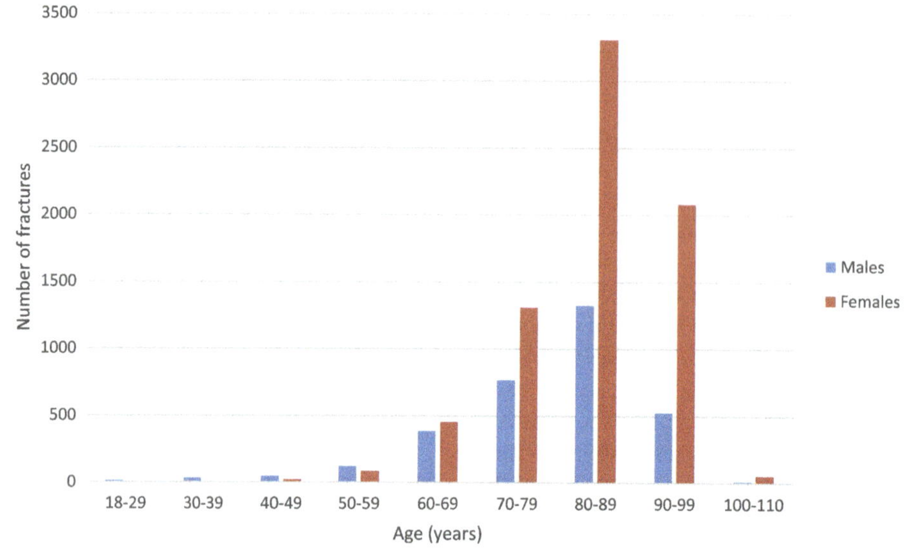

Fig. 1 Distribution of trochanteric and subtrochanteric femoral fractures by age and gender

The location for the trauma was at the patients' current residence or accommodation in 75% ($n = 7631/10249$) of the cases, in a public place in 4.1% ($n = 418/10249$), in a street/road in 3.7% ($n = 378/10249$) or in an unspecified place in 18% ($n = 1822/10249$). The cause of the injury was a fall at the same level (83%, $n = 8796/10548$), an unspecified fall (9.8%, $n = 1034/10548$), a fall from height (4.0%, $n = 420/10548$), a traffic injury (2.0%, $n = 212/10548$) or any other cause (0.8%, $n = 86/10548$). Fractures were most common during the winter months of January and December (Fig. 2).

The fractures were classified according to the ICD-10 code system as trochanteric (S72.1) in 78% ($n = 8260/10548$) and as subtrochanteric (S72.2) in 22% ($n = 2288/10548$) of the cases. In addition, fractures were classified using the AO/OTA classification as 31-A1 in 29% ($n = 3067/10546$), as 31-A2 in 49% ($n = 5191/10546$) and as 31-A3 in 22% ($n = 2288/10546$) of the cases (Fig. 3). The fractured side was equally distributed with 50% ($n = 5253/10548$) involving the right side and 50% ($n = 5295/10548$) involving the left side. Fourteen patients (out of 10,548, 0.1%) had an open fracture and 1.6% ($n = 169/10246$) of the fractures were due to a high-energy trauma. Patient and injury epidemiology data in relation to fracture type are presented in Table 1.

Surgical results

The majority of the patients were operated within 24 h (75%, $n = 4471/5928$), or 36 h (90%, $n = 5354/5928$) from time of the radiograph verifying the fracture to the start of the operation. The operations were performed during night time (22–08 h) in 8.5% ($n = 522/6126$) of the cases. The

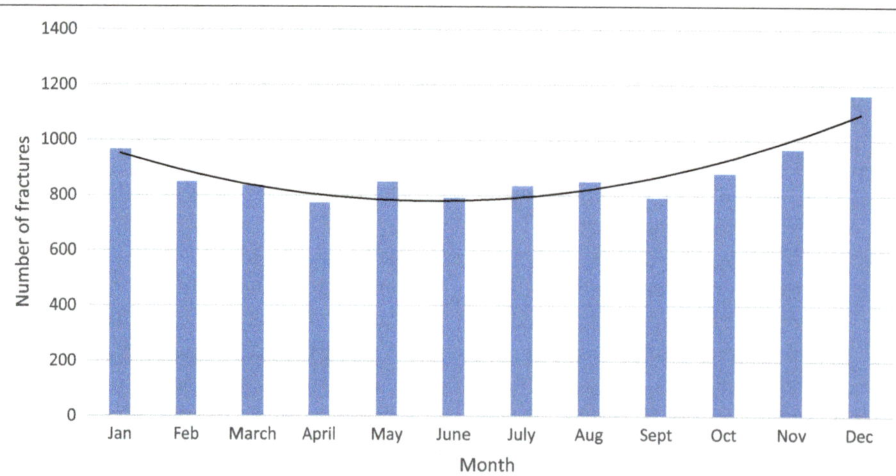

Fig. 2 Monthly distribution of trochanteric and subtrochanteric femoral fractures

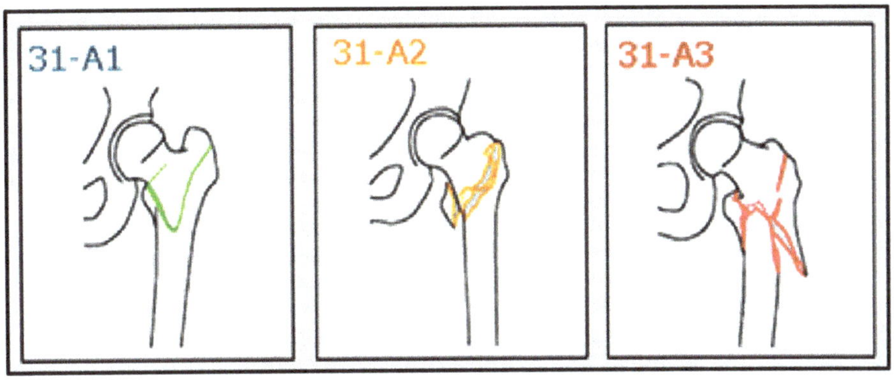

Fig. 3 Fracture groups as presented in the SFR. According to AO/OTA classification of trochanteric and subtrochanteric femoral fractures. The use of the figure in this study has been approved by the SFR: 31-A1 Simple trochanteric fractures. 31-A2 Multifragmented trochanteric fractures. 31-A3 Trochanteric reverse oblique and subtrochanteric fractures.

operations were performed by a specialist in orthopaedic surgery in 62% ($n = 6348/10186$), an orthopaedic registrar in 37% ($n = 3759/10186$) or by any other surgeon in 0.8% ($n = 79/10186$) of the cases. Implants used were: a short antegrade intramedullary nail (42%, $n = 4411/10548$), a plate with sliding hip screw (37%, $n = 3935/10548$), a long antegrade intramedullary nail (18%, $n = 1903/10548$), any other type of plate fixation (1.6%, $n = 167/10548$), a retrograde intramedullary nail (0.6%, $n = 63/10548$), a hip arthroplasty (0.5%, $n = 58/10548$) or other implants (0.1%, $n = 11/10548$). Implants used in relation to fracture type are presented in Fig. 4.

Table 1 Overview of patient and injury epidemiology in relation to fracture type[a]

	31-A1 ($n = 3067$)	31-A2 ($n = 5191$)	31-A3 ($n = 2288$)
Age years, mean (±SD)	82.2 (10.3)	83.2 (9.8)	81.0 (12.0)
% (n=)			
Female gender	65 (1981/3067)	72 (3725/5191)	70 (1610/2288)
Injury location			
At residence	74 (2202/2960)	75 (3816/5069)	73 (1611/2218)
Public place	4.8 (143/2960)	4.6 (233/5069)	4.4 (97/2218)
Street/road	3.5 (103/2960)	3.6 (183/5069)	4.1 (92/2218)
Other	17 (512/2960)	17 (837/5069)	19 (418/2218)
Injury mechanism			
Fall at same level	84 (2561/3067)	84 (4363/5191)	82 (1870/2288)
Unspecified fall	9.7 (299/3067)	10 (532/5191)	8.9 (203/2288)
Fall from height	3.6 (111/3067)	3.4 (179/5191)	5.7 (130/2288)
Traffic	2.4 (74/3067)	1.7 (87/5191)	2.2 (51/2288)
Other	0.7 (22/3067)	0.6 (30/5191)	1.5 (34/2288)
High energy trauma			
Yes	1.4 (43/2971)	1.1 (55/5045)	3.2 (71/2229)
No	97 (2890/2971)	98 (4924/5045)	96 (2134/2229)
Unknown	1.3 (38/2971)	1.3 (66/5045)	1.1 (24/2229)
Open fracture	0 (0)	0.1 (5/5191)	0.4 (9/2288)

Data is presented in relation to the number of available inputs in the register
[a]Fracture type according to the AO/OTA classification:
31-A1 Simple trochanteric fractures
31-A2 Multifragmented trochanteric fractures
31-A3 Trochanteric reverse oblique and subtrochanteric fractures

Mortality

The overall 30-day mortality was 7.7% ($n = 811/10548$) and the 1-year mortality was 26% ($n = 2731/10548$). There was a higher 30-day mortality for males (11%, $n = 355/3231$) compared to females (6.2%, $n = 456/7317$). As was there a higher 1-year mortality for males (32%, $n = 1026/3231$) compared to females (23%, $n = 1705/7317$). One-year mortality for different age-groups is presented in Fig. 5. The 30-day mortality was higher for patients operated > 36 h (9.8%, $n = 56/574$) compared to patients operated ≤24 h (7.8%, $n = 349/4471$) or ≤ 36 h (8.0%, $n = 429/5354$). Operations delayed for surgery > 36 h also had a higher 1-year mortality (31%, $n = 179/574$) compared to operations performed ≤24 h (25%, $n = 1118/4471$) or ≤ 36 h (26%, $n = 1370/5354$). Detailed results on mortality are presented in Table 2.

Discussion

In this observational study of trochanteric and subtrochanteric hip fractures in Sweden during the years 2014 to 2016 the majority of the patients were women (69%) with a high mean age (84 years) and a fracture caused by a fall at the same level at their accommodation. The most common type of fracture according to the AO/OTA classification was a type 31-A2 and the majority of the patients were operated with a short intramedullary nail within 36 h. There was a higher mortality at 30 days and 1 year for males, and for all those who were delayed to surgery > 36 h.

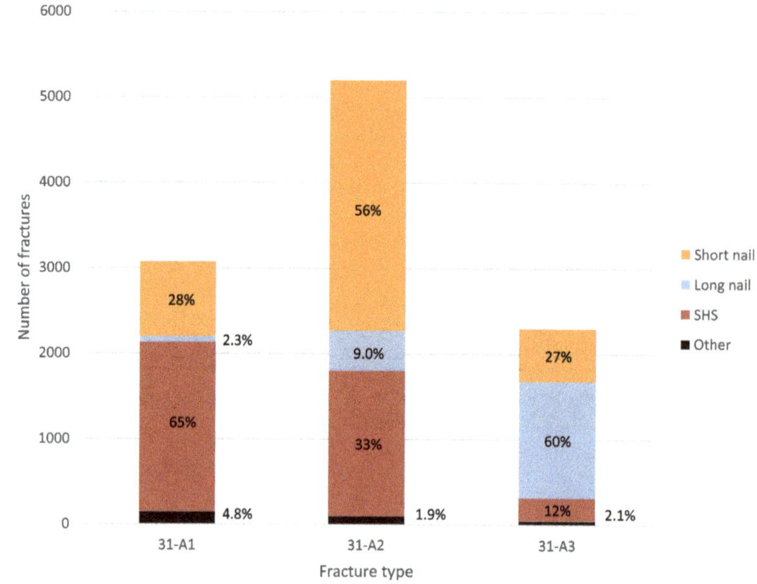

Fig. 4 Fracture type according to the AO/OTA classification in relation to treatment

Epidemiology

Our finding of a higher number of fractures among females is in line with most of the previous studies and has an association with osteoporosis [4, 17–21]. The high age of the patients reflects that there is an increased risk to fall with advanced age, and as these patients often are frail with poor bone-quality there is an increased risk for suffering from a hip fracture even after a low energy fall. Mangram et al. 2014 [17] described that 73% of their trochanteric fracture patients fell at home. Similarly, Haginoa et al. 2017 [6] reported that an indoors simple fall was the trauma mechanism in 80% of their hip fracture patients, and 85% of them were ≥ 90 years old. Interestingly we found that fractures were slightly more common during the winter months of January and December, despite that the majority of them occurred indoors at the patients' accommodation. But this finding is in line with previous studies. Pueyo-Sanchez et al. 2017 [22] reported that in Catalonia, Spain a seasonal variation was observed with more cases in the winter. Similarly, Gronskag et al. 2010 [23] found a seasonal variation in hip fracture incidence among elderly women in Norway, which was characterized by higher fracture rates during the winter months. Finally, Hagino et al. 2017 [6] reported a monthly variation were January had the highest number of patients per month during the observation period.

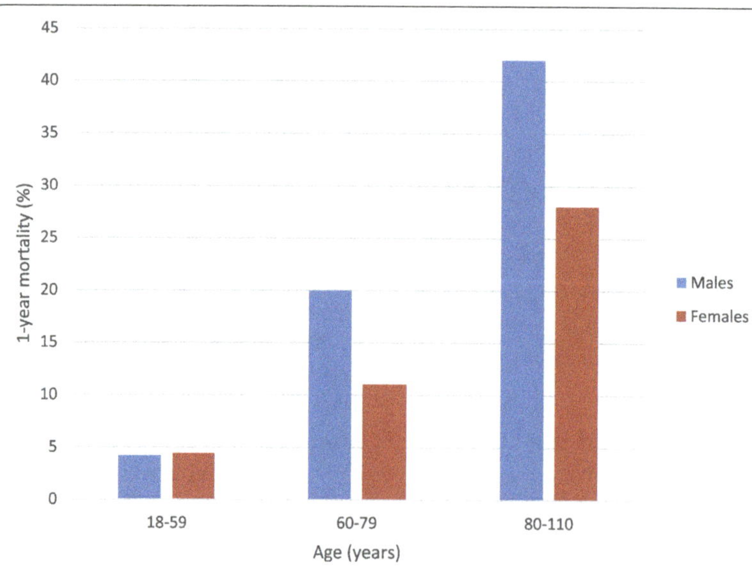

Fig. 5 Comparison of 1-year mortality between males and females for different age-groups

Table 2 Mortality in relation to gender, fracture type and surgical factors

	30-day mortality % (*n*=)	1-year mortality % (*n*=)
All	7.7 (811/10548)	26 (2731/10548)
Gender		
Female	6.2 (456/7317)	23 (1705/7317)
Male	11 (355/3231)	32 (1026/3231)
Fracture type[a]		
31-A1	7.2 (222/3067)	26 (793/3067)
31-A2	8.2 (427/5191)	27 (1389/5191)
31-A3	7.1 (162/228)	24 (548/2288)
Time to surgery		
≤ 24 h	7.8 (349/4471)	25 (1118/4471)
≤ 36 h	8.0 (429/5354)	26 (1370/5354)
> 36 h	9.8 (56/574)	31 (179/574)
Time of surgery start		
08–22	8.2 (460/5604)	26 (1476/5604)
22–08	8.0 (42/522)	24 (126/522)
Implant		
Short intramedullary nail	8.2 (362/4411)	27 (1167/4411)
Long intramedullary nail	6.8 (130/1903)	24 (450/1903)
Plate with sliding hip screw	7.6 (298/3935)	26 (1030/3935)
Other	7.0 (21/299)	28 (84/299)

Data is presented in relation to the number of available inputs in the register
[a]Fracture type according to the AO/OTA classification:
31-A1 Simple trochanteric fractures
31-A2 Multifragmented trochanteric fractures
31-A3 Trochanteric reverse oblique and subtrochanteric fractures

Fracture and treatment characteristics

We found that the AO/OTA type 31-A1 and 31-A2 fractures, which are sometimes referred to as stable, were most common (78%). This finding is similar to Chehade et al. [20] who in 2015 published a prospective consecutive cohort of 743 patients were the majority (60%) were classified as stable trochanteric and only 40% as unstable trochanteric or subtrochanteric fractures. We found that with increasing fracture complexity, the proportion of intramedullary nails was increasing, and also the use of long versus short nails. Previous literature have advocated superiority of intramedullary nails, compared to plate with sliding hip screw, and proposed advantages in the management of unstable trochanteric and subtrochanteric fractures in providing biomechanical stability and improved functional outcome [8, 9, 24–27]. Furthermore, a long nail can offer protection all along the femur, in comparison to a short nail [28–30]. In our observational study we found that although intramedullary nailing was the most commonly used implant overall, the plate with sliding hip screw was commonly used as well, especially for the AO/OTA type 31-A1 fractures (Fig. 4). The "plate versus nail" debate is probably not yet over as the latest Cochrane report comparing intramedullary nails with plate and sliding hip screw concluded that "sliding hip screw appears superior for trochanteric fractures" [31].

Mortality

We found a higher mortality rate in males, despite younger mean age. As a comparison, the expected 1-year mortality for an unselected population of 80 years old in Sweden 2017 was 3.5% for females and 4.8% for males (www.statistikdatabasen.scb.se). In 2010 Kannegaard et al. [32] observed in a nationwide register-based cohort study including more than 41,000 Danish hip fracture patients, increased 1-year mortality in men and that the mean survival time was slightly shorter after trochanteric and subtrochanteric fracture (3.3–3.4 years) compared with other types of hip fractures (3.5–3.8 years). Haentjens et al. [33] performed time-to-event meta-analyses and showed that the relative hazard for all-cause mortality in the first 3 months after a hip fracture was 5.75 in women and 7.95 in men. The majority of our population was operated within 24 h (75%) or 36 h (90%) calculated from the time of the radiograph verifying the fracture to the start of the operation. This is consistent with the current recommendations for the management of hip fractures in many settings, although we still lack an international consensus. Obviously, several factors can affect the postoperative mortality, but the time to surgery is one of the most debated ones. Moja et al. 2012 [34] described in a meta-analysis that a delay to surgery was associated with a significant increase in the risk of death and pressure sores, and recommended that most patients with a hip fracture should be operated within 1 or 2 days. In addition, early fracture fixation and mobilization of these patients decreases the economic burden as it might reduce the overall length of stay, and thus the total cost [35]. On the contrary, a recent prospective cohort study from Lizaur-Utrilla et al. 2018 including 1234 patients who underwent hip fracture surgery suggested that waiting time for the surgery more than 2 days to stabilize patients with active comorbidities at admission was not associated with higher complication or mortality rate. However, the patients who were delayed to surgery due to organizational reasons had a significant higher rate of postoperative complications and 1-year mortality [36]. To be able to operate patients within 24 or 36 h one might need to operate also at nighttime (22:00–8:00 h). We found no relation between mortality and the starting time of the surgery, whether it was performed during daytime or nighttime. Although other studies have defined the nighttime slightly different (16:00–07:00 h) they showed similar results [37, 38].

Strengths of the study

The major strength of this study is the large number of included fractures. The data from the SFR provides prospective data on a national level regardless of local differences in epidemiology, socio-demographics and treatment traditions. The included data is detailed and the register have been well validated [39–41]. Another strength is the mortality data that provides a unique opportunity to integrate epidemiologic data with a relevant outcome measurement.

Limitations of the study

The SFRs coverage during the study period (January 2014 to December 2016) included with increasing number of participating departments by the end of 2016 approximately only 72% of Sweden's orthopaedic departments. However, the remaining clinics that have not yet signed up are mostly smaller units, so in reality the national proportion of excluded fractures is most likely small, but still the incomplete coverage of the SFR as a limitation. Registration of the time for the radiograph confirming the fracture and the start of the operation did not start until 2015. The number of valid inputs in the register on this topic is therefore somewhat limited, but since the total number of valid inputs is large, we still think that the results regarding delay to surgery and timing of the operations are valid indicators and represents true national trends. Another limitation is that due to the descriptive nature of this register study all the results were unadjusted regarding different reasons for delay to surgery, implant choice or co-morbidities of the patients.

Conclusion

Safety measures to prevent fall at elderly patient's accommodation might be a way to reduce the number of trochanteric and subtrochanteric hip fractures. Surgery as soon as possible without delay should be considered to reduce the mortality rate. The selection of surgical methods depends on the fracture complexity.

Abbreviations

AO: Arbeitsgemeinschaft fur Osteosynthesefragen; OTA: Orthopaedic Trauma Association; SFR: Swedish Fracture Register

Acknowledgements

The authors wish to thank Michael Möller, director of the SFR, for valuable contribution.

Authors' contributions

LM, AE: study design and planning. Data analysis. Writing of the manuscript. AB: data collection, data analysis and writing of the manuscript. All authors have read and approved the final manuscript.

Consent for publication

Not applicable.

Competing interests

The authors declare that they have no competing interests.

Author details

[1]Department of Clinical Science and Education, Södersjukhuset, Karolinska Institutet. Department of Orthopaedics, Stockholm South General Hospital, 11883 Stockholm, Sweden. [2]Department of Orthopaedics, Sahlgrenska University Hospital Gothenburg/Mölndal, 431 80 Mölndal, Sweden. [3]Department of Molecular Medicine and Surgery, Karolinska University Hospital, Karolinska Institutet, 17176 Stockholm, Sweden.

References

1. Cooper C, Campion G, Melton LJ 3rd. Hip fractures in the elderly: a world-wide projection. Osteoporos Int. 1992;2(6):285–9.
2. Cheng SY, Levy AR, Lefaivre KA, Guy P, Kuramoto L, Sobolev B. Geographic trends in incidence of hip fractures: a comprehensive literature review. Osteoporos Int. 2011;22(10):2575–86.
3. Gullberg B, Johnell O, Kanis JA. World-wide projections for hip fracture. Osteoporos Int. 1997;7(5):407–13.
4. Brunner LC, Eshilian-Oates L, Kuo TY. Hip fractures in adults. Am Fam Physician. 2003;67(3):537–42.
5. Endo Y, Aharonoff GB, Zuckerman JD, Egol KA, Koval KJ. Gender differences in patients with hip fracture: a greater risk of morbidity and mortality in men. J Orthop Trauma. 2005;19(1):29–35.
6. Hagino H, Endo N, Harada A, Iwamoto J, Mashiba T, Mori S, et al. Survey of hip fractures in Japan: recent trends in prevalence and treatment. J Orthop Sci. 2017;22(5):909–14.
7. Matsuo M, Yamagami T, Higuchi A. Impact of age on postoperative complication rates among elderly patients with hip fracture: a retrospective matched study. J Anesth. 2018;32(3):452–6.
8. Anglen JO, Weinstein JN. Nail or plate fixation of intertrochanteric hip fractures: changing pattern of practice. A review of the American Board of Orthopaedic Surgery Database. J Bone Joint Surg Am. 2008;90(4):700–7.
9. Matre K, Havelin LI, Gjertsen JE, Vinje T, Espehaug B, Fevang JM. Sliding hip screw versus IM nail in reverse oblique trochanteric and subtrochanteric fractures. A study of 2716 patients in the Norwegian hip fracture register. Injury. 2013;44(6):735–42.
10. Uzoigwe CE, Burnand HG, Cheesman CL, Aghedo DO, Faizi M, Middleton RG. Early and ultra-early surgery in hip fracture patients improves survival. Injury. 2013;44(6):726–9.
11. Colais P, Di Martino M, Fusco D, Perucci CA, Davoli M. The effect of early surgery after hip fracture on 1-year mortality. BMC Geriatr. 2015;15:141.
12. Aqil A, Hossain F, Sheikh H, Aderinto J, Whitwell G, Kapoor H. Achieving hip fracture surgery within 36 hours: an investigation of risk factors to surgical delay and recommendations for practice. J Orthop Traumatol. 2016;17(3): 207–13.
13. Lizaur-Utrilla A, Martinez-Mendez D, Collados-Maestre I, Miralles-Munoz FA, Marco-Gomez L, Lopez-Prats FA. Early surgery within 2 days for hip fracture is not reliable as healthcare quality indicator. Injury. 2016;47(7):1530–5.
14. Bergdahl C, Ekholm C, Wennergren D, Nilsson F, Moller M. Epidemiology and patho-anatomical pattern of 2,011 humeral fractures: data from the Swedish fracture register. BMC Musculoskelet Disord. 2016;17:159.
15. Kihlstrom C, Moller M, Lonn K, Wolf O. Clavicle fractures: epidemiology, classification and treatment of 2 422 fractures in the Swedish fracture register; an observational study. BMC Musculoskelet Disord. 2017;18(1):82.
16. Müller ME, Nazarian, S., Koch, P. and Schatzker, J. (1990) The comprehensive classification of fractures of long bones/AO classification of fractures. Springer-Verlag, Berlin, Heidelberg. https://doi.org/10.1007/978-3-642-61261-9.
17. Mangram A, Moeser P, Corneille MG, Prokuski LJ, Zhou N, Sohn J, et al. Geriatric trauma hip fractures: is there a difference in outcomes based on fracture patterns? World J Emerg Surg: WJES. 2014;9(1):59.
18. Diaz AR, Navas PZ. Risk factors for trochanteric and femoral neck fracture. Rev Esp Cir Ortop Traumatol. 2018;62(2):134–41.

19. Carow J, Carow JB, Coburn M, Kim BS, Bucking B, Bliemel C, et al. Mortality and cardiorespiratory complications in trochanteric femoral fractures: a ten year retrospective analysis. Int Orthop. 2017;41(11):2371–80.
20. Chehade MJ, Carbone T, Awwad D, Taylor A, Wildenauer C, Ramasamy B, et al. Influence of fracture stability on early patient mortality and reoperation after Pertrochanteric and intertrochanteric hip fractures. J Orthop Trauma. 2015;29(12):538–43.
21. Buecking B, Bliemel C, Struewer J, Eschbach D, Ruchholtz S, Muller T. Use of the Gamma3 nail in a teaching hospital for trochanteric fractures: mechanical complications, functional outcomes, and quality of life. BMC research notes. 2012;5:651.
22. Pueyo-Sanchez MJ, Larrosa M, Suris X, Casado E, Auleda J, Fuste J, et al. Secular trend in the incidence of hip fracture in Catalonia, Spain, 2003-2014. Age Ageing. 2017;46(2):324–8.
23. Gronskag AB, Forsmo S, Romundstad P, Langhammer A, Schei B. Incidence and seasonal variation in hip fracture incidence among elderly women in Norway. The HUNT study. Bone. 2010;46(5):1294–8.
24. Schneider K, Oh JK, Zderic I, Stoffel K, Richards RG, Wolf S, et al. What is the underlying mechanism for the failure mode observed in the proximal femoral locking compression plate? A biomechanical study. Injury. 2015; 46(8):1483–90.
25. Tucker A, Donnelly KJ, Rowan C, McDonald S, Foster AP. Is the best plate a nail? A review of 3230 unstable intertrochanteric fractures of the proximal femur. J Orthop Trauma. 2018;32(2):53–60.
26. Zhu Q, Xu X, Yang X, Chen X, Wang L, Liu C, et al. Intramedullary nails versus sliding hip screws for AO/OTA 31-A2 trochanteric fractures in adults: a meta-analysis. Int J Surg. 2017;43:67–74.
27. Vermesan D, Prejbeanu R, Poenaru DV, Petrescu H, Apostol E, Inchingolo F, et al. Do intramedullary implants improve survival in elderly patients with trochanteric fractures? A retrospective study. La Clinica terapeutica. 2015; 166(3):e140–5.
28. Hsu CE, Shih CM, Wang CC, Huang KC. Lateral femoral wall thickness. A reliable predictor of post-operative lateral wall fracture in intertrochanteric fractures. Bone Joint J. 2013;95-b(8):1134–8.
29. Mittal R, Banerjee S. Proximal femoral fractures: principles of management and review of literature. J Clin Orthop Trauma. 2012;3(1):15–23.
30. Haidukewych GJ. Intertrochanteric fractures: ten tips to improve results. J Bone Joint Surg Am. 2009;91(3):712–9.
31. Parker MJ, Handoll HH. Gamma and other cephalocondylic intramedullary nails versus extramedullary implants for extracapsular hip fractures in adults. Cochrane Database Syst Rev. 2010;9:Cd000093.
32. Kannegaard PN, van der Mark S, Eiken P, Abrahamsen B. Excess mortality in men compared with women following a hip fracture. National analysis of comedications, comorbidity and survival. Age Ageing. 2010;39(2):203–9.
33. Haentjens P, Magaziner J, Colon-Emeric CS, Vanderschueren D, Milisen K, Velkeniers B, et al. Meta-analysis: excess mortality after hip fracture among older women and men. Ann Intern Med. 2010;152(6):380–90.
34. Moja L, Piatti A, Pecoraro V, Ricci C, Virgili G, Salanti G, et al. Timing matters in hip fracture surgery: patients operated within 48 hours have better outcomes. A meta-analysis and meta-regression of over 190,000 patients. PLoS One. 2012;7(10):e46175.
35. Siegmeth AW, Gurusamy K, Parker MJ. Delay to surgery prolongs hospital stay in patients with fractures of the proximal femur. J Bone Joint Surg Br Vol. 2005;87(8):1123–6.
36. Lizaur-Utrilla A, Gonzalez-Navarro B, Vizcaya-Moreno MF, Miralles Munoz FA, Gonzalez-Parreno S, Lopez-Prats FA. Reasons for delaying surgery following hip fractures and its impact on one year mortality. Int Orthop. 2018.
37. Rashid RH, Zubairi AJ, Slote MU, Noordin S. Hip fracture surgery: does time of the day matter? A case-controlled study. Int J Surg. 2013;11(9):923–5.
38. Switzer JA, Bennett RE, Wright DM, Vang S, Anderson CP, Vlasak AJ, et al. Surgical time of day does not affect outcome following hip fracture fixation. Geriatr Orthop Surg Rehabil. 2013;4(4):109–16.
39. Wennergren D, Ekholm C, Sundfeldt M, Karlsson J, Bhandari M, Moller M. High reliability in classification of tibia fractures in the Swedish fracture register. Injury. 2016;47(2):478–82.
40. Juto H, Gartner Nilsson M, Moller M, Wennergren D, Morberg P. Evaluating non-responders of a survey in the Swedish fracture register: no indication of different functional result. BMC Musculoskelet Disord. 2017;18(1):278.
41. Wennergren D, Stjernstrom S, Moller M, Sundfeldt M, Ekholm C. Validity of humerus fracture classification in the Swedish fracture register. BMC Musculoskelet Disord. 2017;18(1):251.

14

Treatment of displaced transverse fractures of the patella: modified tension band wiring technique with or without augmented circumferential cerclage wire fixation

Tien-Yu Yang[1,2], Tsan-Wen Huang[1,2], Po-Yao Chuang[1,2] and Kuo-Chin Huang[1,2,3*]

Abstract

Background: Displaced transverse fractures of the body of the patella are usually associated with disruption of extensor mechanism and should be fixed surgically. The most common method is a tension band wiring (TBW) technique. Some surgeons concurrently employ an augmented circumferential cerclage wiring (ACCW) technique to help fracture stabilization and aid in fracture healing; however, its role and effect on the treatment outcomes is unclear.

Methods: We performed a STROBE-compliant retrospective observational cohort study on all cases of acute closed patella fracture that were treated at our institution between 2006 and 2012. Of 185 episodes, 72 (38.9%) were eligible for this study according to our inclusion/exclusion criteria. We classified these subjects with AO/OTA type 34-C1.1 or 34-C2 lesions into two groups for analyses: fractures treated with modified TBW and ACCW (group 1, $n = 27$) and those treated with modified TBW alone (group 2, $n = 45$). Plain radiographs were used to evaluate radiographic outcomes and the effect of potential risk factors on fixation failure was analyzed by subgroup comparisons.

Results: Our results revealed that there were no significant differences in the rates of fixation failure ($P = 0.620$), nonunion ($P = 0.620$), and revision surgery ($P = 0.620$) between the groups. Although not statistically significant, there was a trend towards a positive risk association between fixation failure and age distribution > 60 years (10.0% vs. 0.0%, $P = 0.124$; OR = 8.0, $P = 0.168$) and > 70 years (9.4% vs. 2.5%, $P = 0.321$; OR = 4.0, $P = 0.237$) and the superficial level of the K-wires (12.0% vs. 1.5%, $P = 0.117$; OR = 6.3, $P = 0.121$). Regarding those modified TBW patients concurrently treated with an ACCW, the potential risk association between fixation failure and the superficial level of the K-wire was prone to increase further (28.6% vs. 0.0%, $P = 0.060$; OR = 18.6, $P = 0.071$).

Conclusions: Concurrent application of an ACCW might be needless and not efficacious to help fracture stabilization and healing in patients having been treated with modified TBW for displaced transverse fractures of the body of the patella. Adherence to correct surgical technique such as putting the K-wires at the proper level and securing control of the both ends of the K-wires may be more important and help in improving outcomes.

Keywords: Patella fracture, Tension band wiring, Circumferential cerclage wiring, Fixation failure, Nonunion

* Correspondence: kc2672@gmail.com
[1]Chang Gung University College of Medicine, Taoyuan, Taiwan
[2]Department of Orthopaedic Surgery, Chang Gung Memorial Hospital, Chiayi, Taiwan
Full list of author information is available at the end of the article

Background

Among all fracture types of the patella, transverse fracture of the body is the most common [1–4]. If displaced, it should be repaired surgically to restore the function of extensor mechanism and aid in fracture healing [5, 6]. Tension band wiring (TBW) technique, one of the most commonly used surgical method in treating a tension fracture [7–10], has a sound biomechanical advantage such that it can convert a tensile force into a compressive force when the joint is brought through a range of motion [11–13]. With appropriate application of this technique to treat the displaced transverse fractures of the patella, the security of fixation would allow early joint mobilization and the prevention of knee stiffness [14, 15]. The rate of fixation failure is not high and serious complications are uncommon [16]. Despite the potential occurrence of subjective complaints due to hardware irritation, TBW remains the gold standard for the treatment of displaced transverse fractures of the patella body [2, 3, 7, 8, 14–17]. At our institution, a modified TBW technique involving bending both ends of the K-wires is used regularly. Using this modified technique, Wu et al. had reported an excellent treatment result with smooth fracture union, good recovery of joint motion, and few complaints of hardware irritation (3%) [15].

Even though the treatment results of TBW for displaced transverse patella fractures are promising, some surgeons recommend that the combination of augmented circumferential cerclage wiring (ACCW) and TBW would lead to a greater strength of fixation and should be better than TBW alone [18–20]. Curtis, in a cadaveric study on the strength of internal fixation for a fractured patella, compared Müller's TBW technique to the Pyrford technique using a cerclage wire and an anterior TBW looping through the quadriceps tendon [21, 22]. He found that all patellae fixed using Müller's technique failed at an applied force of 20 kg or less and none of the specimens fixed by the Pyrford technique failed at 25 kg [22]. Accordingly, we proposed a null hypothesis that concurrent application of an ACCW does not help fracture stabilization and enhance fracture healing in patients having been treated by TBW for their displaced transverse fractures of the body of the patella. Through a retrospective cohort study design, we tested the hypothesis based on the data (evidence) collected and then decided to either reject the null hypothesis or failed to reject it. The purpose of this study was (1) to determine the impact of an ACCW on the radiographic outcomes and (2) to explore the prognostic factors predicting treatment failure (e.g., fixation failure) in these patients.

Methods

Study population and primary/secondary endpoints

This retrospective cohort study included all patients with a diagnosis of displaced transverse fractures of the patella (AO/OTA type 34-C1.1 and 34-C2) who were treated by modified TBW [15] at our institution between January 2006 and June 2012. After obtaining approval from the Institutional Review Board, cases were identified by matching the International Classification of Diseases (ICD), 9th Revision codes specific for closed patella fracture (822.0) in the computerized trauma registry database of the hospital. At this stage, 185 patients with an acute patella fracture were identified and their medical records were reviewed and confirmed by two independent researchers (TYY and KCH). Among them, we excluded patients aged < 18 years, lost to follow up within 3 months after surgery and those with inadequate radiographs, bilateral patella fractures, open or multiple fractures, vertical fractures, complex fractures, and avulsion fractures of the upper or lower pole of the patella. The aggregate number of enrolled patients in this 6.5-year study was 72.

We summarized the collected data at the time of study enrollment, which included demographics (age and gender), AO/OTA fracture types, surgical methods, aftercare program, radiographic results and surgical complications. To clarify the role of an ACCW on treatment outcomes of displaced transverse patella fracture, we classified the enrolled subjects into two groups for further analyses: fractures treated with modified TBW and ACCW (group 1, $n = 27$) and those with modified TBW alone (group 2, $n = 45$). The primary endpoint of this study was to determine the impact of an ACCW on the radiographic results of displaced transverse patella fracture having been treated by modified TBW. For our secondary endpoint, the effect of potential risk factors on fixation failure was analyzed by subgroup comparisons.

Definitions

Level of the K-wires

It was categorized as superficial or deep. Superficial level was defined as the level of the K-wires anterior to the center of the patella. In contrast, we defined the deep level as being in the center of deeper position of the patella.

Distance between the K-wires

It was categorized as narrow or wide. Narrow distance was defined as the distance between the K-wires less than one third of the patella width. In contrast, we defined the wide distance as being equal or more than one third of the patella width.

Fixation failure

It was defined as hardware breakage, nonunion, or redisplacement of fragments from their initial reduced position with gap separation > 2 mm.

Statistical analysis

Variables were compared using univariate analysis. A χ^2 analysis or a Fisher's exact test was used where appropriate for analyzing categorical data. For numerical data, the Wilcoxan rank sum test was utilized for between-group comparisons. Significance was set at $P < 0.05$ (two-sided). Not statistically significant was abbreviated as NS. All statistic analyses were conducted using the Statistical Package for the Social Sciences (SPSS, version 12.0. SPSS Inc., Chicago, IL, USA) and/or the MedCalc Statistical Software (version 9.5, Broekstraat, Mariakerke, Belgium).

Results

According to the inclusion/exclusion criteria, 72 (38.9%) of 185 episodes were eligible for this study and divided into two groups, including the group of fractures treated with modified TBW and ACCW (group 1, $n = 27$) and the group of those treated with modified TBW alone (group 2, $n = 45$). Baseline data on these 72 patients treated with modified TBW for displaced transverse fractures of the patella are shown in Table 1. Age, age distribution, gender, fracture pattern, level of the K-wires, distance between the K-wires, and aftercare such as use of postoperative splint did not differ between the two groups of patients. Regarding the outcome analysis, there were no significant differences in the rates of fixation failure ($P = 0.620$), nonunion ($P = 0.620$), or revision surgery ($P = 0.620$) between the groups (Table 2). In total there were 4 patients (5.6%) having fixation failure, including 2 group-1 patients (7.4%) and 2 group-2 patients (4.4%), respectively. All of them had nonunion but no wire migration and needed revision surgery to restore their extensor mechanism and enhance fracture union. After bone grafting and revision modified TBW surgery focusing on the adjustment of the level of the K-wires and the distance between them, all these fixation failure patients recovered their function of extensor mechanism and had their patella fractures united eventually (Table 3).

Several potential risk factors for fixation failure were analyzed and shown in Table 4. Although not statistically significant, we observed a trend of positive risk association between fixation failure and age distribution > 60 years (10.0% vs. 0.0%, $P = 0.124$; OR = 8.0, $P = 0.168$) and > 70 years (9.4% vs. 2.5%, $P = 0.321$; OR = 4.0, $P = 0.237$) and the superficial level of the K-wires (12.0% vs. 2.1%, $P = 0.117$; OR = 6.3, $P = 0.121$). Regarding those patients concurrently treated with an ACCW, the risk association between fixation failure and the superficial level of the K-wire increased further (28.6% vs. 0.0%, $P = 0.060$; OR = 18.6, $P = 0.071$).

Table 1 Characteristics of patients treated by tension band wiring technique with or without augmented cerclage wire fixation

Variables	Group 1 ($n = 27$)	Group 2 ($n = 45$)	*P* Value
Age (years), mean (range)	61.33 (32–87)	63.73 (25–88)	0.530
Age > 60 years, n (%)			0.341
Yes	13 (48.1)	27 (60.0)	
No	14 (51.9)	18 (40.0)	
Age > 70 years, n (%)			0.807
Yes	11 (40.7)	21 (46.7)	
No	16 (59.3)	24 (53.3)	
Gender, n (%)			0.802
Male	11 (40.7)	16 (35.6)	
Female	16 (59.3)	29 (64.4)	
Fracture pattern, n (%)			0.535
AO/OTA type 34-C2	6 (22.2)	7 (15.6)	
AO/OTA type 34-C1.1	21 (77.8)	38 (84.4)	
Level of the K-wires, n (%)			0.308
Superficial	7 (25.9)	18 (40.0)	
Deep	20 (74.1)	27 (60.0)	
Distance between the K-wires, n (%)			0.085
Narrow	12 (44.4)	30 (66.7)	
Wide	15 (55.6)	15 (33.3)	
Postoperative splinting, n (%)			0.807
Yes	16 (59.3)	24 (53.3)	
No	11 (40.7)	21 (46.7)	

**P* value < 0.05 is significant

Discussion

The decision of the current retrospective cohort study was failure to reject the null hypothesis [23], i.e., there was no sufficient evidence supporting that the concurrent application of an ACCW could provide a better treatment outcome (e.g., less fixation failure) than modified TBW

Table 2 Radiographic results and revision surgery of patients treated by tension band wiring technique with or without augmented cerclage wire fixation

Variables	Group 1 ($n = 27$)	Group 2 ($n = 45$)	*P* Value
Fixation failure, n (%)			0.620
Yes	2 (7.4)	2 (4.4)	
No	25 (92.6)	43 (95.6)	
Nonunion, n (%)			0.620
Yes	2 (7.4)	2 (4.4)	
No	25 (92.6)	43 (95.6)	
Wire migration, n (%)			1.000
Yes	0 (0.0)	0 (0.0)	
No	27 (100.0)	45 (100.0)	
Revision surgery, n (%)			0.620
Yes	2 (7.4)	2 (4.4)	
No	25 (92.6)	43 (95.6)	

**P* value < 0.05 is significant

Table 3 Demographic data of the cases with fixation failure

Variables	Group 1		Group 2	
	Patient 1	Patient 2	Patient 3	Patient 4
Age, years	66	78	73	88
Gender	F	M	F	M
AO/OTA type 34-C2 fracture	N	N	N	N
Superficial level of the K-wires	Y	Y	N	Y
Narrow K-wire distance	Y	N	Y	N
Without postoperative splinting	Y	N	Y	N
K-wire migration	N	N	N	N
Revision surgery	Y	Y	Y	Y
Final union	Y	Y	Y	Y

*P value < 0.05 is significant

alone while treating patients with displaced transverse fractures of the patella. The fixation failure rate in group 1 and group 2 patients was 7.4 and 4.4%, respectively (P = NS). All these fixation failure patients recovered their function of extensor mechanism and had their patella fractures united by bone grafting and revision surgery with modified TBW alone, focusing on the adjustment of the level of the K-wires and the distance between them. Although not statistically significant, prognostic factor analyses showed that there was a trend towards a higher rate of fixation failure in elderly patients (OR ≥ 4.0, P = NS) and those with their K-wires at the superficial level (OR = 6.3, P = NS). Concurrently applying an ACCW did not decrease the risk association between fixation failure and the superficial level of the K-wires (OR = 18.6 and 1.5, both P = NS, in group 1 and group 2 patients, respectively). We, thus, highlight that concurrent application of an ACCW in patients having been treated with modified TBW technique might be not as efficacious as what we had learned from the literature [18–20]. Reviewing the literature showed that all of these clinical articles were categorized as case-series, a study design lacking comparison groups and thus vulnerable to selection bias and easily leading us to an incorrect conclusion [24, 25]. To further clarify the role and effect of concurrent application of an ACCW on the treatment

Table 4 Prognostic factor analyses: subgroup comparisons of the effects of patient characteristics on fixation failure

Variables	Fixation Failure	Union	P Value	OR (95% CI)	P Value
All patients, n (%)	(n = 4)	(n = 68)			
Patient age > 60 years	4 (100.0)	36 (52.9)	0.124	8.0 (0.4–154.6)	0.168
Patient age > 70 years	3 (75.0)	29 (42.6)	0.321	4.0 (0.4–40.8)	0.237
Female patients	2 (50.0)	43 (63.2)	0.628	0.6 (0.1–4.4)	0.599
AO/OTA type 34 C2 fracture	0 (0.0)	13 (19.1)	1.000	0.5 (0.0–9.0)	0.607
Superficial level of the K-wires	3 (75.0)	22 (32.3)	0.117	6.3 (0.6–63.8)	0.121
Narrow K-wire distance	2 (50.0)	40 (58.8)	1.000	0.7 (0.1–5.3)	0.729
Without postoperative splinting	2 (50.0)	30 (44.1)	1.000	1.3 (0.2–9.5)	0.818
Group 1 patients, n (%)	(n = 2)	(n = 25)			
Patient age > 60 years	2 (100.0)	11 (44.0)	0.222	6.3 (0.3–144.7)	0.249
Patient age > 70 years	1 (50.0)	10 (40.0)	1.000	1.5 (0.1–26.9)	0.783
Female patients	1 (50.0)	15 (60.0)	1.000	0.1 (0.0–3.1)	0.212
AO/OTA type 34 C2 fracture	0 (0.0)	6 (24.0)	1.000	0.6 (0.0–14.2)	0.752
Superficial level of the K-wires	2 (100.0)	5 (20.0)	0.060	18.6 (0.8–447.7)	0.071
Narrow K-wire distance	1 (50.0)	11 (44.0)	1.000	1.3 (0.1–22.7)	0.870
Without postoperative splinting	1 (50.0)	10 (40.0)	1.000	1.5 (0.1–26.9)	0.783
Group 2 patients, n (%)	(n = 2)	(n = 43)			
Patient age > 60 years	2 (100.0)	25 (58.1)	0.509	3.6 (0.2–80.1)	0.415
Patient age > 70 years	2 (100.0)	19 (44.2)	0.212	6.3 (0.3–138.6)	0.244
Female patients	1 (50.0)	28 (65.1)	1.000	0.5 (0.0–9.2)	0.667
AO/OTA type 34 C2 fracture	0 (0.0)	7 (16.3)	1.000	1.0 (0.0–22.4)	0.987
Superficial level of the K-wires	1 (50.0)	17 (39.5)	1.000	1.5 (0.1–26.1)	0.769
Narrow K-wire distance	1 (50.0)	29 (67.4)	1.000	0.5 (0.0–8.3)	0.616
Without postoperative splinting	1 (50.0)	20 (66.7)	1.000	1.2 (0.1–19.6)	0.923

*P value < 0.05 is significant

outcomes, a double-blinded prospective randomized controlled trial is, therefore, necessary in the future.

To the best of our knowledge, this is the first report to determine the impact of concurrently applying an ACCW on the treatment outcomes of displaced transverse patella fractures having been fixed by modified TBW. The present study also provides a higher level of evidence than that of previously published articles by others [18–20]. Moreover, our results challenge the concept proposed and propelled by Curtis in 1990 [22]. After comparing Pyrford technique (TBW + ACCW) to Müller's technique (TBW alone) in a cadaveric study, Curtis concluded that the former gave greater strength of fixation and should be recommended. However, nearly all patellae fixed using Müller's TBW technique failed when the distal ends of the K-wire bent, which is also true in clinical scenario [26–29]. Because of the difficulty capturing the tension band by the migrated or bent distal ends of the K-wires, loss of fixation or reduction can occur in as many as 20% of patella fractures treated with Müller's TBW technique [26–29]. Many revised techniques and technologies were, therefore, developed to solve this problem [15, 18–20, 27–30]. Wu's modified TBW technique is one of the simplest and most effective methods [15]. Using this technique in this study, the total fixation failure rate was 5.6% only. It's interesting that concurrently applying an ACCW could not provide a superior result than Wu's modified TBW alone. Considering the potential hazards on patella vascularity and the non-superiority results, we, therefore, recommend that concurrent application of an ACCW may not be required. Adherence to correct surgical technique of modified TBW technique might be more important and help in improving outcomes.

Our results suggested that the level of the K-wires might be one of the most critical surgical pearls in the treatment of patients with displaced transverse fractures of the body of the patella. The TBW design for treating these lesions needs to handle compression and tension without buckling and snapping. When the compression force overcomes bone's ability to handle compression, buckling occur [31]. When the tension force overcomes wires' ability to handle tension, snapping occurs [26–29, 32–34]. The TBW technique should transfer and dissipate these forces. Putting the parallel K-wires at the superficial level (i.e., anterior to the center of the patella) and with a narrow distance between them (i.e., less then one third of the patellar width) might be inadequate to transfer and dissipate the compression force, thus resulting in buckling and cut-through phenomena [32]. Applying the TBW without securing control of the both ends of the K-wires might be inadequate to transfer and dissipate the tension force, thus resulting in snapping and wire migration, bending, or breakage [33, 34]. Our findings indicated that Wu's modified TBW technique could effectively control the both ends of the K-wires, thus eliminate the possibility of wire migration/bending/breakage and then improve the fixation stability. Concurrently applying an ACCW could not further help the current fixation design handle compression and tension forces. Instead, putting the K-wires at the deep level and with wide distance between them might be more helpful for handling these deforming forces.

Osteoporotic bone is at risk for fractures and fixation failure after surgical stabilization [35]. To determine anatomic sites and circumstances under which a fracture may be a consequence of osteoporosis, Warriner et al. developed the osteoporosis attribution scoring (OAS) system and provided an evidence-based continuum of the likelihood of a fracture being associated with osteoporosis. Using the OAS system they categorized patella fracture as a high likelihood of being because of osteoporosis in older Caucasian women but an indeterminate likelihood in younger African-American man [36]. Our results revealed that there was a paradoxical relationship between fixation failure in patella fractures and some osteoporosis risk factors (e.g., aging, gender and bone quality) [37, 38]. We found a trend towards an increased risk of fixation failure in geriatric patients; however, the risk association did not increase with increasing age. Female gender, fracture comminution (AO/OTA type 34-C2) and without use of postoperative splint were not associated with an increased risk of fixation failure. Whatever role osteoporosis might play in the treatment of patella fractures, we believe that refinement of TBW technique and/or technology to successfully handle the deforming forces should be the most critical surgical pearls. The refined technique and/or technology would effectively improve fixation stability, permit early joint motion, enhance fracture healing, promise an excellent treatment outcome, and thus decrease the cost burden on the family and society for that condition.

Our study has several limitations. First, it is retrospective. Second, the number of patients with treatment failure included during the study period was relatively small and the study may have lacked power to detect the statistical differences in all prognostic factors among subsets of patients. The uncommon occurrence of fixation failure in the current study is to be expected because of the excellent results provided with Wu's modified TBW technique [15]. After a consecutive follow-up study lasting for more than 6 years, our results highlighted the importance of adherence to correct modified TBW technique instead of adding an ACCW in treating these patients. Third, there is lack of functional outcome measures in this study. For treatment of displaced transverse fractures of the patella, TBW technique has been a well-documented surgical method. The role of concurrently applying an ACCW to fractured patella having been fixed with TBW is intended to help fracture stabilization. The purpose of this study was therefore to determine the impact of concurrent application of an ACCW on the treatment outcomes (i.e., fixation failure) until bone healing, leaving functional outcome consideration aside. Lastly, only AO/OTA type 34-C1.1 or 34-C2 fractures were included in this investigation. We excluded all complex fractures and avulsion fractures of the proximal or distal pole of the patella in the current work in order to reduce systemic errors and bias to the smallest possible degree.

Conclusion

We concluded that there was no sufficient evidence supporting that the concurrent application of an ACCW could provide a better treatment outcome (e.g., less fixation failure) than Wu's modified TBW alone while treating patients with a displaced transverse fracture of the patella. Wu's modified TBW technique could effectively control the both ends of the K-wires, thus eliminate the possibility of wire migration/bending/breakage and then improve the fixation stability. Putting the K-wires at the deep level and with wide distance between them might effectively transfer and dissipate the compression force, thus decrease the chance of cut-through phenomena and loss of fixation/reduction. Considering the potential hazards on patella vascularity and the non-superiority results, we, therefore, recommend that concurrent application of an ACCW may not be required.

Abbreviations

ACCW: Augmented circumferential cerclage wire; AO/OTA: Arbeitsgemeinschaft für Osteosynthesefragen/Orthopaedic Trauma Association; ICD: International Classification of Diseases; K-wire: Kirschner-wire; NS: not significant; OAS: Osteoporosis Attribution Scoring; OR: odds ratio; SPSS: Statistical Product and Service Solutions; STROBE: Strengthening the Reporting of Observational studies in Epidemiology; TBW: tension band wire

Acknowledgements

We would like to thank Wen-Chi Liang for her assistance with data collection and statistical analysis.

Authors' contributions

TYY and KCH were involved in the study conception and design, data acquisition, analysis, interpretation, and drafting the manuscript. TWH and PYC were involved in data collection, critical review and analysis of results, and editing the manuscript. All authors read and approved the final manuscript.

Competing interests

The authors declare that they have no competing interests.

Author details

[1]Chang Gung University College of Medicine, Taoyuan, Taiwan. [2]Department of Orthopaedic Surgery, Chang Gung Memorial Hospital, Chiayi, Taiwan. [3]Putz City, Taiwan.

References

1. Nummi J. Fracture of the patella. A clinical study of 707 patellar fractures. Ann Chir Gynaecol Fenn Suppl. 1971;179:1–85.
2. Melvin JS, Metha S. Patellar fractures in adults. J Am Acad Orthop Surg. 2011;19(4):198–207.
3. Mao N, Ni H, Ding W, Zhu X, Bai Y, Wang C, et al. Surgical treatment of transverse patella fractures by the cable pin system with a minimally invasive technique. J Trauma Acute Care Surg. 2012;72(4):1056–61.
4. Yang NP, Chan CL, Yu IL, Lee CY, Chou P. Estimated prevalence of orthopaedic fractures in Taiwan: a cross-sectional study based on nationwide insurance data. Injury. 2010;41(12):1266–72.
5. Yamaguchi GT, Zajac FE. A planar model of the knee joint to characterize the knee extensor mechanism. J Biomech. 1989;22(1):1–10.
6. Greisamer RP, Weinstein H. Applied biomechanics of the patella. Clin Orthop Relat Res. 2001;389:9–14.
7. Hung LK, Chan KM, Chow YN, Leung PC. Fractured patella: operative treatment using the tension band principle. Injury. 1985;16(5):343–7.
8. Weber MJ, Janecki CJ, McLeod P, Nelson CL, Thompson JA. Efficacy of various forms of fixation of transverse fractures of the patella. J Bone Joint Surg Am. 1980;62(2):215–20.
9. Chalidis BE, Sachinis NC, Samoladas EP, Dimitriou CG, Pournaras JD. Is tension band wiring technique the "gold standard" for the treatment of olecranon fractures? A long term functional outcome study. J Orthop Surg Res. 2008;3:9.
10. Maranho DA, Pagnano RG, Volpon JB. Tension band wiring for proximal femoral varus osteotomy fixation in children. Medicine (Baltimore). 2014;93(7):e61.
11. Stoffel K, Klaue K, Perren SM. Functional load of plates in fracture fixation in vivo and its correlate in bone healing. Injury. 2000;31(Suppl 2):S-B37–50.
12. Patel VR, Parks BG, Wang Y, Ebert FR, Jinnah RH. Fixation of patella fractures with braided polyester suture: a biomechanical study. Injury. 2000;31(1):1–6.
13. Baran O, Manisali M, Cecen B. Anatomical and biomechanical evaluation of the tension band technique in patellar fractures. Int Orthop. 2009;33(4):1113–7.
14. Lotke PA, Ecker ML. Transverse fractures of the patella. Clin Orthop Relat Res. 1981;158:180–4.
15. Wu CC, Tai CL, Chen WJ. Patellar tension band wiring: a revised technique. Arch Orthop Trauma Surg. 2001;121(1–2):12–6.
16. Hoshino CM, Tran W, Tiberi JV, Black MH, Li BH, Gold SM, et al. Complications following tension-band fixation of patellar fractures with cannulated screws compared with Kirschner wire. J Bone Joint Surg Am. 2013;95(7):653–9.
17. Taylor BC, Mehta S, Castaneda J, French BG, Blanchard C. Plating of patella fractures: techniques and outcomes. J Orthop Trauma. 2014;28(9):e231–5.
18. Agarwala S, Agrawal P, Sobti A. A novel technique of patella fracture fixation facilitating early mobilization and reducing re-operation rates. J Clin Orthop Trauma. 2015;6(3):207–11.
19. Ong TK, Chee EK, Wong CL, Thevarajan K. Fixation of comminuted patellar fracture with combined cerclage and tension band wiring technique. Malaysian Orthop J. 2008;2(2):40–2.
20. Us AK, Kinik H. Self locking tension band technique in transverse patellar fracture. Int Orthop. 1996;20(6):357–8.
21. Müller ME, Allgöwer M, Schneider R, Willenegger H. Manual of internal fixation: techniques recommended by the AO group, Berlin, etc. Springer-Verlag, 2nd edition, 1979.
22. Curtis MJ. Internal fixation for fractures of the patella. A comparison of two methods. J Bone Joint Surgery Br. 1990;72(2):280–2.
23. Lew MJ. Principles: when there should be no difference: how to fail to reject the null hypothesis. Trends in Pharmacol Sci. 2006;27(5):274–8.
24. Abu-Zidan FM, Abbas AK, Hefny AF. Clinical "case series": a concept analysis. Afr Health Sci. 2012;12(4):557–62.
25. Schaafsma F, Verbeek J, Hulshof C, van Dijk F. Caution required when replying on a colleague's advice; a comparison between professional advice and evidence from the literature. BMC Health Serv Res. 2005;5:59.
26. Smith ST, Cramer KE, Karges DE, Watson JT, Moed BR. Early complications in the operative treatment of patella fractures. J Orthop Trauma. 1997;11(3):183–7.
27. Tian Y, Zhou F, Ji H, Zhang Z, Guo Y. Cannulated screw and cable are superior to modified tension band in the treatment of transverse patella fractures. Clin Orthop Relat Res. 2011;469(12):3429–35.

28. Wang CX, Tan L, Qi BC, Hou XF, Huang YL, Zhang HP, et al. A retrospective comparison of the modified tension band technique and the parallel titanium annulated lag screw technique in transverse patella fracture. Chin J Traumatol. 2014;17(4):208–13.
29. Lin T, Liu J, Xiao B, Fu D, Yang S. Comparison of the outcomes of cannulated screws vs. modified tension band wiring fixation techniques in the management of mildly displaced patellar fractures. BMC Musculoskelet Disord. 2015;16(1):282.
30. Lefaivre KA, O'Brien PJ, Broekhuyse HM, Guy P, Blachut PA. Modified tension band technique for patella fractures. Orthop Traumatol Surg Res. 2010;96(5): 579–82.
31. Nagaraja S, Couse TL, Guldberg RE. Trabecular bone microdamage and microstructural stresses under uniaxial compression. J Biomech. 2005;38(4):707–16.
32. Huang TW, Hsieh PH, Huang KC, Huang KC. Suspension suture augmentation for repair of coracoclavicular ligament disruption. Clin Orthop Relat Res. 2009;467(8):2142–8.
33. Mullett JH, Shannon F, Noel J, Lawlor G, Lee TC, O'Rourke SK. K-wire position in tension band wiring of the olecranon: a comparison of two techniques. Injury. 2000;31(6):427–31.
34. Saeed ZM, Trickett RW, Yewlett AD, Matthews TJ. Factors influencing K-wire migration in tension-band wiring of olecranon fractures. J Shoulder Elb Surg. 2014;23(8):1181–6.
35. Cornell CN. Internal fracture fixation in patients with osteoporosis. J Am Acad Orthop Surg. 2003;11(2):109–19.
36. Warriner AH, Patkar NM, Curtis JR, Delzell E, Gary L, Kilgore M, et al. Which fractures are most attributable to osteoporosis? J Clin Epidemiol. 2011;64(1): 46–53.
37. Miller MA, Liu W, Zurakowski D, Smith RM, Harris MB, Vrahas MS. Factors predicting failure of patella fixation. J Trauma Acute Care Surg. 2012;72(4): 1051–5.
38. Böstmann O, Kiviluoto O, Nirhamo J. Comminuted displaced fractures of the patella. Injury. 1981;13(3):196–202.

15

Clinical implications of fracture-associated vascular damage in extremity and pelvic trauma

F. Gilbert[1,7*], C. Schneemann[2], C. J. Scholz[3], R. Kickuth[4], R. H. Meffert[1], R. Wildenauer[2], U. Lorenz[2], R. Kellersmann[5*] and A. Busch[2,6*]

Abstract

Background: Vascular damage in polytrauma patients is associated with high mortality and morbidity. Therefore, specific clinical implications of vascular damage with fractures in major trauma patients are reassessed.

Methods: This comprehensive nine-year retrospective single center cohort study analyzed demography, laboratory, treatment and outcome data from 3689 patients, 64 patients with fracture-associated vascular injuries were identified and were compared to a control group.

Results: Vascular damage occurred in 7% of patients with upper and lower limb and pelvic fractures admitted to the trauma room. Overall survival was 80% in pelvic fracture and 97% in extremity fracture patients and comparable to non-vascular trauma patients. Additional arterial damage required substantial fluid administration and was visible as significantly anemia and disturbed coagulation tests upon admission. Open procedures were done in over 80% of peripheral extremity vascular damage. Endovascular procedures were predominant (87%) in pelvic injury.

Conclusion: Vascular damage is associated with high mortality rates especially in combination with pelvic fractures. Initial anemia, disturbed coagulation tests and the need for extensive pre-clinical fluid substitution were observed in the cohort with vascular damage. Therefore, fast diagnosis and early interventional and surgical procedures are necessary to optimize patient-specific outcome.

Keywords: Fracture-associated vascular damage, Surgical trauma room, Extremity trauma, Pelvic trauma, Endovascular repair, Level of evidence: IV

Background

Trauma is one of the leading causes of death in western countries, and the most frequent one in people below forty [1]. Whenever the body's integrity is compromised by contusion, concussion or fracture, surgical trauma care is necessary for rapid damage control and specific individualized treatment. This remains, a major challenge for clinicians due to varying patterns of injuries and occasional major traumas, requiring urgent, yet highly specialized therapy [2, 3]. Fast, conclusive and complete injury assessment by examination of head and neck, thorax, abdomen, pelvis and the extremities is further supported by computed tomography (CT) and CT-angiography (CTA) [4, 5].

Head and thoracic injuries are found in approximately 50% of all trauma patients and extremity or pelvic fractures in roughly 30% [6]. Additional vascular damage, especially of arteries or venous plexus is acutely life threatening and further reduces time for decision-making and treatment [7]. Vascular damage in combination with fractures is associated with higher mortality and inferior outcome, especially due to rapid and voluminous blood loss into pelvic or femoral soft tissue compartments. Correct diagnosis may be difficult due to low body temperature and masking effects of other injuries [8–10].

* Correspondence: gilbert_f@ukw.de; kellersman_r@ukw.de; Albert.Busch@mri.tum.de
[1]Department of Orthopaedic Trauma, Hand, Plastic and Reconstructive Surgery, University Hospital Würzburg, Würzburg, Germany
[5]Department of Vascular Surgery, Klinikum Fulda, Fulda, Germany
[2]Department for General Visceral, Vascular & Paediatric Surgery, University Hospital Würzburg, Würzburg, Germany

Doppler ultrasound and CTA increase the detection rate, yet incorrect diagnosis remains frequent thus requiring re-examination after initial stabilization [11, 12]. Depending on type and extent of trauma, presentations may be acute bleeding, hemodynamic instability, pulsating tumors, massive hematoma or ischemic and pulseless extremities [13]. Additionally, vasospasm or complete vascular disruption both may mimic ischemia [14].

Despite recognized difficulties in detecting vascular injury in extremity trauma as well as an increased mortality rate in combination with pelvic trauma, limited data about the immediate clinical implications of vascular damage associated with fractures is available. We therefore analyzed thoroughly demography, initial laboratory results, treatment and outcome of extremity and pelvic fracture-associated vascular injuries in a trauma cohort of 64 patients versus a comparable cohort of patients with isolated osseous damage in a nine-year retrospective single-center study was carried out.

Aim of the study:

The aim of this retrospective cohort study was to recognize patterns of injury where vascular damage and fracture occur and also identification of surrogate parameters which may suspect a vascular involvement in major trauma patients. In addition, the influences of concomitant vascular damage to patient's management and outcome were analyzed.

Methods

Facility

A university hospital and level-one trauma center, embedded in the regional trauma network (Traumanetzwerk Nordbayern-Würzburg) was analyzed. A multidisciplinary team provides twenty-four-seven trauma care; following standard operating procedures according to guidelines of the German National Society for Trauma Surgery (DGU) are implemented. Ultrasound, X-ray and multi-slice computed tomography (CT) are available on site in the trauma room. A board-certified vascular surgeon and an interventional radiologist are part of the trauma team.

Patient identification.

A retrospective analysis of all admissions to the surgical trauma room from December 2005 until December 2013 identified 3689 cases, including primary trauma admissions and secondary transfers from other centers.

The initial analysis included trauma mechanism and pattern of injuries, specifically identifying all vascular damages. Additional examination included fractures, immediate vascular, visceral, urologic or pediatric surgery or invasive vascular diagnostics and interventions. Every case with vascular involvement and extremity or pelvic fracture was then analyzed for age, sex, blunt or penetrating trauma, hospital stay, intensive care unit (ICU) stay, number of operations, method of treatment, amputation, death, trauma scores (Glasgow coma scale, GCS; injury severity index, ISS; Revised Injury Severity Classification Score, RISC I), preclinical fluid management and initial laboratory results. Data were available for 100% of patients, except for preclinical fluid management (36.7 and 49.3% for vascular injury group and fracture only group, respectively).

This cohort (vascular injury group) was then subdivided in regard to localization of the fracture, upper/lower extremity or pelvis, and the corresponding vascular damage. Patients with vascular involvement of the head and neck ($N = 36$), i.e. carotid artery dissection, were excluded in this study.

Control group

In order to compare outcome and laboratory results, a control group consisting of 60 major trauma patients with limb/pelvic fractures only and no additional vascular damage, based on CTA, clinical assessment and clinical course, was selected. Inclusion criteria were surgical trauma room admission and fractures without further vascular, visceral, thoracic, spinal or cranial damage.

Statistics

Group comparisons of count data were performed with $\chi 2$ tests when the smallest value in the contingency table was 5 or more, otherwise Fisher's exact test was performed. Normally distributed measurement values (Shapiro-Wilk $p \geq 0.05$) were examined with the Welch two sample t-test, in cases where the normality assumption did not hold (Shapiro-Wilk $p < 0.05$) the Wilcoxon rank sum test was applied. Dependencies between measurement values were examined with linear regression. Endpoint (survival) analyses were performed with Cox regression. P-values < 0.05 were considered significant.

Results

Demographic data

Within the nine-year study period, 3689 patients were admitted to the trauma room. Fractures of the extremities, the pelvis or the shoulder girdle (i.e. clavicula, scapula) were found in 904 patients. A third presented with multiple (≥2) fractures (Additional file 1: Table S1).

Vascular damage associated with a corresponding fracture of the extremities or the pelvis, requiring specific vascular repair, was identified in 64 cases (Fig. 1). Vessel injuries were confined to the arterial system in lower and upper limb, while arterial damage was the reason to treat in 66% in pelvic fractures and venous damage requiring treatment was seen in 34%. The mean age of this cohort was 49 ± 17 years, 78% were male and 94% sustained blunt trauma

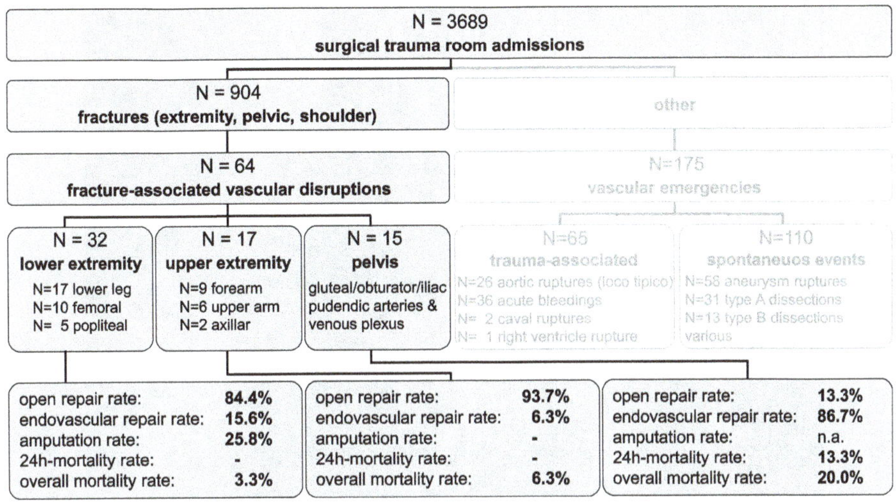

Fig. 1 Demography, treatment and outcome of fracture-associated vascular injury. The chart shows the number (64 + 175 = 239) of vascular involvements in all 3689 surgical trauma room admissions in the study period (2005–2013). 64 cases of fracture-associated vascular disruption involving the upper/lower limb and the pelvis were treated by immediate open or endovascular repair. 175 cases required immediate vascular surgical exploration due to primary vascular emergencies like i.e. trauma-associated aortic rupture and acute bleeding or spontaneous aneurysm rupture or aortic dissection (blurred out)

(79.4% traffic accident; 12.6% fall; 7.9% work-related accident) (Additional file 1: Table S1). The lower limb and its vessels were involved twice as often as upper limb and pelvis, however facture-associated vascular injury occurred at almost same rates in either localization (4.2, 6.2, 6.1% for upper limb, pelvis and lower limb, respectively) (Figs. 2 and 3). All patients had a CTA of the clinically suspected trauma area after exclusion of cerebral hemorrhage by native CT in cases of suspected head trauma. Depending on the treatment strategy, patients were then immediately transferred to the operating room or the angiography suite. A specific trauma mechanism could not be linked to vascular damage.

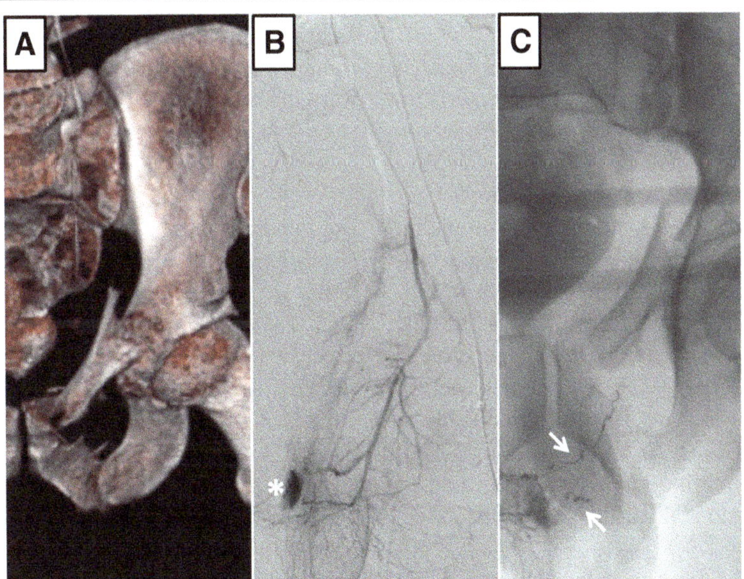

Fig. 2 Pelvic fracture with associated arterial bleeding and consecutive embolization. The figure shows a 3D-reconstruction of a pelvic CT, with a type C pelvic fracture and destruction of the superior and inferior pubic rami at the time of trauma room admission in a hemodynamic unstable patient (**a**). CTA was suggestive of pelvic arterial bleeding and immediate angiography was indicated. Digital subtraction angiography (DSA) (**b**) revealed arterial bleeding from branches of the obturator artery with pooling of contrast agent around the symphysis (*). Super-selective microcoil embolization (arrows) of the feeding vessels helped to control the bleeding and stabilize the patient (**c**)

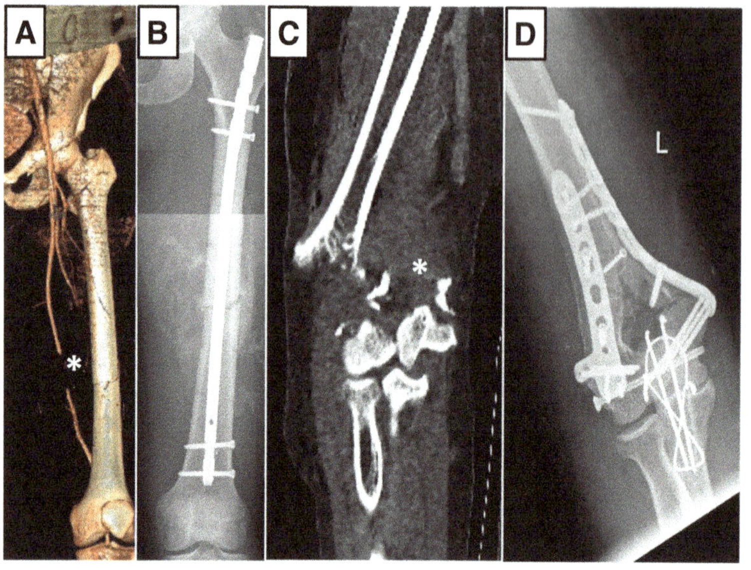

Fig. 3 Extremity fractures with associated vascular damage. 3D-reconstruction (**a**) of the initial CT of a patient after motorcycle accident with closed femoral shaft fracture and disruption of the superficial femoral artery (★) with active bleeding palpable as pulsatile femoral mass (signal loss of soft tissue contrast agent pooling due to 3D-reconstruction sequence). Of note, fracture lines (**a**) indicate medial translocation of the osseous fragment towards the artery, probably causative of arterial rupture. Initial treatment included immediate open arterial reconstruction with vein graft interposition and external stabilization and after 12 days intramedullary nail repair (**b**). CTA with active pooling of contrast agent (*) from the brachial artery in a patient after fall with a grade IIIb open fracture of the humeral shaft (**c**). Initial treatment included patch plasty of the brachial artery, external fixation and fasciotomy of the forearm compartments. After 10 days the elbow joint was reconstructed with open reduction and plate fixation, an olecranon osteotomy was performed for better joint visualization

In total, 239 (6.5%) cases of all trauma room admissions had vascular implications that required immediate vascular repair (Fig. 1).

Laboratory results

Comparing this group with a similar non-vascular trauma group, no differences in baseline characteristics were seen (Additional file 1: Table S1). However, fracture-associated arterial damage and consecutive blood loss into the surrounding soft tissues seriously aggravated the initial clinical presentation. Hemoglobin levels, a surrogate marker of blood loss, and prothrombin time (Quick) as well as activated partial thromboplastin time (PTT) were significantly lower in the vascular trauma group. Concordantly fibrinogen was at the lower limit (Table 1). These effects were pronounced in the pelvis and the lower extremity (Additional file 2: Table S2). Markers of cellular stress and disintegration, lactate, myoglobin and creatine kinase were elevated in both groups, yet showed no statistically significant difference (Table 1).

Subsequent analysis of the pre-clinical fluid administration revealed a significantly higher need of total volume to secure safe transport (Table 1). As expected, the total volume correlated inversely with the initial hemoglobin measurement at admission ($p < 0.001$). Regression analysis revealed lowering of the hemoglobin-value by 1 mg/dl with every 200 ml of fluids administered. This effect was four times stronger in the vascular trauma group (Additional file 3: Table S3). Unfortunately, initial blood pressure measurements and reports about tourniquet or pelvic clamp usage were not available. A drop in fibrinogen by 1 g/L was associated with roughly 700 ml of fluid administration. No significant values were detected in both groups, yet the observed trends suggest a stronger effect with additional vascular damage (Additional file 3: Table S3).

Outcome analysis

No differences were seen in mortality rates between patients with extremity fracture only and such with associated vascular damage (Table 2). In both groups overall survival was over 90% and death, if any, was due to accompanying head injury, thoracic injury or prolonged course of disease with septic complications. However, a notably high immediate mortality rate (≤24 h) of 13.3% and overall mortality rate of 20% was associated with pelvic fracture with vascular damage. These could, however, not be related to a specific fracture type or vessel involvement (66% arterial/33% venous).

Fracture-associated vascular disruption resulted in longer hospital stay, longer ICU stay and a higher number of revision surgery after the initial procedure for bleeding control and primary fixation (Table 2). Also, the lower extremity amputation rate was significantly higher.

Table 1 Laboratory results and pre-clinical fluid administratio

	Hemoglobin (mg/dl)	Quick (%)	PTT (s)	Fibrinogen (g/l)	Lactate (mmol/l)	Myoglobin (μg/l)	Creatine kinase (U/l)	Crystallines (ml)	Colloids (ml)	Total volume (ml)
Vascular injury group	9.95 ± 2.6	59.2 ± 21.6	41.9 ± 25.2	1.7 ± 0.9	2.1 ± 1.2	1356 ± 1441	393 ± 316	1000 ± 741	500 ± 0	1500 ± 1112
Fracture only group	11.67 ± 2.6	78.0 ± 19.3	35.3 ± 20.7	2.2 ± 0.6	1.8 ± 0.9	855 ± 856	372 ± 337	1000 ± 0	500 ± 0	1000 ± 741
P	0.0004	0.0002	0.002	0.003	0.24	0.24	0.77	0.09	0.64	0.03

The table shows the mean ± standard deviation (SD) or median ± median absolute deviation (MAD) where appropriate (cristalloides; colloides) for each parameter and the *P*-value for comparison between vascular and control trauma population. Significant *P*-values are shown in bold. (normal ranges: hemoglobin: 11.5-16 g/dL; prothrombin time according to Quick: 70–120%; activated partial thromboplastin time, PTT: 25–36 s; fibrinogen: 1.6–4.0 g/L; lactate: < 0.5 mmol/L; Myoglobin: < 55 μg/L; creatin kinase: < 170 U/L)

Table 2 Outcome parameters and trauma scores of vascular and control trauma populations

	Overall survival	Hospital stay (d)	ICU stay (d)	Operations (number)	Amputation (leg)	GCS	ISS	RISC I
Vascular injury group	92.5%	36.0 ± 22.1	15.0 ± 14.8	6.0 ± 4.7	25.8%	13.2 ± 3.3	23.4 ± 13.8	81.5 ± 25.1
Fracture only group	91.3%	21.5 ± 13	7.2 ± 7.3	2.9 ± 2.4	–	13.3 ± 3.5	22.7 ± 14.2	86.2 ± 23.1
Effect size Effect type	0.486 hazard	12.5 median diff	5.5 median	2	8.32	0	0	−1.9
Test type	ratio Cox regression	Wilcox-Test	diff Wilcox-Test	median diff Wilcox-Test	odds ratio Fisher's exact-t	median diff Wilcox-Test	median diff Wilcox-Test	median diff Wilcox-Test
P	0.28	0.00002	0.009	0.000003	0.03	0.8	0.74	0.3

The table shows the comparison of the vascular trauma group to the fracture only group, indicating mean ± SD, effect size, effect type and the type of test used, along with their significance. Significant *P*-values are shown in bold. (*GCS*,Glasgow Coma Scale, *ISS* Injury Severity Index, *RISC I*,Revised Injury Severity Classification Score)

Two amputations were due to primary subtotal above-the-knee amputation during trauma, five were due to severe soft tissue damage and one was due to prolonged ischemia after complicated pelvic fracture with iliac artery occlusion. No upper extremity amputation occurred. The grade of soft tissue damage was, however, comparable for lower and upper extremities (grade IIIC according to Gustilo/Anderson in >70% of cases). Compartment release had to be done in eight lower and one upper extremity, these cases did not correlate with subsequent need for amputation. These implications were not reflected by either of the trauma scores GCS, ISS or RISC I (Table 2).

Vascular surgical and interventional endovascular means were applied for bleeding control. Open surgical procedures included autologous vein interposition, patch plasty, ligature as well as direct suture and were the method of choice in both extremities (Figs. 1 and 3). Pelvic fracture associated bleedings were mostly treated by endovascular coiling or covered stent implantation in one case (Figs. 1 and 2).

Discussion

Fracture-associated vascular injury of the limbs and especially the pelvis may have severe consequence for the patient. Accurate detection, early treatment and supportive therapy determine the outcome [15].

Mechanisms of vascular trauma include blunt trauma (external force or through fracture fragments), sharp trauma or strain which might lead to disruption or intima damage leading to ischemia (Fig. 3) [16, 17]. Presentation is thus hemorrhage or ischemia, a phenomenon best described for supracondylar humeral fracture or knee trauma [18–20]. The initial clinical symptoms, especially hemodynamic instability, were not available retrospectively in our cohort. Nevertheless, the established algorithm of local CT-angiography in case of suspected severe fracture of the pelvis and the extremities provided good results, since all patients with vascular injury were identified immediately and no late amputations due to ischemia occurred [5, 12, 21].

In 3–9% of fractures a concomitant vascular damage is reported varying due to regional and socioeconomic factors [10, 22–24]. In this single-center cohort we identified an accompanying vascular damage in 7% of the fractures. Required treatments were very heterogeneous, for the fracture-associated vascular injury as well as vascular incidents in general (Fig. 1). Unfortunately, most publications are case reports or case series focusing on a specific entity or treatment, thus not catering for the need for more general data analysis [25]. No conclusive pattern of injury for consecutive vascular damage could be identified in our cohort, in fact, vascular damage has to be expected regardless of the fracture localization, the impact of trauma or any trauma scores (Table 2).

This data displays a similar incidence of vascular injury in upper/lower extremity and pelvic fractures. Nevertheless, outcomes such as higher immediate mortality in pelvic fractures and significant amputation rates for the lower extremity are area-specific (Fig. 1 and Table 2). The management is considerably influenced by the degree of tissue damage and occasional primary subtotal amputation. Of 15 pelvic fractures, 4 were classified stable while the rest were type B/C fractures (Pennal and Tile classification) possibly yielding additional rupture of the venous plexus. Patients with fractures and vascular injuries also show a longer hospital stay and higher number of operative procedures (Table 2). Elevated immediate mortality in the fracture only group was due to the higher rate of multiple fractures, suggestive of more severely trauma (Table 2 and Additional file 2: Table S2). The additional severity of vascular damage to multi-injured patients is currently not reflected by any trauma score (Table 2).

This study demonstrates the effect of additional vascular damage on the admission laboratory data (Table 1 and Additional file 2:Table S2 and Additional file 3: Table S3). The presented results show similar trends in overall, as well as entitiy-specific analysis (Additional file 2: Table S2). Low hemoglobin, and altered coagulation were, however, associated with an increased need of fluid in the preclinical course. Thus some dilution effect has to be taken into consideration However, the available data in retrospective analysis was not available in all patients, and results have to be interpreted carefully. Nevertheless, substantial fluid administration and low initial hemoglobin, i.e. by rapid blood gas analysis, may raise the attention to direct diagnostics to identifying vascular damage. Trauma-induced coagulation defect is a severe co-morbidity, strongly associated with an increased mortality [26]. Early therapy might also include platelet-directed treatments [27, 28].

Ever since the late stages of World War II, where ligation of arteries and veins was the treatment of choice, surgical and technical abilities have evolved towards a diversified armamentarium, significantly increasing limb salvage and survival rates, nowadays enabling individualized care [29, 30]. Especially rapid endovascular repair for bleeding control has evolved as primary option for certain clinical entities of vascular injury, like embolization in pelvic bleeding, stentgraft implantation in aortic transection or thoracic outlet vessel breach [22, 25, 31, 32]. However, mangled extremities remain a domain of open vascular repair (Fig. 1). Open fracture, eventual contamination and massive tissue loss require autologous reconstruction [9, 33, 34].

Conclusion

This retrospective single-center cohort study we could demonstrate that fracture-associated vascular damage occurs in one of fourteen trauma patients, with a specific clinical impact regarding pre-hospital fluid management, eventual early transfusion and coagulation support. A multidisciplinary approach requires trauma and vascular surgery in combination with interventional radiology to guarantee the best possible outcome for overall survival and limb salvage.

Additional files

Additional file 1: Table S1. Baseline characteristics of vascular and control trauma populations. Both populations have a similar size and show no differences in age, sex and trauma type distribution. The number of patients with multiple fractures is slightly higher in the control trauma population.

Additional file 2: Table S2. Laboratory results and total preclinical volume comparison between vascular and control trauma population overall and based on area of fracture. The table shows the mean ± SD or median ± MAD where appropriate for each parameter and the *P*-value for comparison between vascular and control trauma population. Significant *P*-values are shown in bold. (normal ranges: hemoglobin: 11.5-16 g/dL; prothrombin time according to Quick: 70–120%; activated partial thromboplastin time, PTT: 25–36 s; fibrinogen: 1.6–4.0 g/L; lactate: < 0.5 mmol/L).

Additional file 3: Table S3. Preclinical fluid administration in dependence of hemoglobin and fibrinogen. Regression results of indicated parameters against total administered volume are shown for the overall study population as well as both patient groups separately. The effect size corresponds to the average volume of required preclinical fluid administration when the examined parameter value is increased by 1. Significant P-values are shown in bold.

Abbreviations

CT: Computed tomography; CTA: computed tomography angiography; GCS: Glasgow coma scale; ISS: Injury severity index; PTT: Partial thromboplastin time; RISC I: Revised Injury Severity Classification Score

Acknowledgments

We thank S. Duell for administrative help and C. Wagner for help with patient identification in SAP. We especially thank all the nursing and medical staff that makes working in the emergency room possible every day and night.

Funding

This publication was funded by the German Research Foundation (DFG) and the University of Wuerzburg in the funding program Open Access Publishing. Funding includes only the publication fee. No funding for the design of the study, the collection, analysis, and interpretation of data and for writing the manuscript was obtained.

Authors' contributions

FG: made substantial contribution in design an conception of the study, performed acquisition of data and interpretation of data, revisited the manuscript critically CS: performed acquisition of data and interpretation of data CJS: performed acquisition of data and interpretation of data RK: made substantial contribution in design and conception of the study, revisited the manuscript RM: made substantial contribution in design and conception of the study, revisited the manuscript RW: made substantial contribution in design and conception of the study, revisited the manuscript UL: made substantial contribution in design and conception of the study, revisited the manuscript RK: made substantial contribution in design and conception of the study, wrote the manuscript AB: made substantial contribution in design and conception of the study, wrote the manuscript. All authors approved the final version of the manuscript.

Consent for publication

Written informed consent for publication of individual person's data were obtained from every patient.

Competing interests

The authors declare that they have no competing interests.

Author details

[1]Department of Orthopaedic Trauma, Hand, Plastic and Reconstructive Surgery, University Hospital Würzburg, Würzburg, Germany. [2]Department for General Visceral, Vascular & Paediatric Surgery, University Hospital Würzburg, Würzburg, Germany. [3]Core Unit Systems Medicine IZKF, University Hospital Würzburg, Würzburg, Germany. [4]Department of Diagnostic and Interventional Radiology, University Hospital Würzburg, Würzburg, Germany. [5]Department of Vascular Surgery, Klinikum Fulda, Fulda, Germany. [6]Department for Vascular and Endovascular Surgery Klinikum rechts der Isar, Technical University Munich, Munich, Germany. [7]Department of Trauma Hand Plastic and Reconstructive Surgery, University Munich Germany, Julius-Maximilians-University of Würzburg Oberdürrbacherstr, 6 D-, 97080 Würzburg, Germany.

References

1. Bundesamt D-S. https://www.destatis.de/DE/ZahlenFakten/GesellschaftStaat/Gesundheit/Todesursachen/Todesursachen.html.
2. Tiel Groenestege-Kreb D, van Maarseveen O, Leenen L. Trauma team. Br J Anaesth. 2014;113(2):258–65. https://doi.org/10.1093/bja/aeu236 PubMed PMID: 24980423.
3. Wurmb TE, Fruhwald P, Knuepffer J, et al. Application of standard operating procedures accelerates the process of trauma care in patients with multiple injuries. Eur J Emerg Med. 2008;15(6):311–7. https://doi.org/10.1097/MEJ.0b013e3283036ce6 PubMed PMID: 19078832.
4. Wurmb TE, Fruhwald P, Hopfner W, et al. Whole-body multislice computed tomography as the first line diagnostic tool in patients with multiple injuries: the focus on time. J Trauma. 2009;66(3):658–65. https://doi.org/10.1097/TA.0b013e31817de3f4 PubMed PMID: 19276734.
5. Fung Kon Jin PH, Goslings JC, Ponsen KJ, et al. Assessment of a new trauma workflow concept implementing a sliding CT scanner in the trauma room: the effect on workup times. J Trauma. 2008;64(5):1320–6. https://doi.org/10.1097/TA.0b013e318059b9ae PubMed PMID: 18469657.
6. Sektion Notfall- & Intensivmedizin SNdDGfrUDAT. Jahresbericht 2015. 2015.
7. Hupp T, Eisele R. Traumatic injuries to the extremities including bone and blood vessel damage: priorities, triage and interdisciplinary management. Gefässchirurgie. 2002;7(4):202–7. https://doi.org/10.1007/s00772-002-0242-7.
8. Scalea TM, DuBose J, Moore EE, et al. Western trauma association critical decisions in trauma: management of the mangled extremity. J Trauma Acute Care Surg. 2012;72(1):86–93. https://doi.org/10.1097/TA.0b013e318241ed70 PubMed PMID: 22310120.
9. Rozycki GS, Tremblay LN, Feliciano DV, et al. Blunt vascular trauma in the extremity: diagnosis, management, and outcome. J Trauma. 2003; 55(5):814–24. https://doi.org/10.1097/01.TA.0000087807.44105.AE PubMed PMID: 14608150.
10. Marzi I, Lustenberger T. Management of Bleeding Pelvic Fractures. Scandinavian journal of surgery. 2014;103(2):104–11. https://doi.org/10.1177/1457496914525604 PubMed PMID: 24737854.
11. Seamon MJ, Smoger D, Torres DM, et al. A prospective validation of a current practice: the detection of extremity vascular injury with CT angiography. J Trauma 2009;67(2):238–243; discussion 243-4. doi: https://doi.org/10.1097/TA.0b013e3181a51bf9. PubMed PMID: 19667874.
12. Luo W, Hosseini H, Zderic V, et al. Detection and localization of peripheral vascular bleeding using Doppler ultrasound. J Emerg Med. 2011;41(1):64–73. https://doi.org/10.1016/j.jemermed.2010.01.001 PubMed PMID: 20189743.

13. Halvorson JJ, Anz A, Langfitt M, et al. Vascular injury associated with extremity trauma: initial diagnosis and management. J Am Acad Orthop Surg. 2011;19(8):495–504 PubMed PMID: 21807917.
14. Shah SR, Wearden PD, Gaines BA. Pediatric peripheral vascular injuries: a review of our experience. J Surg Res. 2009;153(1):162–6. https://doi.org/10.1016/j.jss.2008.03.006 PubMed PMID: 18541266.
15. Albert B, Gilbert F, Schneemann C, Kickuth R, Meffert R, Kellersmann R, Wildenauer R, Lorenz U. Klinische Implikationen bei Fraktur-assoziierten Gefäßschäden im Schockraum. 134. München: Kongress Deutsche Gesellschaft für Chirurgie ICM; 2017. p. 284. https://goo.gl/Qs3hdH.
16. Linder F, Vollmar J. [The current status of treatment of arterial injuries and their sequelae]. Chirurg 1965;36:55–63. PubMed PMID: 14265784.
17. Larcan A, Fieve G. Louis Sencert, vascular surgeon (1878–1924). J Mal Vasc. 1986;11(Suppl B):68–74 PubMed PMID: 3519817.
18. Wegmann H, Eberl R, Kraus T, et al. The impact of arterial vessel injuries associated with pediatric supracondylar humeral fractures. J Trauma Acute Care Surg. 2014;77(2):381–5. https://doi.org/10.1097/TA.0000000000000306 PubMed PMID: 25058268.
19. Parker S, Handa A, Deakin M, et al. Knee dislocation and vascular injury: 4 year experience at a UK major trauma Centre and vascular hub. Injury. 2015. https://doi.org/10.1016/j.injury.2015.11.014 PubMed PMID: 26652226.
20. Xu YQ, Li Q, Shen TG, et al. Early diagnosis and treatment of trauma in knee joints accompanied with popliteal vascular injury. Int J Clin Exp Med. 2015; 8(6):9421–9 PubMed PMID: 26309604; PubMed Central PMCID: PMCPMC4538002.
21. Linder F, Mani K, Juhlin C, et al. Routine whole body CT of high energy trauma patients leads to excessive radiation exposure. Scand J Trauma Resusc Emerg Med. 2016;24(1):7. https://doi.org/10.1186/s13049-016-0199-2 PubMed PMID: 26817669; PubMed Central PMCID: PMCPMC4729033.
22. Hauschild O, Aghayev E, von Heyden J, et al. Angioembolization for pelvic hemorrhage control: results from the German pelvic injury register. J Trauma Acute Care Surg. 2012;73(3):679–84. https://doi.org/10.1097/TA.0b013e318253b5ba PubMed PMID: 22710767.
23. Poyhonen R, Suominen V, Uurto I, et al. Non-iatrogenic civilian vascular trauma in a well-defined geographical region in Finland. Eur J Trauma Emerg Surg. 2015;41(5):545–9. https://doi.org/10.1007/s00068-014-0460-1 PubMed PMID: 26037992.
24. Galyfos G, Kerasidis S, Stefanidis G, et al. Iatrogenic and non-iatrogenic arterial injuries in an urban level I trauma Centre in Greece. Int Angiol. 2015; 25 PubMed PMID: 26406965.
25. Lustenberger T, Wutzler S, Stormann P, et al. The role of angio-embolization in the acute treatment concept of severe pelvic ring injuries. Injury. 2015; 46(Suppl 4):S33–8. https://doi.org/10.1016/S0020-1383(15)30016-4 PubMed PMID: 26542864.
26. Gando S, Hayakawa M. Pathophysiology of trauma-induced coagulopathy and Management of Critical Bleeding Requiring Massive Transfusion. Semin Thromb Hemost. 2016;42(2):155–65. https://doi.org/10.1055/s-0035-1564831. PubMed PMID: 26716498.
27. Ramsey MT, Fabian TC, Shahan CP, Sharpe JP, Mabry SE, Weinberg JA, Croce MA, Jennings LK. A prospective study of platelet function in trauma patients. J Trauma Acute Care Surg. 2016. https://doi.org/10.1097/TA.0000000000001017. PubMed PMID: 26895088.
28. Fachgesellschaften. AdWM. S3 – Leitlinie Polytrauma/ Schwerverletzten-Behandlung. online publication. 2011 valid till 2016-06-30;AWMF RegNr 012/019.
29. Barr J, Cherry KJ, Rich NM. Vascular surgery in world war II: the shift to repairing arteries. Ann Surg. 2016;263(3):615–20. https://doi.org/10.1097/SLA.0000000000001181 PubMed PMID: 25719811.
30. De BM, Simeone FA. Battle injuries of the arteries in world war II; an analysis of 2,471 cases. Ann Surg. 1946;123:534–79 PubMed PMID: 21024586.
31. Serra R, de Franciscis S, Grande R, et al. Endovascular repair for acute traumatic transection of the descending thoracic aorta: experience of a single centre with a 12-years follow up. J Cardiothorac Surg. 2015;10(1):171. https://doi.org/10.1186/s13019-015-0388-5 PubMed PMID: 26590963; PubMed Central PMCID: PMCPMC4655082.
32. Sinha S, Patterson BO, Ma J, et al. Systematic review and meta-analysis of open surgical and endovascular management of thoracic outlet vascular injuries. Journal of vascular surgery : official publication, the Society for Vascular Surgery [and] International Society for Cardiovascular Surgery. North American Chapter. 2013;57(2):547–567 e8. https://doi.org/10.1016/j.jvs.2012.10.077 PubMed PMID: 23337863.
33. The Lower Extremity Vascular Repairs Outcome Group; Fortuna G, DuBose J, Mendelsberg R, Inaba, K, Haider A, Joseph B, Skarupa D, Selleck MJ, O'Callaghan T, Charlton-Ouw K. Contemporary outcomes of lower extremity vascular repairs extending below the knee: a multicenter retrospective study. J Trauma Acute Care Surg. 2016. https://doi.org/10.1097/TA.0000000000000996. PubMed PMID: 26885995.
34. Scott AR, Gilani R, Tapia NM, et al. Endovascular management of traumatic peripheral arterial injuries. J Surg Res. 2015;199(2):557–63. https://doi.org/10.1016/j.jss.2015.04.086 PubMed PMID: 26115809.

16

Why tibial plateau fractures are overlooked

Cecilie Mullerup Kiel[1,2*], Kim Lyngby Mikkelsen[2] and Michael Rindom Krogsgaard[1,2]

Abstract

Background: Tibial plateau fractures (TPFs) are sometimes overlooked in the emergency room (ER). Using a national register covering 18 years we aimed to find out why and to evaluate if use of a specific radiographic decision rule, Pittsburgh Knee Rules (PKRs), could have reduced the number of overlooked TPFs.

Methods: Medical records for 137 patients, prospectively registered during 18 years by the Danish Patient Compensation Association (DPCA) (a national register), were studied. The inclusion criterion was a delayed diagnosis of a fracture in the knee following a trauma. Case records, legal assessments, and evaluations by specialist doctors were reviewed, and the consequences of the delayed diagnosis for outcome and treatment were registered.

Results: Only 58 patients (42%) had been evaluated according to PKRs. In 53 patient cases, the fracture was not diagnosed on radiographs obtained at the first medical contact. However, in 84% of these cases, the fracture was visible or was suspected by retrospective evaluation. 50 out of 79 patients, for whom X-rays were not obtained, were candidates for radiographs according to PKRs, 17 cases lacked information to evaluate by PKRs and 12 cases were not candidates. In 53% of all cases, it was evaluated that the fracture position had worsened at the time of diagnosis. A significant disability compensation was granted in 36% of cases due to the delayed identification of fractures, totaling 841,000 EUR.

Conclusions: The major reasons for overlooking TPFs were 1) difficulty in recognizing the fractures on X-rays and 2) that X-ray decision rules were not employed. Two thirds of the patients, for whom a radiograph had not been prescribed, would have had an X-ray, if the PKRs had been used. Overlooking TPFs significantly increased patient disability in one third of cases. We recommend that healthcare professionals in the ER use X-ray decision rules in addition to clinical examination to avoid overlooking TPFs. When standard radiographs are evaluated as normal in patients that are clinically suspect of a TPF, oblique X-rays, magnetic resonance imaging (MRI) or Computed Tomography (CT)-scan should be considered.

Keywords: Tibial plateau fracture, Magnetic resonance imaging (MRI), X-rays, Pittsburgh knee rules, Clinical decision rules, Knee fracture

Background

Knee fractures account for about 6% of all trauma admissions to hospitals [1]. Tibial plateau fractures (TPFs, Fig. 1) comprise 1% of fractures in all age groups [2] and 8% in the elderly population [3]. The incidence of TPFs in Denmark is 10.3 per 100,000 annually [2]. The fractures can be difficult to recognize on standard radiographs [4], since the uninjured joint surface is often projected on top of the fractured part of the tibiae plateau in the anterior-posterior, and side views. TPFs are one of the most common radiological pathologies to be overlooked by doctors [5]. However, to the best of our knowledge there are only two studies addressing overlooked TPFs. The first [6] focused on overlooked fractures of the anterior tibial plateau, whereas the other [7] described eight overlooked osteoporotic fractures in elderly patients.

The Pittsburgh Knee Rules (PKRs) and similar decision-making rules were developed to improve accuracy in the use of X-ray imaging in cases of acute knee injuries. PKRs have a sensitivity close to 100% [8–13] and an inter-observer agreement of 0.71 [9]. Additionally, it has been demonstrated that the use of PKRs reduces the number of X-ray images obtained at hospitals by

* Correspondence: cecilie.m.kiel@gmail.com
[1]Section for Sports Traumatology M51, Bispebjerg-Frederiksberg Hospital (Part of IOC Research Center Copenhagen), University of Copenhagen, Bispebjerg Bakke 23, DK-2400 Copenhagen, NV, Denmark
[2]Danish Patient Compensation Association, Kalvebod Brygge 45, 1560 Copenhagen, NV, Denmark

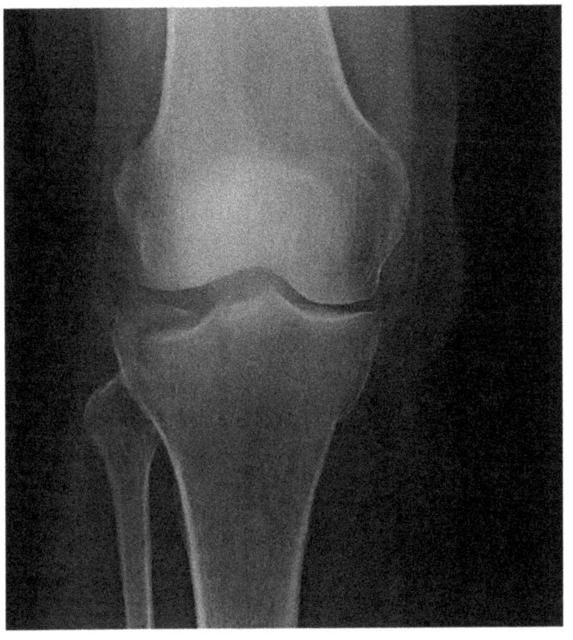

Fig. 1 X-ray imaging of a lateral tibial plateau fracture. From https://commons.wikimedia.org/wiki/File:Tibial_Plateau_Fracture.jpg

30–78% [12, 14]. It is unknown if failure to obtain X-ray images at the primary healthcare contact for a knee injury is an underlying cause of overlooking TPFs. The objectives of this study were 1) to analyze why TPFs were overlooked in Denmark during an 18-year period, 2) to study the consequences of a delayed diagnosis for treatment and patient outcome, and 3) to evaluate if diagnosis of TPFs could have been established by use of PKRs.

Methods

Type of clinical study

This is a retrospective, descriptive study of prospectively collected cases of overlooked TPFs in Denmark 1996–2013 from the Danish Patient Compensation Association (DPCA). DPCA is a national public body, to which any patient or healthcare professional who experiences malpractice or complications in connection with treatment in the Danish healthcare system (private or public) can freely submit a compensation claim. Healthcare professionals are legally obligated to inform the patient about DPCA if this is suspected. The system is a "no fault" scheme, where no individual is blamed, and it focuses only on compensation. Information about the DPCA is described in [15], which also explains how claims are approved or rejected. A person's disability is expressed in % according to a table from the National Board of Industrial Injuries in Denmark. "Additional disability" involves the extra disability (expressed in %) caused by treatment malpractice. Additional disability of < 5% is regarded as insignificant and is not compensated.

Inclusion criterion

We included claims of delayed diagnosis of a fracture in the knee following a knee trauma (defined as a blunt trauma, a fall, a twist of the knee, or other injuries). The trauma had to be referable to an exact date to be included. Cases with a diagnostic delay of less than 24 h were excluded.

Clinical information on date of injury, first contact with medical care, date of correct diagnosis, trauma mechanism, patient age at the time of injury, diagnostic modalities used at first contact with medical care, side of injured knee, fracture classification according to ICD10 [16], treatment, outcome (expressed as disability %), and eventual monetary compensation for additional disability was manually collected from the included patients' records.

Decision rules

Several decision rules exist to establish the indication for radiography of the knee. However, the PKRs were chosen in this study due to the high inter-observer agreement and sensitivity of these rules. The PKRs state that a radiograph of the knee is indicated following a fall or blunt trauma if the patient is younger than 12 or older than 50 years of age, or if the patient is unable to walk four weight-bearing steps (see flow chart of the decision rules in Fig. 2).

Hence, to evaluate the use of PKRs in our cases, the medical records were examined for patient age, evidence of trauma mechanism, and the patient's ability to walk four weight-bearing steps at first medical contact. We defined that patients had not been able to walk four weight-bearing steps if this was specifically stated in the records, or if the patient was discharged with crutches.

The DPCA evaluation of the compensation claims included evaluation by orthopedic surgeons of the patient history and the clinical examination of the knee at the first medical contact. Moreover, it was evaluated whether the fracture was in fact visible on radiographs obtained at the first medical contact. Based on information about the following course, the orthopedic surgeon deemed if the fracture position had worsened during the period of diagnostic delay. At the time when no further change in the condition was expected, it was evaluated, based on specific medical examination, if the diagnostic delay had caused additional disability. Depressed fractures were regarded as displaced.

Data handling

The use of personal data, including healthcare data, is protected by the Danish Act on Processing of Personal Data [15]. The study was therefore performed under the

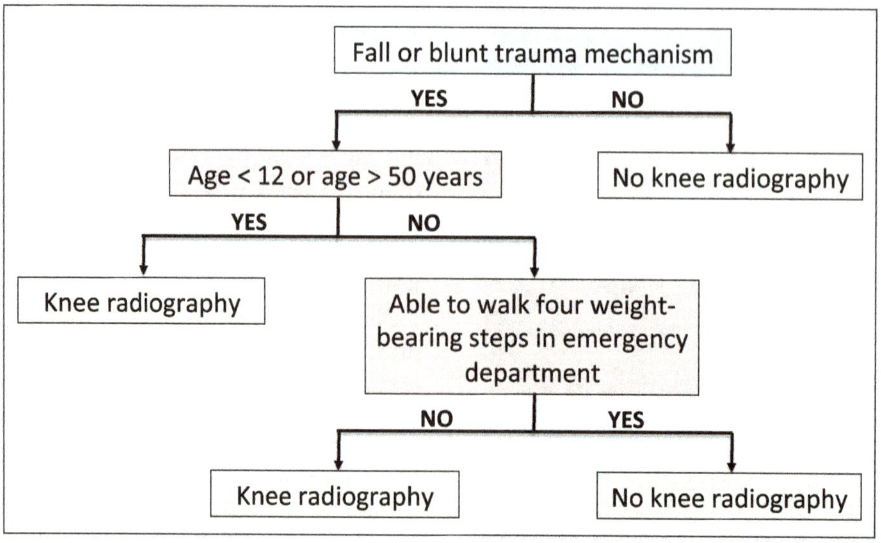

Fig. 2 Flowchart of the Pittsburgh Knee Rules

general permission for data collection to the Danish Patient Compensation Agency (2012–42-0325), and no further approval was necessary, as the data leaving the DPCA were anonymous. Ethical approval was not necessary, as the patients were not contacted.

Results

A total of 156 cases met the inclusion criterion, but19 cases were excluded, leaving 137 cases for the study. The reasons for exclusion were double registration (9 cases), absence of trauma to the knee (7 cases), and that the fracture was not a TPF (one torus fracture, one patella fracture and one epiphysiolysis). Of the included cases, 64 cases (47%) involved fractures to the right knee, 72 cases (53%) to the left knee, and one case involved a patient with fractures in both knees. 65% of fractures were located in the lateral tibia condyle. Fracture displacement was seen in 78% of cases, 21% of fractures were not displaced, and in one fracture displacement could not be determined with certainty. Displacement ranged between 3 and 20 mm.

In 35% of the cases, it was documented if the patient could walk four weight-bearing steps at the first point of medical contact, while in 54% of cases, this was not documented. 8% of the patients could not be mobilized due to multi-trauma (see Fig. 3).

According to the information in the medical records, the PKRs had been followed in 42% of cases and had not been followed in 41% of the cases. In 17% there was not enough information to evaluate if PKRs had been followed. The correlation between whether PKRs had been followed and if weigh-bearing was documented in the patients file is shown in Fig. 4.

Fracture types according to ICD-10 are presented in Table 1.

X-ray images were obtained for 53 patients (39%) at the first medical contact, and not obtained in 79 of cases (58%). In three cases there were radiographs from abroad, and in two cases radiographs were performed within 24 h after the initial medical contact. In 50 of the 79 un-imaged cases, X-ray imaging would have been indicated by the PKRs. In 12 cases the PKRs would not have indicated x-ray imagining and in 17 cases we do not have sufficient information to evaluate if PKRs would yield an X-ray examination or not. We estimate that if PKRs had been used in all cases, the number of overlooked knee fractures would have been reduced by 36%.

Thirteen of the undiagnosed fractures were discovered at radiological conference within a few days after the first medical contact. X-ray images had been obtained

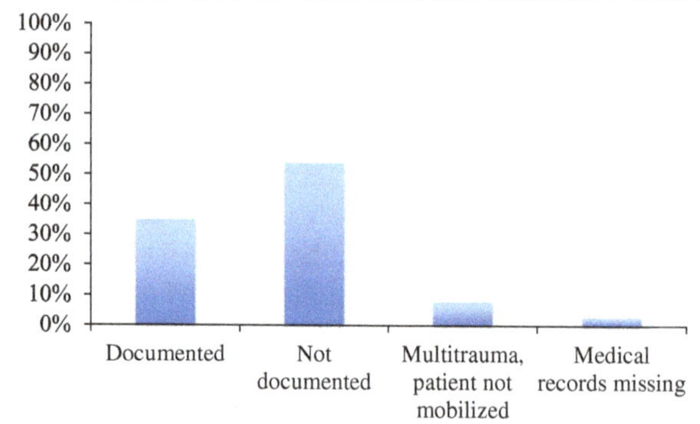

Fig. 3 Bar chart showing the distribution of patients divided into four categories depending on whether or not weigh-bearing was documented, whether the patient suffered from multi-trauma preventing mobilization, and whether the medical record was missing relevant data

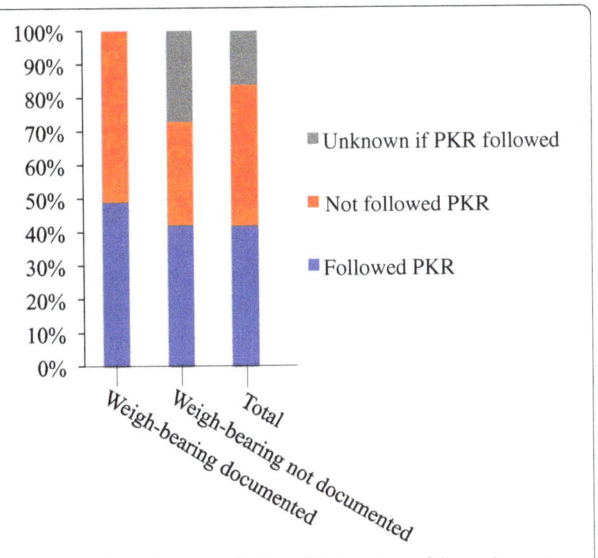

Fig. 4 Bar chart showing whether PKRs had been followed or not and the correlation to documentation of weight-bearing ability

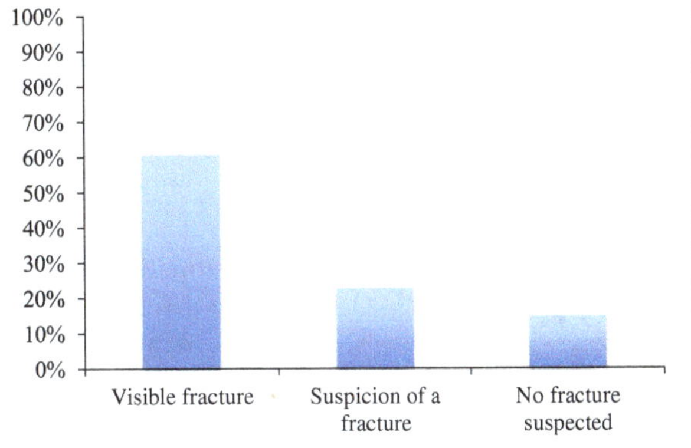

Fig. 5 Bar chart showing whether a fracture was evaluated to be visible or not at retrospective evaluation

for four patients abroad, with fractures visible in two out of three cases, while the X-ray images were not available in the fourth case. Retrospective evaluation of all X-ray images available at first medical contact was performed at the DPCA by orthopedic specialists. As seen in Fig. 5, 61% of fractures were evaluated as visible, in 23% there was suspicion of a fracture, and in 15% of cases fractures were not visible or suspected. Original X-ray images were missing in one case.

The mechanism of trauma was blunt in 40% of cases and a fall in 49% of cases, and by other mechanisms in 11%. In 78% of the cases, it was a junior doctor or resident doctor who was the responsible healthcare providing individual. In one case, a radiologist was responsible, in 7% of cases general practitioners provided healthcare, and in 15% of cases, specialist doctors were responsible. The average delay of diagnosis was 75 days (range: 1–536). Eight patients had a delay of four days or less. In 53% of cases, it was evaluated that the fracture position had worsened as a consequence of the diagnostic delay. Overlooking the fracture at the primary medical contact resulted in no additional disability in 52% of the cases. In 13% of cases, the patient had less than 5% additional disability, whereas in 35% of cases, the additional disability was 5% or more. Only seven patients received monetary compensation for additional loss of work ability caused by the diagnostic delay. The total compensation was equivalent to 841,000 EUR.

Table 2 lists the modalities that were used to establish the diagnosis.

In most cases, a new treatment was initiated after the fracture had been diagnosed (see Table 3).

Table 1 Details of the overlooked fractures. Seven patients had two diagnoses

Diagnose code ICD-10	Number of fractures
DS821 - Fractura partis proximalis tibiae	10
DS821A - Fractura condyli tibiae (Y-fracture)	3
DS821B - Fractura condyli tibiae lateralis	93
DS821C - Fractura condyli tibiae medialis	16
DS821D - Fractura eminentiae intercondyloideae tibiae	22

Discussion

The major underlying reasons for undiagnosed TPFs included difficulty in recognizing the fractures on X-rays and that radiographs were not taken because PKRs (or similar rules) were not employed at the first medical contact. In 84% of the cases, where an X-ray image was obtained in the ER at first medical contact, the fracture was visible or suspected at retrospective evaluation of the X-rays. Anterior tibial plateau fractures can be hard to recognize in anterior-posterior as well as lateral projections [6]. TPFs can be overlooked on normal X-ray images due to the anatomy of the tibial plateau, which causes a distortion in radiography, underestimating

Table 2 Methods to establish the diagnosis

Diagnostic measure	N	%
X-rays	78	55.7
MR	44	30.7
CT	5	3.6
Knee arthroscopy	4	2.9
Knee arthroscopy + X-rays	3	2.1
X-rays + CT	3	2.1
X-rays + MRI	3	2.1
MRI + CT	1	0.7

Table 3 Treatment after the fracture had been diagnosed

Treatment changed	80%
Surgical treatment optimal, but too late to perform	6%
No change of treatment	13%
Patient refused suggested change in treatment	1%

anterior surface depression and overestimating posterior surface depression [17]. Osteoporotic fractures of the tibial plateau can be misdiagnosed, because primary X-ray images often look normal for 2–3 weeks, until an area of sclerosis is formed by collapse of cancellous bone in the tibial plateau [7]. It also affects the diagnostic sensitivity how the patient is positioned, since the only evidence of a TPF can be the presence of a fat/fluid level in the suprapatellar recess in the lateral projection, provided that the patient is positioned horizontally [4, 17]. Oblique projections should be considered in addition to standard projections when TPFs are suspected but not confirmed by standard AP- and lateral X-rays, as adding oblique knee views increases the sensitivity from 79 to 85% [18].

MRI-scan is considered the state-of-the-art for detection of occult fractures [19], and this or a CT-scan should be considered in patient cases with a clinical suspicion of a TPF and where X-ray images are normal even though CT-scans are fast and provide a detailed view of the fracture pattern and articular surface [4], MRI-scans are better suited for accurately displaying occult fractures and for visualizing soft tissue injuries, which often occur along with the fractures [20].

We found that for 50 patients an X-ray would have been indicated if PKRs had been followed. Even though TPFs can be difficult to identify on standard X-ray images, most of these fractures would likely have been discovered at the first medical contact, if the principles of the PKRs had been followed (and radiographs been obtained) in addition to the clinical examination in the ER setting. Figures from the Danish National Patient Register (extracted from the register's website) show that between 2005 and 2013 a total of 8797 patients were discharged with a fracture of the proximal tibiae. Of these, 1489 were coded as tibial plateau fractures, and of the 7308 fractures that did not have a detailed coding, we estimate that half were TPFs. This entails that about 5000 TPFs occurred in Denmark during these 9 years. A study on the epidemiology of TPFs from Aalborg University hospital in Denmark supports this conclusion as it evaluated the incidence of TPFs to be 10.3 per 100,000 citizens annually [2]. The dark number (patients who have not claimed a case at DCPA) is unknown, but it is assessed that only 15–85% of all patients eligible for compensation, claim their case [15]. Overlooking a fracture is regarded as a grave mistake among patients, and we have estimated the dark number to be 100% of the registered cases in our study. From this it can be estimated that 3.9% of all TPFs in Denmark were not diagnosed at first medical contact. An implication of this finding may thus be that decision rules (such as PKRs) should be mandatory to employ in addition to clinical examination to triage knee trauma patients correctly. Additionally, these decision rules may also help minimize the number of X-ray images to be captured in the ER by identifying clinically relevant cases for X-ray examination [8, 9, 11–14, 21]. Not only would this save personnel time and ER resources, but it would also lower the overall patient exposure to X-rays. The finding that 12 patients (15% of the patients for whom an X-ray image was not obtained) would not have been offered X-ray imaging, if PKRs had been used, could be interpreted as low sensitivity of PKRs. However, in all of these 12 cases the trauma mechanism was not a blunt trauma or a fall, but in most cases a twist, and in principle the PKRs do not apply with these trauma mechanisms. In addition, these 12 patients were a very selective group, as they were not clinically suspected to have a fracture. Therefore, our findings do not conflict with the generally accepted 94–100% sensitivity of PKRs to identify TPFs [14].

In 7% of the examined cases, it was evaluated that surgical intervention would have been indicated, if fractures had been discovered at the first medical contact, which in most cases most likely would have resulted in a superior outcome. In 80% of patients the treatment was changed following diagnosis of their fracture, and many of these patients would likely have had a shorter rehabilitation period, if the fracture had been diagnosed at first medical contact. The finding that 36% of the patients in our study had an additional disability of 5% or more because the primary diagnosis of their fracture was missed, underlines that overlooking a TPF has a significant negative effect on patient outcome.

Limitations to the study

A limitation of this study is that the specialist consultants who performed the retrospective viewing of the X-ray images in most cases knew what they were looking for, which might have interfered with their evaluation of whether a fracture could have been diagnosed at first medical contact or not. Also, our study underestimates the true incidence of overlooked TPFs, since only patients who file a claim are registered in the DPCA database, as addressed in our discussion.

Conclusion

The most important underlying reasons for overlooking TPFs in the ER setting of Danish hospitals were 1) that TPFs were not identified on X-rays and 2) X-rays were not taken, because decision rules for indication of knee X-rays had not been followed in the ER setting. If a fracture is clinically suspected in case of normal AP and lateral X-rays, oblique projections should be considered. However, MRI or CT-scans are more sensitive and should be performed if clinical suspicion persists. To prevent a potential fracture from displacement, the patient should be immobilized with a fixed knee brace and disabled from bearing weight until a final diagnosis has been reached.

We estimated that if PKRs had been used in all patients, the number of overlooked knee fractures would have been reduced by 36%. As overlooking a TPF often results in additional disability for the patient, it would be beneficial if healthcare staff in the ERs used clinical decision rules in addition to the clinical examination. This holds the potential to save personnel time, hospital resources, and lower the overall patient exposure to X-rays.

Abbreviations

CT: Computed Tomography; DPCA: Danish Patient Compensation Association; ER: Emergency Room; MRI : Magnetic Resonance Imaging; PKRs: Pittsburgh Knee Rules; TPF: Tibia Plateau Fracture

Acknowledgements

We thank Associate Professor Andreas H. Laustsen (Technical University of Denmark) for proof-reading.

Funding

This research did not receive any economical funding.

Authors' contributions

MK and KL designed the study. KL ran the algorithm to find the relevant medical cases. CK performed the background research, subtracted the relevant data from the medical records, and interpreted the data. CK and MK wrote the paper. All authors discussed the results and implications and commented on the manuscript at all stages. All authors read and approved the final manuscript.

Consent for publication

Not applicable.

Competing interests

The authors declare that they have no competing interests.

References

1. Ebrahimzadeh MH, Birjandinejad A, Moradi A, Fathi Choghadeh M, Rezazadeh J, Omidi-Kashani F. Clinical instability of the knee and functional differences following tibial plateau fractures versus distal femoral fractures. Trauma Mon. 2015;20(1):e21635.
2. Elsoe R, Larsen P, Nielsen NP, Swenne J, Rasmussen S, Ostgaard SE. Population-based epidemiology of Tibial plateau fractures. Orthopedics. 2015;38(9):e780–6.
3. Frattini M, Vaienti E, Soncini G, Pogliacomi F. Tibial plateau fractures in elderly patients. Chir Organi Mov. 2009;93(3):109–14.
4. Dennan S. Difficulties in the radiological diagnosis and evaluation of tibial plateau fractures. Radiography. 2004;10:151–8.
5. Sprivulis P, Frazer A, Waring A. Same-day X-ray reporting is not needed in well-supervised emergency departments. Emerg Med (Fremantle). 2001; 13(2):194–7.
6. Maheshwari J, Pandey VK, Mhaskar VA. Anterior tibial plateau fracture: an often missed injury. Indian J Orthop. 2014;48(5):507–10.
7. Prasad N, Murray JM, Kumar D, Davies SG. Insufficiency fracture of the tibial plateau: an often missed diagnosis. Acta Orthop Belg. 2006;72(5):587–91.
8. Seaberg DC, Yealy DM, Lukens T, Auble T, Mathias S. Multicenter comparison of two clinical decision rules for the use of radiography in acute, high-risk knee injuries. Ann Emerg Med. 1998;32(1):8–13.
9. Cheung TC, Tank Y, Breederveld RS, Tuinebreijer WE, de Lange-de Klerk ES, Derksen RJ. Diagnostic accuracy and reproducibility of the Ottawa knee rule vs the Pittsburgh decision rule. Am J Emerg Med. 2013;31(4):641–5.
10. Bachmann LM, Haberzeth S, Steurer J, Ter RG. The accuracy of the Ottawa knee rule to rule out knee fractures (structured abstract). Ann Intern Med. 2004;140(2):121–4.
11. Hawley C, Rosenblatt R. Ottawa and Pittsburgh rules for acute knee injuries. J Fam Pract. 1998;47(4):254–5.
12. Konan S, Zang TT, Tamimi N, Haddad FS. Can the Ottawa and Pittsburgh rules reduce requests for radiography in patients referred to acute knee clinics? Ann R Coll Surg Engl. 2013;95(3):188–91.
13. Richman PB, McCuskey CF, Nashed A, Fuchs S, Petrik R, Imperato M, Hollander JE. Performance of two clinical decision rules for knee radiography. J Emerg Med. 1997;15(4):459–63.
14. Seaberg DC, Jackson R. Clinical decision rule for knee radiographs. Am J Emerg Med. 1994;12(5):541–3.
15. Tilma J, Norgaard M, Mikkelsen KL, Johnsen SP. Existing data sources for clinical epidemiology: the Danish patient compensation association database. Clin Epidemiol. 2015;7:347–53.
16. Trifork Medical. . In: Diagnosekoder. http://www.diagnosekoder.dk/. Accessed Jan 2018.
17. Newberg AH, Greenstein R. Radiographic evaluation of tibial plateau fractures. Radiology. 1978;126(2):319–23.
18. Gray SD, Kaplan PA, Dussault RG, Omary RA, Campbell SE, Chrisman HB, Futterer SF, McGraw JK, Keats TE, Hillman BJ. Acute knee trauma: how many plain film views are necessary for the initial examination? Skelet Radiol. 1997;26(5):298–302.
19. Hegenscheid K, Puls R, Rosenberg C. Imaging strategies for knee injuries. Radiologe. 2012;52(11):980–6.
20. Xu Y, Li Q, Su P, Shen T, Zhu Y. MDCT and MRI for the diagnosis of complex fractures of the tibial plateau: a case control study. Exp Ther Med. 2014;7(1): 199–203.
21. Tandeter HB, Shvartzman P. Acute knee injuries: use of decision rules for selective radiograph ordering. Am Fam Physician. 1999;60(9):2599–608.

17

The use of bidirectional rapid reductor in minimally invasive treatment of bicondylar tibial plateau fractures: preliminary radiographic and clinical results

Hengrui Chang[1,2†], Zhanle Zheng[1,2†], Yiyang Yu[1,2], Jiasheng Shao[1,2] and Yingze Zhang[1,2*]

Abstract

Background: Minimally invasive treatment of complex tibial plateau fracture represents one of the most challenging problems in orthopedic surgery. We intended to describe the percutaneous surgery involving an originally designed traction device which might facilitate the closed reduction for bicondylar tibial plateau fractures. Further, to assess the clinical outcomes of this minimally invasive technique.

Methods: Between December 2015 and July 2016, Twenty-one patients, mean age 43.71 ± 13.80 years, suffering from a bicondylar tibial plateau fracture (AO/OTA 41-type C) were included. All fractures were firstly reduced by skeletal traction with the aid of bidirectional rapid reductor, and residual depressed fragments were treated with minimally invasive bone tamp reduction. We then evaluated at a minimum follow-up of one year: (1) the rate of complications, (2) the radiographic outcomes (the amount of depression, tibial plateau widening, tibial plateau angle and posterior slope angle) and (3) the clinical outcome (Rasmussen scoring system).

Results: All patients had their fractures healed without secondary displacement. No instrument-related complications occurred during operation. Post-operatively, superficial infection was found in two patients and donor-site morbidity was found in one patient. We observed a < 5 mm step-off in 100% of patients and a < 5 mm plateau widening in 95.5% of patients. Three patients were considered indicative of malalignment with TPA > 90° or PSA > 15°. At last evaluation, the Rasmussen clinical score was excellent in 11 patients (52.3%), good in 9 (42.9%) and fair in 1 (4.8%), and the radiological score was excellent in seven patients (33.3%), good in 14 (66.7%).

Conclusions: The bidirectional rapid reductor facilitates the minimally invasive treatment of bicondylar tibial plateau fracture. The patients exhibited excellent functional recovery. These results should be validated with a larger group of patients and longer period results.

Keywords: Tibial plateau fractures, Minimally invasive, Traction reduction, Compression bolt, Internal fixation

* Correspondence: drzhangyz2016@sina.com
†Hengrui Chang and Zhanle Zheng contributed equally to this work.
[1]Department of Orthopaedic Surgery, the Third Hospital of Hebei Medical University, NO.139 Ziqiang Road, Shijiazhuang, Hebei 050051, People's Republic of China
[2]Key laboratory of biomechanics of Hebei Province, Shijiazhuang, Hebei 050051, People's Republic of China

Background

Bicondylar tibial plateau fractures (AO/OTA type C) represent 20.4% of all proximal tibial fractures [1, 2]. Because of articular comminution and the frequent occurrence soft-tissue injuries, clinical management still remains challenging for traumatic surgeons [3–5]. Traditional open reduction and internal fixation (ORIF) requires extensive soft tissue dissection, which may lead to numerous soft-tissue complications [6–8]. The Ilizarov technique allows a better choice of closed reduction and fixation which does not necessitate excessive soft-tissue stripping [9]. Today, this technique is being widely used in open and comminuted tibial plateau fractures. However, the external fixation method has its theoretical risks, including pins infection, neurovascular injury, deep venous thrombosis, scar problems, and limitation of joint movement [9, 10]. Besides, frequent management of the circular frame was inconvenient for both patients and doctors.

Recently, several studies have advocated the use of an indirect reduction technique with the aid of knee arthroscopy in tibial plateau fractures. Short- to medium-term clinical outcomes have shown various advantages over ORIF in terms of minimally invasive procedure, accurate reduction monitoring and precise evaluation of intra-articular pathologies [3, 11, 12]. We found this technique to have several limitations. The evidence-based systematic review showed that the majority of included patients had Schatzker type I to III fractures, which suggested that ARIF might have difficulties in managing complex tibial plateau fractures [13]. Lacking of effective traction instruments, varus or valgus malalignment could be hardly reduced through indirect way, especially when knee joint dislocation existed.

Based on the historical experience, the key factor of minimally invasive treatment for such injuries, we considered, was effective and persistent traction which allowed closed restoration of lower extremity alignment during operation. The primary goal of the present study was to describe a percutaneous surgery involving an originally designed traction device which might facilitate the closed reduction for high-energy tibial plateau fractures. Further, we evaluated the safety of the surgery and analyzed the clinical satisfaction at a minimum follow-up of 1 year after surgery.

Methods

Between December 2015 and July 2016, 78 patients with tibial plateau fractures were admitted to our emergency department. For this study, skeletally mature patients with an acute, closed, bicondylar tibial plateau fractures (AO/OTA type C) were included in this study. The exclusion criteria were: skeletally immature patients, pathological fractures, concomitant ipsilateral distal femoral fractures, significant pre-existing degenerative joint disease, patients requiring intensive care or with severe systemic illness.

We identified 21 patients meeting the inclusion/exclusion criteria (Fig. 1a, b). Of the 21 patients included, there were 15 men and 6 women, with 3 left knee injuries and 18 right knee injuries. The average age in this series was 43.7 ± 13.8 years (range 21–67). Most injuries were the results of high-energy trauma including a fall from a height (eight patients), an electric bicycle collision (three patients), an automobile collision (nine patients) and a crushing accident (one patient). 6 patients were associated with other skeletal injuries, and none of which occurred around the injured knee. Basic information, including sex, age, mechanism of injury, and injured side, were gathered from all patients and concluded in Table 1.

During the hospitalization, all patients were treated with transcalcaneus traction for primary alignment maintaining and pain alleviation. Definite treatment was delayed until the soft tissue conditions had improved. Full approval from local Ethics Committee (KE 2016–001-2) was received for this study and all subjects enrolled were confirmed to provide informed consent.

Surgical protocol

Positioning

Patients were in supine position on the radiolucent operating table with a tourniquet placed around the proximal thigh. The tourniquet was inflated to 300 mmHg once the closed traction was complete. Disinfectant preparation covered from proximal 2/3 femoral until to the distal end of lower extremity of injured side. Meanwhile, the anterior superior iliac spine (ASIS) and its surrounding area were also under preparation for the purpose of autogenous bone grafts acquirement. A rolled sheet was placed under the affected knee joint to maintain knee flexion at 30 degrees.

Closed reduction in bidirectional rapid reductor

The bidirectional rapid reductor is composed of a folding scaffold, connecting rods made of carbon fiber, two traction bows and Kirschner wires (Fig. 2a). All components were able to be packed up into a customized instrument box and were convenient to be sterilized. Two 2.5 mm Kirschner wires were firstly inserted through distal tibia and superior femoral condyle, then, each Kirschner wire was attached to a traction bow (Fig. 3a, b). The carbon fiber rod connected the proximal traction bow to the scaffold which straddled the lower leg and distal traction bow was attached to the rotary handle located on the scaffold (Fig. 3c, d). The scaffold maintained a traction position during the operation. The length of the connection rod could be adjusted to accommodate different patients.

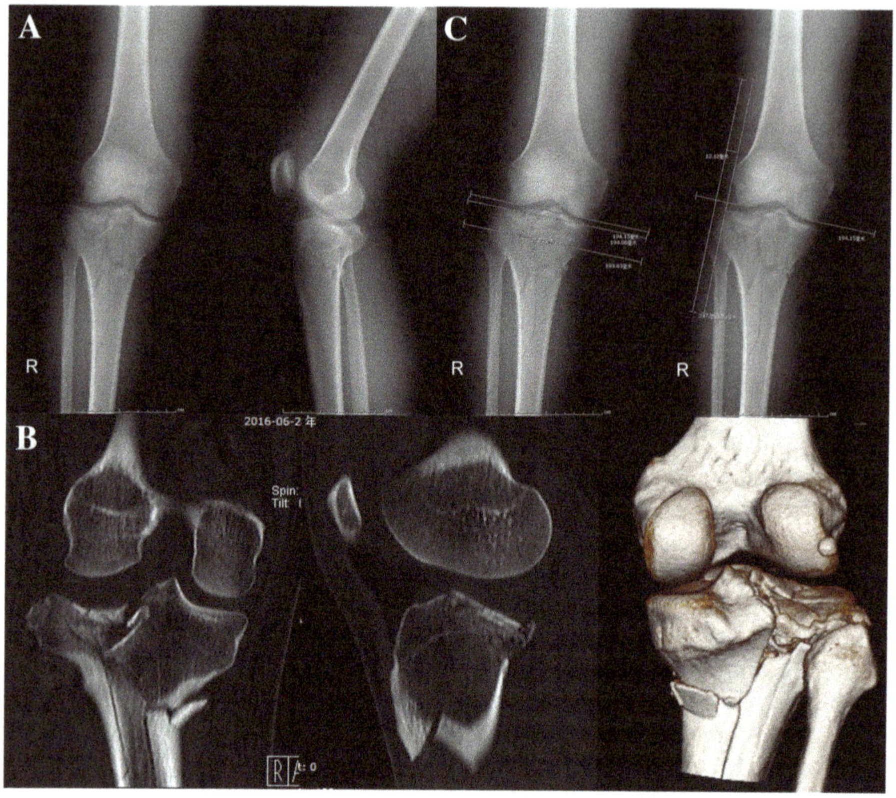

Fig. 1 A 34-year-old male sustained a closed complex tibial plateau fracture after automobile collision. Preoperative X-ray images (**a**), preoperative CT images (**b**) and preoperative radiological measurement of articular depression (25.0 mm) and plateau widening(12.12 mm) (**c**)

Bidirectional rapid reductor was finished assembling all in the sterile field.

After confirming that all parts of the reductor were securely joined, a closed-loop traction system was formed by connecting the distal femur, knee joint and distal tibia to the reductor (Fig. 4a). Rotate the handle in a clockwise direction and, as a result, the whole extension force will fall on the distal end of tibia. In the mean time, a counterforce came into being above the knee joint due to the obstruction caused by connecting rod and scaffold. Through ligamentotaxis and skeletal traction, the tibial plateau's widening, tibial length as well as varus or valgus angulation could be primarily corrected under fluoroscopic guidance. After achieving satisfactory reduction, as revealed by C-arm examination both on anteroposterior (AP) and lateral views, the reductor could sustain the lower extremity in a reduction position. The whole traction process was achieved on the operating table and no special positioning of patient was needed, which largely facilitated the placement of fluoroscopy monitors.

Elevation of depressed articular fragments

For patients with articular depression, care must be taken to locate the orientation of depressed fragments based on preoperative x-rays and CT scan. A 2.5 mm K-wire was chosen as a guide for creation of a tunnel. The ideal entry point was 2 cm below the centre of tibia tubercle, slightly medial or lateral to the long axis of tibia which depends on the location of depressed fragments. Mostly, the medial approach was used for the management of lateral plateau depression. A longitudinal 3 cm skin incision was made on the medial aspect of the tibia around the K-wire. Then, a cortex portal was made, and the depressed fragments was elevated with a customized bone tamp via the inferior transosseous tunnel created by step drills. The whole reduction process is performed with gentle tapping of the bone tamp under the inspection of AP and lateral views of fluoroscopy (Fig. 4b). Percutaneous reduction was optimized until intraoperative fluoroscopy suggested satisfactory articular reconstruction without a remaining articular depression. Subsequently, the Autogenous bone graft harvested from the iliac crest was then inserted into the bone tunnel to support the subchondral bone and articular surface (Fig. 4c).

Internal fixation

Once the reduction was obtained, minimally invasive percutaneous plate osteosynthesis (MIPPO) was performed using pre-contoured locking compression plate (LCP)

Table 1 Patient demographics and outcomes, $N = 21$

Case	Age ranges	Sex	Side	AO/OTA classification	Mechanism of injury	Soft-tissue Injuries	Associated skeletal injuries (side)	Follow-up (Months)	Clinical Result (Rasmussen Score)	Radiological Result (Rasmussen Score)
1	35–45	M	R	41-C2	Fall from a height	None	None	20	29	18
2	45–55	M	R	41-C3	Electric bicycle collision	Lateral meniscal tear	None	20	30	14
3	45–55	M	L	41-C3	Fall from a height	Lateral meniscal tear ACL avulsion fracture PCL partial tear	None-	20	30	12
4	55–65	F	R	41-C3	Fall from a height	Lateral meniscal tear	None	19	24	14
5	55–65	F	R	41-C2	Automobile collision	None	Femoral neck fractures (R)	19	28	16
6	30–40	M	R	41-C1	Automobile collision	None	Distal radius fracture (L)	18	30	16
7	60–70	F	R	41-C1	Fall from a height	Medial meniscal tear	None	18	26	18
8	35–45	M	R	41-C1	Automobile collision	None	None	17	27	18
9	45–55	M	L	41-C3	Electric bicycle collision	ACL partial tear	None	17	30	16
10	25–35	M	R	41-C1	Automobile collision	None	Radial fracture (R)	17	28	18
11	45–55	M	R	41-C3	Fall from a height	Lateral meniscal tear Medial meniscal tear	Calcaneal fracture (R)	17	26	14
12	20–30	M	R	41-C2	Automobile collision	None	None	17	24	14
13	35–45	F	R	41-C1	Fall from a height	None	None	17	26	16
14	40–50	M	R	41-C3	Automobile collision	Lateral meniscal tear	None	16	26	14
15	15–25	M	R	41-C3	Automobile collision	Lateral meniscal tear	Ankle fracture (R)	15	30	18
16	30–40	M	L	41-C3	Fall from a height	None	None	15	29	18
17	55–65	M	R	41-C1	Automobile collision	None	None	14	26	16
18	25–35	F	R	41-C2	Automobile collision	None	None	14	30	18
19	30–40	M	R	41-C3	Crushing accident	None	None	13	24	14
20	55–65	F	R	41-C3	Fall from a height	Lateral meniscal tear Medial meniscal tear	Tibial fracture (L)	12	19	14
21	20–30	M	R	41-C2	Electric bicycle collision	None	None	12	26	14

ACL anterior Cruciate ligament, *MCL* medial collateral ligament, *M* male, *F* female, *R* right, *L* left

Table 2 X-ray measurement of the 21 tibial plateau fractures

	Tibial Plateau Depression (mm)	Tibial Plateau Widening (mm)	Tibial Plateau Angle (°)	Posterior Slope Angle (°)
Preoperation	8.42 ± 8.43	8.06 ± 6.57	NA	NA
Postoperation	1.35 ± 1.59	1.88 ± 1.92	87.86 ± 2.57°	9.76 ± 3.70°
The last follow-up	1.65 ± 1.92	2.05 ± 2.05	87.76 ± 2.98°	10.29 ± 3.41°
p Value	$P^1 < 0.01$; $P^2 = 0.55$	$P^2 < 0.01$; $P^2 = 0.79$	$P^2 = 0.91$	$P^2 = 0.64$

NA not available
P^1 p value of the comparison of pre- and post-operative variables
P^2 p value of the comparison of post-operative and the last follow-up variables

designed for proximal tibia (WEGO, Wei Hai city, PR China). In all cases, dual plate fixation was used medially and laterally, and no additional plate was needed. Subsequently, one or two compression bolts designed with special slot (WEGO, Wei Hai city, PR China) would be inserted through the most proximal holes of two plates (Fig. 2b), which permitted further restoration of the tibial plateaus' width. Once the nut passed through the slot, the bolt's tail could be easily broken off at this constricted area with appropriate size left. Care was taken to ensure the alignment was not changed on the AP views when tightening the left screws.

Arthroscopic evaluation

Following the optimal fixation, the bidirectional reductor was disassembled and arthroscopic examination was then performed using gravity inflow and without incision sutured. The heamarthrosis was drained and any osteochondral fragments were removed. Previous reconstruction of the articular surface and soft tissue injury was then evaluated (Fig. 4d, e).

Postoperative management

Immediate non-weight bearing joint motion was encouraged as the pain subsided. Based on general condition and post-operative X-ray examinations, progress weight-bearing usually started with crutches at 8 weeks. Peri- and post-operative complications such as wound infection, thrombosis, compartment syndrome, donor site pain and joint stiffness were recorded. Independent knee assessments were carried out post-operatively using the Rasmussen's clinical and radiologic scores after a mean duration of follow up of 16.5 months (range, 12 to 20 months). The amount of fragment depression, plateau widening, TPA (tibial plateau angle) and PSA (posterior slope angle) were measured on the preoperative, postoperative radiographs and at the time of the latest follow-up on the basis of X-ray measurement (Fig. 5a, b).

Statistical methods

Statistical analysis was performed using IBM SPSS Statistics 21 (SPSS Inc., Chicago, IL). Data are presented as mean values ± SD for continuous variables. The normality of the distribution of the parameters was tested using the Kolmogoroff-Smirnoff test. Continuous variables with non-normal distribution were analyzed using the Mann-Whitney U test (preoperative/postoperative/follow-up radiological outcomes). All tests were 2-sided and a P value of < 0.05 was considered significant.

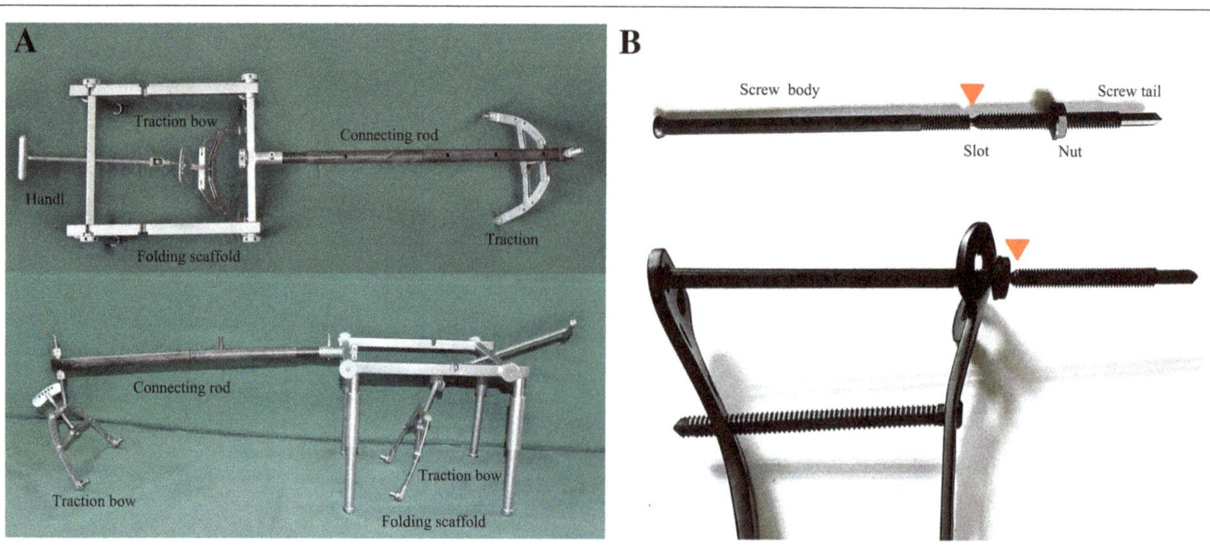

Fig. 2 The general view of the bidirectional rapid reductor (**a**) and slot-designed compression bolt (**b**). The compression bolts consist of nuts and slot-designed area (arrow)

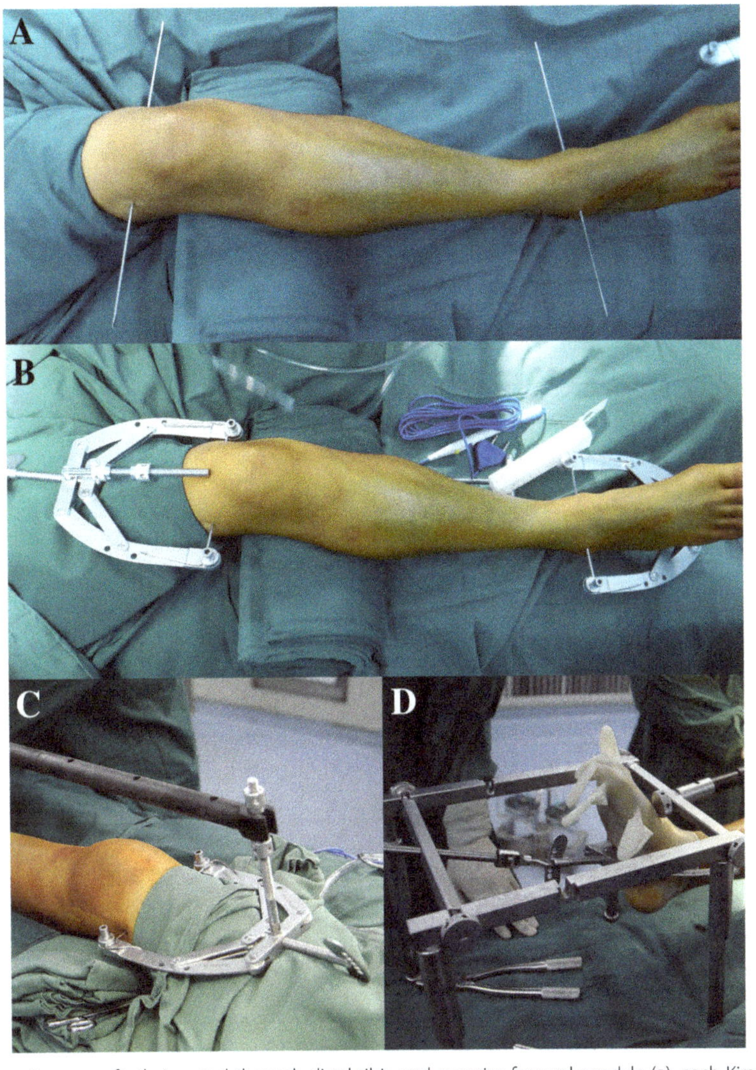

Fig. 3 Two 2.5 mm Kirschner wires were firstly inserted through distal tibia and superior femoral condyle (**a**), each Kirschner wire was attached to a traction bow (**b**), The carbon fiber rod connected the proximal traction bow to the scaffold which straddled the lower leg (**c**), the distal traction bow was attached to the rotary handle located on the scaffold (**d**)

Results

Six patients suffered from OTA/AO 41-C1, 5 from 41-C2 and 10 from 41-C3 fractures. With the help of rapid reductor, all 21 cases of bicondylar tibial plateau fractures were reduced in a closed fashion, and none converted to open reduction. The average operation time was 100 min (excluding the time of arthroscopic examination, range 50 to 150 min, SD 29.4). The average blood loss was 135 mL (range 80 to 300 min, SD 58.1). Through arthroscopy, an intra-articular diffusion of cancellous bone debris was observed in three patients. The fragments were all removed using nucleus pulposus clamps and were not registered as a complication. Two cases with high energy fractures developed superficial infections, which delayed the wound healing, and were managed with a course of oral antibiotics for a week. There were no episodes of wound dehiscence, deep venous thrombosis or compartment syndrome at the time of hospital discharge. No patient subsequently developed deep infection, osteomyelitis or joint stiffness at follow-ups. One patients who received autogenous bone grafts sustained donor-site morbidities. However, this patient did not require further intervention for pain relieve because of their well tolerance of the pain. No other adverse outcomes were occurred during follow-up.

In 16 of 21 fractures, autogeneous bone grafts were implanted to provide mechanical support for the reduced fragments. Associated soft tissue injuries were common, occurring in 9 (42.9%) patients. Arthroscopy revealed tears of the lateral meniscus alone ($n = 5$), the medial meniscus alone ($n = 1$), or a combination of both meniscus ($n = 2$). There were three lateral meniscal

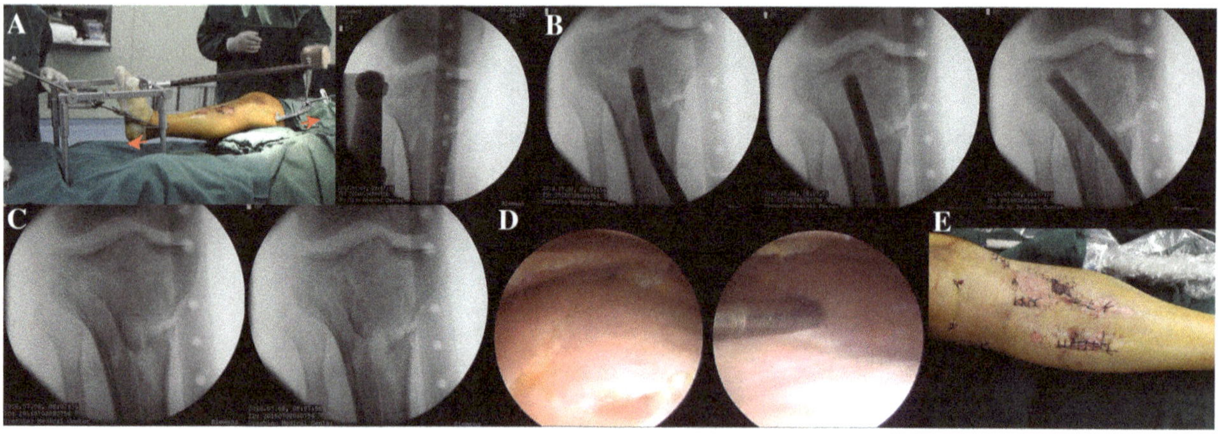

Fig. 4 Intraoperative process of the newly proposed treatment. Demonstration of the interaction forces acting on the distal tibia and superior femoral condyle (**a**, arrow), percutaneous reduction of the depressed fragments (**b**), the insertion of autogenous bone graft to support the articular surface (**c**), After reduction and internal fixation under fluoroscopic visualization, arthroscopy revealed a nearly anatomic reduction of lateral articular (**d**), Seven minimal incisions after the operation, four for percutaneous insertion of plates, one for indirect reduction of depressed fragments and two for arthroscopic inspection (**e**)

repairs and five partial meniscectomy performed. One partial meniscal tears required conservative treatment. There was one partial ACL (anterior cruciate ligament) ruptures, one partial PCL (posterior cruciate ligament) ruptures, and one avulsion fracture of PCL. Considering the displacement was minimal, the eminence avulsion and other incomplete ligament injuries were all treated with the immediate cast-brace fixation. Using the distal tip of probe (length = 3 mm) as reference, arthroscopy showed a persistent > 3 mm fracture depression in three patients and a > 3 mm fracture gap in one patient. However, in these cases, all the displacement was less than 6

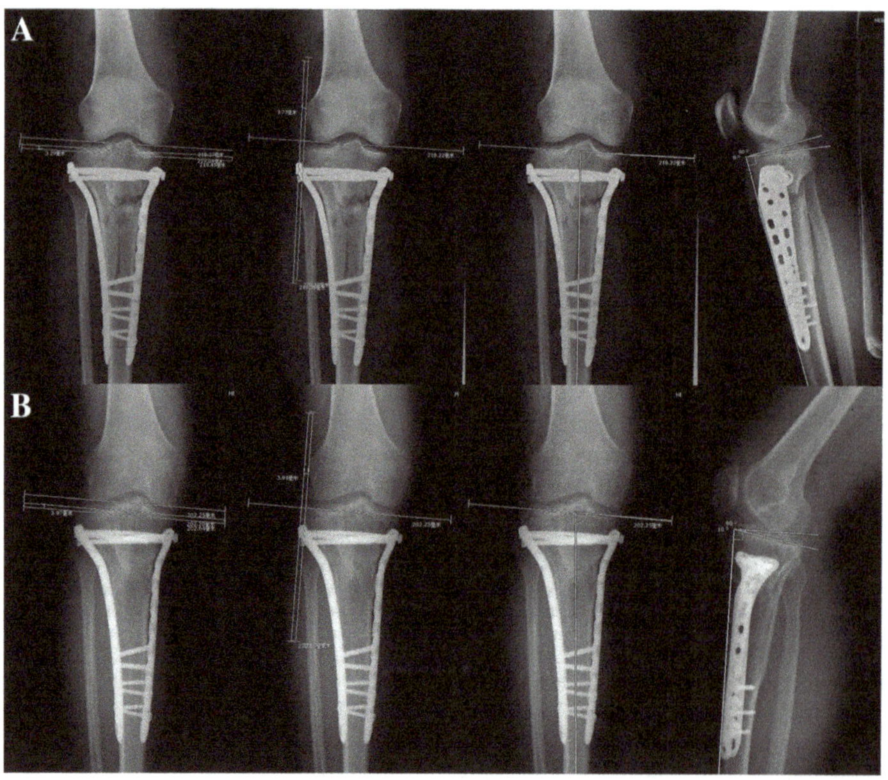

Fig. 5 The postoperative measurements of step-off (3.29 mm), plateau widening (3.73 mm), TPA (87°) and PSA (8°) (**a**). At the last follow-up, the radiological measurements the step-off (3.97 mm), plateau widening (3.94 mm), TPA (85°) and PSA (10°) (**b**)

mm (twice the length of probe tip) and without further intervention.

All 21 patients were followed up at a mean of 16.5 ± 2.5 months (range, 12 to 20 months) postoperatively. At last follow-up, all patients had healed their fractures with no loss of reduction. The mean depressed step-off of the lateral joint decreased from 8.42 ± 8.43 mm (0–26.60 mm) pre-operatively to 1.35 ± 1.59 mm (0–4.49 mm) post-operatively ($p < 0.01$). The mean lateral plateau widening decreased from 8.06 ± 6.57 mm (0–29.35 mm) pre-operatively to 1.88 ± 1.92 mm (0–5.4 mm) post-operatively ($p < 0.01$). The mean TPA and PSA were 87.86 ± 2.57° and 9.76 ± 3.70°, respectively. We observed a ≤ 2 mm step-off in 68.2% (15/22) of patients and a > 2–5 mm step-off in 100% of patients. We also observed a < 5 mm plateau widening in 95.5% of patients with only one patient having a widening > 5 mm (5.4 mm). 3 cases (14.3%) of malalignment of proximal tibia were identified in this group, two of which involved in coronal plane (TPA: 92°; 94°) and one in sagittal plane (PSA: 16°). These radiological results were stable until the last follow up after surgery. We found a mean lateral step-off of 1.65 ± 1.92 mm ($p = 0.55$), plateau widening of 2.05 ± 2.05 mm ($p = 0.79$), TPA of 87.76 ± 2.98° ($p = 0.91$) and PSA of 10.29 ± 3.41° ($p = 0.64$) (Table 2). Finally, the mean radiographic Rasmussen score was 15.71 ± 1.93 (12–18), with seven patients (33.3%) rated as excellent and 14 patients (66.7%) rated as good.

The mean Rasmussen clinical score was 27.05 ± 2.84 (19–30). Eleven patients (52.3%) were classified as excellent, nine (42.9%) were classified as grade good, one (4.8%) were classified as fair. The patient who was rated as fair had residual depression of 4.5 mm of the lateral tibial plateau, with mild valgus deformity (TPA: 94°). This patient complained of intense, constant pain around the lateral compartment after activity. The range of motion at last follow-up was mean flexion 129.29 ± 8.70° (115–140°) and mean extension 1.95 ± 3.47 (0–11°) (Fig. 6).

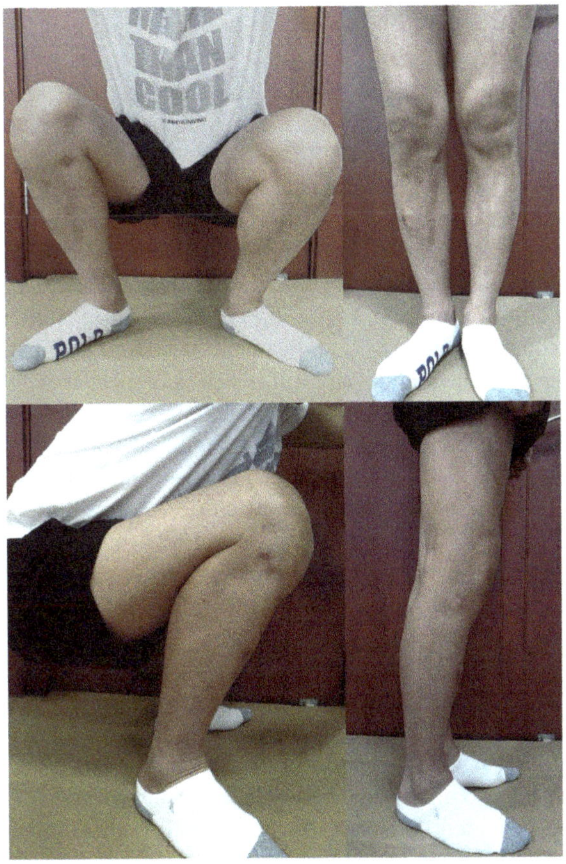

Fig. 6 Pictures of the knee function of the case demonstrated in Figs. 1, 4 and 5 at the final review 13 months after the accident

Discussion

In the present study, we treated 21 bicondylar tibial plateau fractures with bidirectional traction device and slot-designed compression bolts in a minimally invasive manner. The rapid reductor could not only efficiently reduce the fracture but also maintained it in an anatomical position. Anatomic or nearly anatomic reduction of the articular surface, tibial plateau width, TPA and PSA was achieved in most cases. This minimally invasive procedure offered advantages of low soft-tissue related complications and less operation time. The technique itself was safe without any instrument-related adverse case. All fractures healed well and satisfactory functional recovery was identified in the majority of the patients.

Given the soft tissue damage and comminuted fracture pattern of OTA/AO type C tibial plateau fractures, surgical treatment has been associated with a high complication rate, specifically postoperative deep wound infection [5, 14]. Previous studies have shown that long-term outcome depended more on the stability of the knee and that less extensive operations might lead to satisfactory results [15, 16]. Unfortunately, alignment and stability were not easily controlled in the treatment of complex fractures of the tibial plateau, particularly when minimally invasive surgery was required. Some surgeons preferred to use a fracture table or other skin traction device to treat tibial plateau fractures in a closed way. However, its function on managing articular depression was limited [17, 18]. Ilizarov fixation allowed distraction, which aided reduction of the peri-articular fragments when applied along the lower limb. Clinical studies showed good long-term functional results in high-energy tibial plateau fractures [9, 19]. However, frequent pin-site infections and potential risk of later limitation of movement have been notified even in experienced hands [9, 20, 21]. The overall incidence of pin-site infection was reported to be 23.9 to 53.3% [9, 10, 22, 23].

Besides, postoperative adjustment of the external fixation required additional workload both for patients and doctors.

Different from skin traction, the bidirectional traction device could generate enormous longitudinal force applied on the distal end of tibia. Meanwhile, an equivalent counterforce came into being because of the obstruction by the connection rod. This is what so called "bidrectional traction" [24]. The closed-loop traction system could able to maintain the lower limb in a traction condition from the beginning to the end of surgery. Through skeletal traction, ligamentotaxis and soft-tissue (capsule, ligaments and muscles) compression, the widening displacement and malalignment could be partially reduced in a closed way. Compared with manual traction or distractor, the traction force generated by the rapid reductor was much more effective, sustained and symmetrical. Instead of arthrotomy, traction-based reduction was easier to perform which resulted in shorter operative time and less blood loss. In the present study, the average operative time and blood loss were 100 min and 135 ml, respectively. By the method, all 21 AO/OTA type C fractures gained satisfactory reduction initially.

We elevated any depressed segments with a customized bone tamp under the guidance of fluoroscopy. The methods mentioned above was similar to the "Medial Approach" technique which was firstly adopted by Levy et al. [25]. Benefit from the compression of tensive soft-tissue, the tibial plateau remained stable and was unlikely to be wider when depressed fragment was elevated to its anatomic position. With the application of intraoperative arthroscopy, we were able to demonstrate that fracture reduction was successful in 82% patients leaving a fracture depression or gap < 3 mm, Finally, our radiological outcomes are promising as we obtained a ≤ 2 mm step-off in 68.2% (15/22) of patients and a > 2–5 mm step-off in 100% of patients.

As another study putted, we also acknowledged that the depressed fragments could not always be anatomically restored especially when the articular was severely damaged [3]. This could be handled with meticulous pre-operative preparation and careful manipulation maybe with frequent X-ray exposure at first. Therefore, surgeons should take notice of the necessity of radiation protection. Krause et al. recommended arthroscopy should be indicated in comminuted tibial plateau fractures [4]. In this study, the articular reconstruction visualized by arthroscopy was consistent with fluoroscopic results. Although a residual step-off or fracture gap was existed in four cases, we decided no further management at the sacrifice of further soft-tissue stripping and longer operation time.

Slot-designed compression bolt was another key instrument which had dual functions of both reduction and fixation. We once applied the same technique in managing calcaneal fractures and received satisfactory outcomes [26–28]. In fact, the laterally displaced fragments were difficult to reduce simply by traction. The compression bolt which played as the bridge of lateral and medial plate could provide efficient compression force to further restore the width of tibial plateau. When the nut was tightened, the compression force did not act on the bone facet directly, but on the dual plates and then transmitted to tibial plateau. The mechanical transmission avoided stress concentration and hardware-related complications including osteoclasia and osteolysis. The unique slotted design facilitated the removal of the distal part of screw without a residual tail left, which decreased the risk of hardware irritation beneath skin. Meanwhile, the compression force generated by the bolts lasted for a long time until the fracture was healed which was crucial for preventing further displacement when early mobilization and weight bearing carried on. The radiological results in the present study were stable until the last follow up without any case of loss of reduction or alignment.

Using the Rasmussen criteria for radiographic assessment, excellent to good outcome was achieved in all our cases, which is comparable to the similar series treated with Ilizarov technique (90 to 100%) [22, 29]. When applying the Rasmussen clinical rating system, the average score in our study was 27.1 and excellent to good outcome was achieved in 95% patients. According to the same rating system, Barbary et al. reported a similar functional result of 93% good to excellent satisfaction after the Ilizarov treatment [29]. In a series of 59 complex plateau fractures, Catagni et al. reported a result of 96.6% good to excellent satisfaction after Ilizarov fixation [10]. Based on these evidences, we suggested that the percutaneous treatment, according to our technique of rapid reductor, could achieve similar clinical results compared with Ilizarov technique. Complications in the current series were minimal because of the obviation of traditional arthrotomy and easier manipulation. No case of joint stiffness, pin tract infection, deep infection or other severe event happened.

Some limitations to this study should be acknowledged. First, this study reports a small series of patients with bicondylar tibial plateau fractures. Besides, there was no control group with which to compare our results. However, the goal of our study was to describe and evaluate a novel technique which was originally developed in our department. Second, the inclusion criteria for this study were, however, focusing on bicondylar tibial fracture (AO/OTA type C). Actually, with the aid of bidirectional rapid reductor, this percutaneous technique could be applied for all types of tibial plateau fractures (Schatzker type I to VI). Another limitation was that the duration of follow-up in our protocol was short with the mean time of 16.5 months. We were not able to provide data concerning mid-term or long-term complication such as the traumatic arthritis related to this technique.

Conclusion

Our observations suggest that the bidirectional rapid reductor facilitates the minimally invasive treatment for bicondylar tibial plateau fractures. This novel technique required limited soft-tissue exposure which was typically suitable for high-energy related fractures. The patients exhibited excellent functional recovery. However further comparatives studies with a higher number of patients and longer follow-up are needed to confirm our short-term data.

Abbreviations

ACL: Anterior cruciate ligament; LCP: Locking compression plate; MIPPO: Minimally invasive percutaneous plate osteosynthesis; ORIF: Open reduction and internal fixation; PCL: Posterior cruciate ligament; PSA: Posterior slope angle; TPA: Tibial plateau angle

Acknowledgment

Not Applicable.

Funding

This research did not receive any specific grant from funding agencies in the public, commercial, or not-for-profit sectors.

Authors' contributions

YZZ designed the trial. HRC and YYY contributed to manuscript drafting and interpretation of data. ZLZ and JSS contributed to data collation and statistic analysis. YZZ and ZLZ contributed to the clinical treatment. All authors have read and approved the final manuscript.

Competing interests

The authors declare that they have no competing interests.

References

1. Zhang YZ. Fractures of the tibia/fibula. In: Zhang YZ, ed. Clinical Epidemiology of Orthopaedic Trauma. New York: Thieme Medical Publishers; 2016. p. 253–255.
2. Marsh JL, Slongo TF, Agel J, et al. Fracture and dislocation classification compendium - 2007: Orthopaedic trauma association classification, database and outcomes committee. J Orthop Trauma. 2007;21:S1–133.
3. Chan YS, Yuan LJ, Hung SS, Wang CJ, Yu SW, Chen CY, Chao EK, Lee MS. Arthroscopic-assisted reduction with bilateral buttress plate fixation of complex tibial plateau fractures. Arthroscopy. 2003;19(9):974–84.
4. Krause M, Preiss A, Meenen NM, Madert J, Frosch KH. "Fracturoscopy" is superior to fluoroscopy in the articular reconstruction of complex Tibial plateau fractures-an arthroscopy assisted fracture reduction technique. J Orthop Trauma. 2016;30(8):437.
5. Moore TM, Patzakis MJ, Harvey JP. Tibial plateau fractures: definition, demographics, treatment rationale, and long-term results of closed traction management or operative reduction. J Orthop Trauma. 1987;1(2):97.
6. Chiu CH, Cheng CY, Tsai MC, Chang SS, Chen AC, Chen YJ, Chan YS. Arthroscopy-assisted reduction of posteromedial tibial plateau fractures with buttress plate and cannulated screw construct. Arthroscopy. 2013;29(8):1346–54.
7. Stokel EA, Sadasivan KK. Tibial plateau fractures: standardized evaluation of operative results. Orthopedics. 1991;14(3):263–70.
8. Young MJ, Barrack RL. Complications of internal fixation of tibial plateau fractures. Orthop Rev. 1994;23(2):149.
9. Keightley AJ, Nawaz SZ, Jacob JT, Unnithan A, Elliott DS, Khaleel A. Ilizarov management of Schatzker IV to VI fractures of the tibial plateau: 105 fractures at a mean follow-up of 7.8 years. Bone Joint J. 2015;97-B:1693.
10. Catagni MA, Ottaviani G, Maggioni M. Treatment strategies for complex fractures of the tibial plateau with external circular fixation and limited internal fixation. J Trauma Acute Care Surg. 2007;63:1043–53.
11. Ohdera T, Tokunaga M, Hiroshima S, Yoshimoto E, Tokunaga J, Kobayashi A. Arthroscopic management of tibial plateau fractures--comparison with open reduction method. Arch Orthop Trauma Surg. 2003;123(9):489–93.
12. Rossi R, Bonasia DE, Blonna D, Assom M, Castoldi F. Prospective follow-up of a simple arthroscopic-assisted technique for lateral tibial plateau fractures: results at 5 years. Knee. 2008;15(5):378–83.
13. Chen XZ, Liu CG, Chen Y, Wang LQ, Zhu QZ, Lin P. Arthroscopy-assisted surgery for tibial plateau fractures. Arthroscopy. 2015;31(1):143–53.
14. Barei DP, Nork SE, Mills WJ, Coles CP, Henley MB, Benirschke SK. Functional outcomes of severe bicondylar tibial plateau fractures treated with dual incisions and medial and lateral plates. J Bone Joint Surg (Am Vol). 2006; 88(8):1713–21.
15. Marsh JL, Smith ST, Do TT. External fixation and limited internal fixation for complex fractures of the tibial plateau. J Bone Joint Surg (Am Vol). 1995; 77(5):661.
16. Watson JT, Coufal C. Treatment of complex lateral plateau fractures using Ilizarov techniques. Clin Orthop Relat Res. 1998;353(353):97–106.
17. Duwelius PJ, Connolly JF. Closed reduction of tibial plateau fractures. A comparison of functional and roentgenographic end results. Clin Orthop Relat Res. 1988;230(230):116.
18. Koval KJ, Sanders R, Borrelli J, Helfet D, Dipasquale T, Mast JW. Indirect reduction and percutaneous screw fixation of displaced tibial plateau fractures. J Orthop Trauma. 1992;6(3):340–6.
19. Morgan SJ, Jeray KJ, Saliman LH, Miller HJ, Williams AE, Tanner SL, Smith WR, Broderick JS. Open reduction and internal fixation compared with circular fixator application for bicondylar tibial plateau fractures. Results of a multicenter, prospective, randomized clinical trial. J Bone Joint Surg Am. 2006;88:2613–23.
20. Britten S, Ghoz A, Duffield B, Giannoudis PV. Ilizarov fixator pin site care: the role of crusts in the prevention of infection. Injury. 2013;44:1275.
21. Laible C, Earl-Royal E, Davidovitch R, Walsh M, Egol KA. Infection after spanning external fixation for high-energy tibial plateau fractures: is pin site-plate overlap a problem? J Orthop Trauma. 2012;26:92–7.
22. Telmo R, Carl E, Eriksson BI, Jon K, Lars N. The Ilizarov external fixator-a useful alternative for the treatment of proximal tibial fractures a prospective observational study of 30 consecutive patients. BMC Musculoskelet Disord. 2013;14:11.
23. Ferreira N, Marais LC. Bicondylar tibial plateau fractures treated with fine-wire circular external fixation. Strateg Trauma Limb Reconstr. 2014;9(1):25–32.
24. Wei C, Tao Z, Wang J, Bo L, Hou Z, Zhang Y. Minimally invasive treatment of displaced femoral shaft fractures with a rapid reductor and intramedullary nail fixation. Int Orthop. 2016;40(1):167–72.
25. Levy BA, Herrera DA, Macdonald P, Cole PA. The medial approach for arthroscopic-assisted fixation of lateral tibial plateau fractures: patient selection and mid- to long-term results. J Orthop Trauma. 2014;2(3 Suppl):201–5.
26. Wang Q, Chen W, Su Y, Pan J, Zhang Q, Peng A, Wu X, Wang P, Zhang Y. Minimally invasive treatment of calcaneal fracture by percutaneous leverage, anatomical plate, and compression bolts--the clinical evaluation of cohort of 156 patients. J Trauma. 2010;69(6):1515–22.
27. Zhang T, Su Y, Chen W, Zhang Q, Wu Z, Zhang Y. Displaced intra-articular calcaneal fractures treated in a minimally invasive fashion: longitudinal approach versus sinus tarsi approach. J Bone Joint Surg (Am Vol). 2014;96(4): 302–9.

Suboptimal outcomes after closed reduction and internal fixation of displaced femoral neck fractures in middle-aged patients: is internal fixation adequate in this age group?

Cheng-Tzu Wang[1], Jia-Wan Chen[2], Karl Wu[1,2], Chiang-Sang Chen[1], Wen-Chih Chen[1], Jwo-Luen Pao[1], Chih-Hung Chang[1] and Tsung-Yu Lan[1,2*]

Abstract

Background: There have been many studies regarding nongeriatric femoral neck fractures (FNFs), which included patients of a wide age range (between 20 and 60 years old). We aimed to determine whether internal fixation provided acceptable outcomes for middle-aged patients with displaced FNFs, and identify predictors of successful internal fixation.

Methods: A total of 117 patients, aged 50–60 years and who underwent closed reduction and unilateral internal fixation using cannulated screws, were included. The outcomes were classified as either "complications" (varus malunion, femoral neck shortening, non-union/early collapse, avascular necrosis, or arthroplasty during the follow-up) or "optimal outcomes" (no complications). Patients with displaced FNFs (Garden stages III–IV, $n = 69$) were categorized according to whether they experienced acceptable or unacceptable reduction. We evaluated whether patients' clinical characteristics could predict optimal outcomes.

Results: Patients with displaced FNFs generally experienced complications (84.1%). Twenty-two percent of patients experienced optimal outcomes when acceptable reduction was achieved. Patients with unacceptable reductions experienced complications. Optimal outcomes were positively associated with Pauwels' type II fracture (OR: 8.67, $p = 0.025$) and negatively associated with excessive alcohol consumption ($p = 0.045$).

Conclusions: Compared with the younger age group, complication rates are higher in middle-aged patients with displaced FNFs treated using cannulated screws. If internal fixation is to be used for a displaced FNF, patient selection is essential. Care must be taken to avoid selecting patients with excessive alcohol consumption, while successful internal fixation may be more likely for patients with Pauwels' type II fracture.

Keywords: Femoral neck fracture, Internal fixation, Middle-aged patients

* Correspondence: gbwsh0130@gmail.com
[1]Department of Orthopaedic Surgery, Far Eastern Memorial Hospital, No. 21, Sec. 2, Nanya S. Rd., Banciao Dist, New Taipei City 220, Taiwan
[2]Department of Mechanical Engineering, Oriental Institute of Technology, New Taipei City, Taiwan

Background

Femoral neck fractures (FNFs) are an important health concern, with multiple causes, such as trauma, malignancy, and bone metabolism disorders. The possibility of stress fractures should be especially considered in athletes and recreational runners without a history of trauma, as the rare fracture pattern of FNFs might easily be missed on radiography and is best detected by magnetic resonance imaging (MRI) [1, 2]. Displaced FNFs are difficult to treat, which result in a high rate of complications (e.g., non-union and osteonecrosis) [3, 4]. Age has traditionally been considered an important factor for treatment selection, as closed or open reduction with internal fixation is favored for younger patients, because it preserves the femoral head and cartilage. In contrast, primary arthroplasty is preferred to allow elderly patients to regain their daily functioning [5]. However, the optimal treatment for middle-aged patients is unclear as existing comorbidities and osteoporosis must be considered. Previous studies regarding nongeriatric FNFs included patients with a wide age range, between 20 and 60 years [3, 6–8]. We hypothesized that it might mimic the higher failure rate of middle-aged patients. In addition, national health policies and insurance coverage can significantly influence clinical decision-making. Thus, treatment of FNFs in middle-aged patients is complicated, and only a few studies have evaluated the outcomes of displaced FNFs treated using internal fixation. Therefore, this study aimed to evaluate the outcomes of displaced FNFs after closed reduction and internal fixation among middle-aged patients, and to identify factors that predict successful internal fixation and optimal outcomes.

Methods

Patients

This single-center retrospective study evaluated data from 161 middle-aged patients (50–60 years old) with isolated FNFs that were treated using cannulated screws between 2005 and 2014. Since there has been no consensus about the optimal implant for displaced FNFs, patients treated with other implants, including sliding-hip screw (22 patients) and Kowles pins (10 patients) were not included. We hope that simplification of the implant will minimize the selection bias. The patients' medical records were used to collect data regarding age, sex, mechanism of injury, comorbidities, smoking, and alcohol use.

DSM-IV-TR (Diagnostic and Statistical Manual of Mental Disorders, 4th Edition, Text Revision) criteria were applied for evaluation of alcohol use disorder. In our cohort, patients who met the criteria for "alcohol abuse" or "alcohol dependence" were categorized under "excessive alcohol consumption" [9]. Patients with (1) a delayed surgery > 6 h after diagnosis; (2) malignancy or a pathological fracture; (3) a bone metabolism disorder that could affect fracture healing; (4) end-stage renal disease; (5) multiple fractures requiring ipsilateral femoral shaft fixation; (6) a follow-up period < 2 years; and (7) inappropriate or incomplete radiographs were excluded. Thus, 117 patients were considered eligible for the present study.

Surgery

Fractures were classified as undisplaced (Garden stages I–II, $n = 48$) or displaced (Garden stages III–IV, $n = 69$). We used Pauwels' classification to determine whether vertical shearing force significantly influenced internal fixation failure for displaced fractures. All fractures were managed by senior attending surgeons or fellowship-trained orthopedic traumatologists. Patients underwent closed reduction and unilateral internal fixation with cannulated screws, using the lateral approach through a small incision. The first implant was inserted inferiorly along the calcar, and the two other implants were placed superiorly to create a triangular configuration. The implants were inserted deep enough to ensure stability through subchondral bone purchase. The distance between the screw tip and the femoral head border was < 10 mm in all cases (8.1 ± 3.5 mm). Surgeries were performed as soon as possible after the diagnosis, generally within < 6 h at our center. To prevent the bias of delayed surgery, the cases involving surgery > 6 h after the diagnosis were excluded from the present study. Open reduction or capsulotomy was not performed. The patients were not allowed to bear weight for ≥8 weeks after the surgery until they exhibited radiographic evidence of callus formation. After evidence of bony union was detected, touch-down weight bearing with a walker was initiated and the level of ambulation was gradually increased. Follow-up radiography was performed at least twice during the first postoperative month, and then the frequency was decreased to monthly. Patients were followed up for ≥2 years (range: 2–8 years).

Radiographic Assessment & Outcomes

Preoperative radiographs were taken in patients at the time of admission; the immediate postoperative film was obtained within hours after surgery; and follow-up images were taken in every visit in our outpatient department. Fracture union was defined as a visible callus bridging the fracture site present within 6 months of surgery [6].

Each radiograph was evaluated twice in a blinded fashion by a single author (CT Wang); then, an additional senior staff (TY Lan) repeated the assessments to ensure reliability. To resolve concerns with inter-observer reliability, we used SPSS (Version 22, SPSS Inc., Chicago, Illinois) to determine the intra-class correlation coefficient.

The outcomes were classified as either "optimal outcomes" or "complications". Optimal outcomes were defined as bony union with < 5° varus and < 5 mm femoral neck shortening [7, 8, 10], osteonecrosis, and subsequent arthroplasty. Complications were defined as > 5° varus malunion or shortening > 5 mm of the femoral neck [7, 8, 10], non-union/early collapse, avascular necrosis (AVN) of the femoral head/neck after union, or arthroplasty during follow-up. Varus malunion and femoral neck shortening were evaluated based on a comparison to the radiographs of the contralateral hip. Regarding the quantitative assessment of femoral neck shortening, we used the method described by Zlowodzki et al. [7, 10]. Because the degree of shortening or varus collapse may change during the follow-up period, assessment was performed on post-operative films, but the last follow-up radiograph (at least 2 years after surgery) was used for the final decision.

Non-union/early collapse was defined as re-displacement of the fracture site requiring an additional surgery during any follow-up radiographic examination, or the absence of radiographic evidence of union at 6 months after surgery [6, 10]. AVN was identified using magnetic resonance imaging or radiography and the advanced Ficat stages (Ficat III/IV).

We counted all complications in patients with co-existing conditions, such as AVN in a patient with varus malunion, non-union/early collapse requiring arthroplasty to regain mobility, or arthroplasty to address osteoarthritis several years after varus malunion.

Data analysis

The data were categorized according to reduction quality, and the displaced group was divided into a group with acceptable reduction ($n = 50$) or unacceptable reduction ($n = 19$), based on the immediate postoperative radiographs. Acceptable reduction was defined as < 5 mm displacement on the antero-posterior and lateral plain radiograph, ≤5° varus to 25° valgus on the antero-posterior plain radiograph, and ≤ 10° on the lateral plain radiograph [6, 11].

We also evaluated the acceptable reduction group to observe any differences according to Pauwels' type, smoking, alcohol consumption, or diabetes mellitus, and to identify predictors of optimal outcomes. Variables were compared using the Chi-square test or Fisher's exact test, as appropriate, and p-values of < 0.05 were considered statistically significant. We used SPSS software (Version 22, SPSS Inc., Chicago, Illinois) throughout.

Results

Patients had a mean age of 55.4 years (range: 50–60 years) and included 43 men (36.7%). Forty-eight patients had Garden stages I–II (the non-displaced group), and 69 patients had Garden stages III–IV (the displaced group) (Table 1). The mechanisms of injury were simple fall in 72 patients, fall-from-height in 28 patients, and vehicle accident in 17 patients. There was no statistical difference in gender and mechanism of injury between the groups.

Table 1 The outcomes and complications according to the Garden classification

	Non-displaced	Displaced	*P*-value*
All patients (male:female)	48 (13:35)	69 (30:39)	N/A
Optimal outcomes	45 (93.7%)	11 (15.9%)	0.001
Complications	3 (6.3%)	58 (84.1%)	
Varus malunion/shortening	0	27 (39.1%)	0.001
Avascular necrosis	1 (2.1%)	10 (14.5%)	0.026
Non-union/early collapse	2 (4.2%)	23 (33.3%)	0.001
Shift to arthroplasty	3 (6.3%)	26 (37.7%)	0.001

*P-values were calculated using Fisher's exact test

The non-displaced group had an extremely high success rate (93.8%, $n = 40$), with only 2 cases of non-union/early collapse and 1 case that developed osteonecrosis after bony union. No varus malunion or femoral neck shortening was identified in the undisplaced group.

The displaced group had a high complication rate, and optimal outcomes were only achieved in 11 patients (15.9%). The complications during a minimum follow-up of 2 years included non-union/early collapse (33.3%, $n = 23$) and AVN after bony union (14.5%, $n = 10$). Many cases were converted to arthroplasty (37.7%, $n = 26$) because of major complications, which typically involved non-union/early collapse early after surgery or the progression of AVN later after surgery. The displaced group had a union rate of 66.7%, although most of these cases developed femoral neck shortening or varus malunion (27 patients, 39.1% of the displaced group). Two patients underwent revisional ORIF and, subsequently, achieved bony union with varus and shortening.

Acceptable reduction was achieved in 72.5% ($n = 50$) of the cases with displaced fractures (Table 2), although only 22% of these patients ($n = 11$) experienced anatomical union without early collapse or AVN. Thus, the complication rate was 78% when good reduction was

Table 2 Characteristics of the displaced group according to reduction quality

	Acceptable	Unacceptable	*P*-value*
All patients (male:female)	50 (22:28)	19 (8:11)	N/A
Optimal outcomes	11 (22%)	0	0.028
Complications	39 (78%)	19 (100%)	
Varus malunion/shortening	15 (30%)	12 (63.2%)	0.007†
Avascular necrosis	8 (16%)	2 (10.5%)	0.715
Non-union/early collapse	17 (34%)	6 (31.5%)	0.773†
Shift to arthroplasty	18 (36%)	8 (42.1%)	0.640†

*P-values calculated using the chi-square test
†P-values calculated using the Fisher's exact test

initially achieved. Varus malunion or femoral neck shortening occurred in 15 patients, and 6 patients initially had anatomical union but, subsequently, developed AVN after several years (mean: 2 years, range: 1–6 years). Subsequent arthroplasty was performed in 18 patients, which accounted for 36% of patients who achieved acceptable reduction but, eventually, required arthroplasty. Seventeen of these cases involved non-union/early collapse.

None of the patients in the unacceptable reduction group achieved optimal outcomes, and this outcome was significantly poorer than the optimal rate of 22% in the acceptable group ($p = 0.028$). The varus malunion rate was significantly higher in the unacceptable reduction group (63.2% vs. 30%, $p = 0.007$). The rates of AVN with subsequent arthroplasty were high in both groups, and the difference was not statistically significant ($p = 0.715$) (Table 2).

Most patients who achieved optimal outcomes in the acceptable reduction group had Pauwels' type II fractures (91%). The odds ratio for optimal outcomes among Pauwels' type II fractures was 8.67 ($p = 0.025$) (Table 3). Patients with complications were more likely to smoke (25.6%), excessively consume alcohol (28.2%), and have diabetes mellitus (17.9%), compared to patients that did not experience complications. Only excessive alcohol consumption significantly predicted poor outcomes in the present study ($p = 0.045$) (Table 4).

Table 4 Outcomes in the acceptable reduction group according to smoking, alcohol consumption, and diabetes

	Optimal outcomes	Complications	*P*-value*
Smoking	2 (18.1%)	10 (25.6%)	0.472
Alcohol consumption	0	11 (28.2%)	0.045
Diabetes mellitus	1 (9%)	7 (17.9%)	0.430

*P-values were calculated using Fisher's exact test

Discussion

Internal fixation is the gold standard treatment for non-displaced fractures in young and elderly patients, because it provides optimal outcomes [12, 13]. Our results support this approach, as 93.8% of that patient group experienced optimal outcome without complications. However, the failure rate for displaced fractures is much higher than that for non-displaced fractures, and displaced fractures are frequently complicated by AVN and non-union [3, 4]. Non-union of FNFs represents an early mechanical failure before bony union is achieved, and this complication is considered catastrophic because it necessitates revisional surgery (Fig. 1). Barnes et al. have reported an increased age-related risk of non-union [14], and Parker et al. have reported that their 50–60-year-old patients commonly experienced displacement (30%) and non-union (13.5%) [3]. In contrast, a study of young patients with displaced FNFs (15–50 years old) revealed a non-union rate of only 8%, and the authors concluded that this result was influenced by fracture displacement and reduction quality [15]. In comparison with the younger group, we observed a relatively high non-union rate (34%) among middle-aged patients in the present study, which might imply that a wide range of "young patients" is inadequate.

Table 3 Outcomes in the acceptable reduction group according to Pauwels' classification

	Optimal outcomes	Complications
Pauwels' I	0	4 (100%)
Pauwels' II	10 (34.5%)*	19 (65.5%)
Pauwels' III	1 (5.8%)	16 (94.2%)[a]

*The odds ratio for optimal outcomes in the Pauwels' II group was 8.57 ($p = 0.025$ using Fisher's exact test)
[a]Note the high complication rate in the Pauwels' III group

Although AVN is not an urgent problem, it can lead to chronic hip pain and subsequent arthroplasty. The incidence of AVN is higher among displaced FNFs than in undisplaced FNFs [3, 16]. Furthermore, a prospective study from 2009 revealed a relatively high rate of AVN among young patients (< 60 years old: 20.5%, > 80 years old: 12.5%) [4]. The benefit of decompression of the capsule to relieve pressure in femoral neck fractures remains unclear. This treatment is not completely supported in the current literature, and many studies reported no significant difference in patient outcomes with capsulotomy [17–20]. The present study revealed an AVN rate of 16% among patients with good reduction, although we failed to identify a significant association between AVN development and reduction quality.

Relatively minor complications, such as varus malunion and neck shortening, can also lead to unsatisfactory outcomes. Although it is generally not necessary to perform arthroplasty for varus malunion or shortening, problematic complications can emerge during long-term follow-up, such as hip impingement, loss of hip motion, arthrosis, and labral lesions. Concomitant screw back-out can also cause hip irritation and a limping gait. Zlowodzki et al. found, in an observational cohort study, that femoral neck shortening had the greatest adverse effect on the SF-36 physical functioning score [7], and Zielinski et al. reported that femoral neck shortening can impair gait velocity [21]. Thus, novel devices have been developed to prevent neck shortening, and implants with a locked side plate may be a solution to the fractured neck sliding along multiple cancellous screws. However, the use of locking devices for FNFs remains controversial, as a retrospective study from 2014 revealed catastrophic outcomes among patients who received locking devices, which may have been related

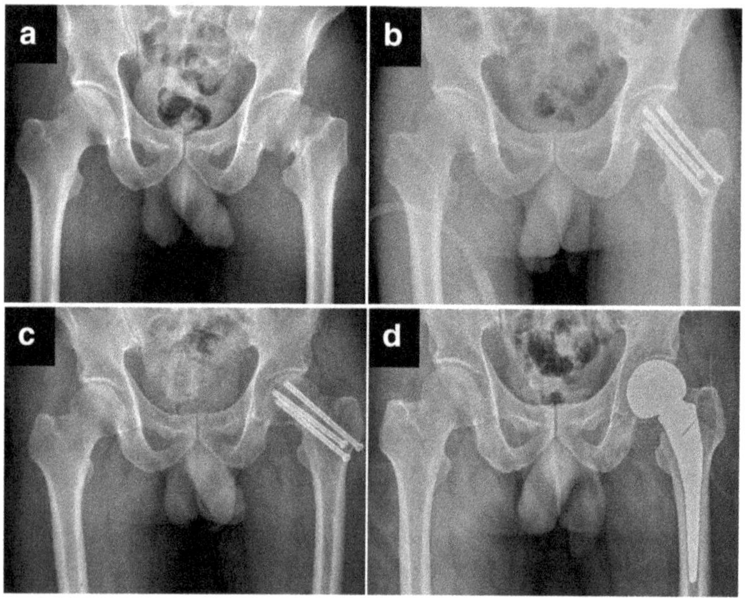

Fig. 1 A typical clinical course of failed internal fixation in middle-aged patient. **a** A 56-year-old male patient with history of alcohol consumption sustained a left displaced femoral neck fracture. **b** Three cannulated screws were applied within 6 h and acceptable reduction was achieved. **c** Postoperative 6 months, there was still non-union with screw backout. **d** Screws were removed and hemiarthroplasty was performed. The case highlighted a common but catastrophic course of middle-aged patients with FNFs, even good reduction was achieved during primary fixation

to decreased micromotion at the fracture site [22]. In the present study, most patients with varus malunion or shortening developed an asymmetric gait and required walking aids or shoe lifts. Thus, even when fracture healing was achieved without non-union or AVN, patients still experienced complications because of femoral neck malunion or shortening.

Unlike sex, underlying disease, osteoporosis, and fracture pattern, adequate reduction and stable fixation are controllable factors in the treatment of displaced FNFs. Good reduction and adequate fixation are associated with successful treatment of young patients [23]. Haidukewych et al. reported that good reduction helped prevent AVN and non-union among 15–50-year-old patients [15]. Our study revealed that intraoperative acceptable reduction is considered a basic requirement for achieving optimal outcomes; none of our patients with unacceptable reduction achieved optimal outcomes. However, even acceptable reduction was achieved for displaced fractures, most of the cases (18 patients, 36%) subsequently underwent either bipolar hemiarthroplasty (13 cases) or total hip replacement (5 cases). In addition, 15 patients who experienced minor complications (e.g., varus malunion and neck shortening) experienced chronic hip pain and gait disturbance that necessitated the long-term use of walking aids or shoe lifts.

Pauwels' type III fractures have a high complication rate because of the dominant vertical shearing force. Some clinicians suggest using a sliding hip screw for unstable fracture patterns. Deneka et al. reported that a sliding hip screw with a de-rotation screw provides superior outcomes for unstable fractures, compared to parallel cancellous screws [24]. In contrast, Clark et al. did not detect any difference between cases of subcapital fractures that were treated using a sliding hip screw or three cancellous screws in a triangular configuration [25]. A more recent study revealed inconclusive results regarding the "gold standard" of internal fixation for displaced FNFs, and the authors noted that fixation strength did not appear to be affected by subcapital or transervical patterns for the parallel cancellous screws or the sliding hip screw [26]. In the present study, all patients received parallel cancellous screws, and none received sliding hip screws. Nevertheless, we observed an extremely high complication rate for Pauwels' type III fractures (16/17, 94.2%), even when acceptable reduction was achieved. The choice of the implant device depends on multiple factors and is not always clear; however, in hindsight, sliding hip screws and an additional de-rotation may provide more biomechanical stability to overcome vertical shearing force.

The present study revealed a notable association between optimal outcomes and Pauwels' type II fractures (Table 3), as 91% (10/11) of the patients with optimal outcomes had Pauwels' type II fractures. Furthermore, the odds ratio for optimal outcomes with Pauwels' type II fractures was 8.67 ($p = 0.025$). This is likely because it is ideal to have the implant's axis perpendicular to the fracture line, and we believe that the compression force from parallel screws in Pauwels' type II fractures provides optimum efficiency (vs. type I and type III cases), which can promote fracture healing and bone consolidation. Furthermore, excessive alcohol consumption has been identified as a risk factor for suboptimal outcomes in previous reports [6], and our findings support this relationship among middle-aged patients. For example, 28% of the patients with complications in the acceptable reduction group reported excessive alcohol consumption, and none of the patients who achieved optimal outcomes reported excessive alcohol consumption. We believed that the concurrent physiological and psychological problems associated with alcohol abuse may lead to poor compliance and a high failure rate. Therefore, it is essential to consider the high risk in these patients, and other treatment options should be considered if surgery is indicated in these patients.

Besides internal fixation, primary arthroplasty has been advocated for displaced FNFs by many studies. Swart et al. found that primary total hip arthroplasty (THA) can be a cost-effective treatment for displaced FNFs among 45–65-year-old patients [27]. Rogmark et al. found that patient treated with arthroplasty have superior outcomes compared with those treated by internal fixation if there is no major complication [28]. Similarly, a national survey published in 2013 reported that patients treated with THA have less pain and better satisfaction compared with those treated with hemiarthroplasty or internal fixation [29]. However, the clinical judgement between internal fixation and arthroplasty is limited in countries with strict national health insurance programs. For example, Taiwanese patients are not covered for arthroplasty until the age of 60 years. Therefore, some middle-aged patients with high failure rate, such as Pauwels' III fracture with excessive alcohol consumption, have no alternative but to receive a primary internal fixation and an unavoidable revision surgery.

The present study has several limitations. First, we did not include patients who received sliding hip screws, and it is possible that the specific implants could have influenced our findings, although there is no consensus regarding the ideal implant(s) for each fracture pattern. Furthermore, patients were not treated using open reduction, which may have increased the rate of unacceptable reductions and number of cases with suboptimal outcomes. Moreover, we identified several potentially significant prognostic factors, although the small sample size limited the power of the analyses and findings. Therefore, larger studies are needed to validate and expand on our findings.

In conclusion, the present study revealed an unacceptably high complication rate among middle-aged patients who underwent internal fixation for displaced FNFs, even when acceptable reduction was achieved. Thus, the overall rate of subsequent arthroplasty was high, especially in cases with non-union and AVN. Moreover, even when fracture union is achieved without AVN, varus malunion and shortening can lead to adverse outcomes. Although primary arthroplasty is another choice of treatment, the longevity of the prosthesis is still a major concern. If internal fixation is to be used for a displaced FNF, patient selection is essential to achieving optimal outcomes. Care must be taken to avoid selecting patients with excessive alcohol consumption, while successful internal fixation may be more likely for patients with Pauwels' type II fracture.

Acknowledgements
This work was supported by grants from the Far Eastern Memorial Hospital (FEMH-2018-C-044). We greatly thank all the members of FEMH Orthopaedic Department of Surgery for their assistance.

Funding
This study was supported by grants from the Far Eastern Memorial Hospital (FEMH-2018-C-044). No other financial associations that may be relevant or seen as relevant to the submitted manuscript.

Authors' contributions
W-CT and L-TY participated in the study design, in collecting the data, the statistical analyses and drafting of the manuscript. C-JW, W-K, C-CS, participated in the study design, data acquisition and manuscript revision. C-WC, P-JL and C-CH advised and assisted drafting of the manuscript, also helped to revise the manuscript. All authors read and approved the final manuscript.

Competing interests
The authors declare that they have no competing interests.

References

1. Maden C, Robbins A, Volpin A, Biz C, Konan S. Outcome of surgical management of stress fractures in high demand individuals. Br J Hosp Med (Lond). 2018;79:26–30.
2. Biz C, Berizzi A, Crimì A, Marcato C, Trovarelli G, Ruggieri P. Management and treatment of femoral neck stress fractures in recreational runners: a report of four cases and review of the literature. Acta Biomed. 2017;88(4 -S):96–106.
3. Parker MJ, Raghavan R, Gurusamy K. Incidence of fracture-healing complications after femoral neck fractures. Clin Orthop Relat Res. 2007;458:175–9.
4. Loizou CL, Parker MJ. Avascular necrosis after internal fixation of intracapsular hip fractures: a study of the outcome for 1023 patients. Injury. 2009;40:1143–6.
5. Bhandari M, Devereaux PJ, Tornetta P 3rd, Swiontkowski MF, Berry DJ, Haidukewych G, et al. Operative management of displaced femoral neck fractures in elderly patients. An international survey J Bone Joint Surg Am. 2005;87:2122–30.
6. Huang TW, Hsu WH, Peng KT, Lee CY. Effect of integrity of the posterior cortex in displaced femoral neck fractures on outcome after surgical fixation in young adults. Injury. 2011;42:217–22.
7. Zlowodzki M, Brink O, Switzer J, Wingerter S, Woodall J Jr, Petrisor BA, et al. The effect of shortening and varus collapse of the femoral neck on function after fixation of intracapsular fracture of the hip. a multi-center cohort study J Bone Joint Surg Br. 2008;90:1487–94.
8. Stockton DJ, Lefaivre KA, Deakin DE, Osterhoff G, Yamada A, Broekhuyse HM, et al. Incidence, magnitude, and predictors of shortening in young femoral neck fractures. Injury. 2015;29:293–8.
9. Diagnostic and Statistical Manual of Mental Disorders, 4th edition. Text revision (DSM–IV-TR). In: American Psychiatric Association; 2000.

10. Zlowodzki M, Ayieni O, Petrisor BA, Bhandari M. Femoral neck shortening after fracture fixation with multiple cancellous screws: incidence and effect on function. J Orthop Trauma. 2008;64:163–9.
11. Lindequist S, Tornkvist H. Quality of reduction and cortical screw support in femoral neck fractures. An analysis of 72 fractures with a new computerized measuring method. J Orthop Trauma. 1995;9:215–21.
12. Chen WC, Yu SW, Tseng IC, Su JY, Tu YK, Chen WJ. Treatment of undisplaced femoral neck fractures in the elderly. J Trauma. 2005;58:1035–9.
13. Conn KS, Parker MJ. Undisplaced intracapsular hip fractures: results of internal fixation in 375 patients. Clin Orthop Relat Res. 2004;421:249–54.
14. Barnes R, Brown JT, Garden RS, Nicoll EA. Subcapital fractures of the femur: a prospective review. J Bone Joint Surg Br. 1976;58:2–24.
15. Haidukewych GJ, Rothwell WS, Jacofsky DJ, Torchia ME, Berry DJ. Operative treatment of femoral neck fractures in patients between the ages of fifteen and fifty years. J Bone Joint Surg Am. 2004;86-A:1711–6.
16. Nikolopoulos KE, Papadakis SA, Kateros KT, Themistocleous GS, Vlamis JA, Papagelopoulos PJ, et al. Long-term outcome of patients with avascular necrosis, after internal fixation of femoral neck fractures. Injury. 2003;34:525–8.
17. Bonnaire F, Schaefer DJ, Kuner EH. Hemarthrosis and hip joint pressure in femoral neck fractures. Clin Orthop Relat Res. 1998;353:148–55.
18. Harper WM, Barnes MR, Gregg PJ. Femoral head blood flow in femoral neck fractures. An analysis using intra-osseous pressure measurement. J Bone Joint Surg Br. 1991;73:73–5.
19. Maruenda JI, Barrios C, Gomar-Sancho F. Intracapsular hip pressure after femoral neck fracture. Clin Orthop Relat Res. 1997;340:172–80.
20. Florschutz AV, Langford JR, Haidukewych GJ, Koval KJ. Femoral neck fractures: current management. J OrthopTrauma. 2015;29:121–9.
21. Zielinski SM, Keijsers NL, Praet SF, Heetveld MJ, Bhandari M, Wilssens JP, et al. FAITH trial investigators. Femoral neck shortening after internal fixation of a femoral neck fracture. Orthopedics. 2013;36:e849–58.
22. Thien R, Herman A, Kedem P, Chechik A, Shazar N. Osteosynthesis of unstable intracapsular femoral neck fracture by dynamic locking plate or screw fixation: early results. J Orthop Trauma. 2014;28:70–6.
23. Manninger J, Kazar G, Fekete G, Fekete K, Frenyo S, Gyarfas F, et al. Significance of urgent (within 6 h) internal fixation in the management of fractures of the neck of the femur. Injury. 1989;20:101–5.
24. Deneka DA, Simonian PT, Stankewich CJ, Eckert D, Chapman JR, Tencer AF. Biomechanical comparison of internal fixation techniques for the treatment of unstable basicervical femoral neck fractures. J Orthop Trauma. 1997;11:337–43.
25. Clark DI, Crofts CE, Saleh M. Femoral neck fracture fixation. Comparison of a sliding screw with lag screws. J Bone Joint Surg Br. 1990;72:797–800.
26. Michalis P, Paul R, Peter VG. Biomechanical rationale for implant choices in femoral neck fracture fixation in the non-elderly. Injury. 2015;46:445–52.
27. Swart E, Roulette P, Leas D, Bozic KJ, Karunakar M. ORIF or arthroplasty for displaced femoral neck fractures in patients younger than 65 years old: an economic decision analysis. J Bone Joint Surg Am. 2017;99:65–75.
28. Rogmark C, Carlsson A, Johnell O, Sembo I. A prospective randomised trial of intimal fixation versus arthroplasty for displaced fractures of the neck of the femur. Functional outcome for 450 patients at two years. J Bone Joint Surg Br. 2002;84:183S.
29. Leonardsson O, Rolfson O, Hommel A, Garellick G, Åkesson K, Rogmark C. Patient-reported outcome after displaced femoral neck fracture: a national survey of 4467 patients. J Bone Joint Surg[Am] 2013;95-A:1693–1699.

19

Association between stress fracture incidence and predicted body fat in United States Army Basic Combat Training recruits

Joseph J. Knapik*, Marilyn A. Sharp and Scott J. Montain

Abstract

Background: A stress fracture (SF) is a highly debilitating injury commonly experienced in United States Army Basic Combat Training (BCT). Body fat (BF) may be associated with this injury but previous investigations (in athletes) have largely used SF self-reports and lacked sufficient statistical power. This investigation developed an equation to estimate %BF and used that equation to examine the relationship between %BF and SF risk in BCT recruits.

Methods: Data for the %BF predictive equation involved 349 recruits with BF obtained from dual-energy X-ray absorptiometry. %BF was estimated using body mass index (BMI, weight/height^2), age (yr), and sex in the entire population of BCT recruits over an 11-year period ($n = 583{,}651$). Medical information was obtained on these recruits to determine SF occurrence. Recruits were separated into deciles of estimated %BF and the risk of SFs determined in each decile.

Results: The equation was %BF = – 7.53 + 1.43 • BMI + 0.13 • age – 14.73 • sex, with sex either 1 for men or 0 for women ($r = 0.88$, standard error of estimate = 4.2%BF). Among the men, SF risk increased at the higher and lower %BF deciles: compared to men in the mean %BF decile, the risk of a SF for men in the first (lowest %BF) and tenth (highest %BF) decile were 1.27 (95%confidence interval (95%CI) = 1.17–1.40) and 1.15 (95%CI = 1.05–1.26) times higher, respectively. Among women, SF risk was only elevated in the first %BF decile with risk 1.20 (95%CI = 1.09–1.32) times higher compared to the mean %BF decile.

Conclusions: Low %BF was associated with higher SF risk in BCT; higher %BF was associated with higher SF risk among men but not women.

Keywords: Stress fracture, Military personnel, Body fat, Age, Gender, Body mass index, Height, Weight, Race/ethnicity

Background

A stress fracture (SF) is a serious and debilitating injury commonly seen in United States (US) Army Basic Combat Training (BCT). Previous studies found medically diagnosed SF incidence in BCT to range from 0.8 to 5.1% for men and 1.1 to 18.0% among women [1–7]. SFs often require removal from BCT and supervised rehabilitation that lasts an average of 62 days [8]. Well researched factors increasing susceptibility to SFs in BCT include female gender [2, 3, 9, 10, 11], older age [9, 12, 13], and race/ethnicity other than black [2, 9, 12–15]. The association between SF risk and physical characteristics like height, weight, and body mass index (BMI) is not clear because results were mixed in the various investigations [9, 14, 16–21]. No study to date has examined the association between SF risk and body fat (BF) in BCT, but there have been several investigations examining this association in athletes [22–25]. However, in most of these investigations [22–24] SFs were self-reported and all [22–25] involved few athletes with SFs ($n \leq 31$) suggesting low statistical power.

BMI is generally taken as a surrogate for BF since it has a close relationship to %BF with correlations on the order of 0.7 [26–28]. However, a particular absolute BMI level does not reflect the same level of body fat in men and women. Examination of the data in a previous BCT study showed that for the same BMI, women had 13 to 15% more BF [26]. Multiple regression equations that

* Correspondence: joseph.j.knapik.ctr@mail.mil
US Army Research Institute of Environmental Medicine, 10 General Greene Ave, Natick, MA 01760, USA

have included age, sex, and/or race/ethnicity in addition to BMI have shown improved ability to predict %BF with correlation ranging from 0.81 to 0.91 [28–33].

This investigation examines the ability of BMI, age, sex, and race to predict %BF in a cohort of recruits in BCT. After developing and validating a %BF predictive equation, this investigation uses that equation to examine the association between %BF and SF risk in the entire population of US Army recruits attending BCT over an 11-year period. A specific %BF equation developed using military recruits would appear to be the most appropriate to examine this relationship in BCT. Based on previous studies [28–34] it was hypothesized that an equation using BMI, age, sex, and race/ethnicity should produce a correlation with a direct measure of %BF in the range of 0.81 to 0.91. It was also hypothesized that both high and low %BF would increase the risk of SFs based on studies that have observed this relationship between BMI and %BF [9, 35].

Methods

This study involved a secondary analysis of data from past investigations that was approved by Human Subjects Protection Office of the US Army Research Institute of Environmental Medicine. Four legacy databases were used, one to develop a %BF prediction equation and the others to apply this predictive equation to examine the relationship between %BF and SF risk. The database used to develop the %BF predictive equation contained date of birth, height, weight, sex, race/ethnicity, and percent body fat (%BF) on 180 male and 169 female BCT recruits. [36] Height was measured with a stadiometer (Model GPM, Seritex Inc., Carlstadt, NJ) and weight with a digital scale (Model 770, Seca Corp., Columbia MD) with subjects in T-shirts, shorts, underclothing, and socks. Date of birth, sex, and race/ethnicity were self-reported. Body fat (BF) was measured with dual-energy X-ray absorptiometry (DXA, Model DPXL, Lunar Corp., Madison WI) [36]. Scanning with the DXA began at the head and progressed in 1-cm segments to the feet with the machine set to the faster 10-min scanning speed. The Lunar software (version 3.6) was used to provide %BF for each participant. Coefficients of variation for measuring fat mass using DXA have ranged from 0.8 to 5.0% [37].

A database of all recruits attending BCT between 1997 and 2007 was compiled from three databases by the Armed Forces Health Surveillance Branch (AFHSB) of the Defense Health Agency. The first of these databases was the Defense Manpower Data Center (DMDC) Master Personnel File which was searched from January 1997 to December 2007 (11-year period) to identify individuals based on their first demographic record (indicating entry into the Army), with a rank of private (E1) to specialist (E4), and 17 to 35 years of age. DMDC database also provided birth year and race/ethnicity. The second AFHSB database was the Defense Medical Surveillance System which provided the injury data on recruits identified in the DMDC database. Specific International Classification of Diseases, Version 9, Clinical Modification (ICD-9) codes were searched for the inclusive time from each recruit's first DMDC record to 10 weeks after the first DMDC record. This covered the period of BCT plus time in the reception station (where recruits are initially in-processed). SF cases were recruits with the occurrence of an ICD-9 code for pathological fractures or SFs (ICD-9 codes 733.1–733.19 and 733.93–733.98). Pathological fracture codes were included because, prior to 2001, there was no ICD-9 code specifically for SFs and the 733.1–733.19 series contained the codes that clinicians in military facilities were instructed to use for this purpose. It was previously shown that use of the pathological fracture codes rapidly declined shortly after the SF codes were introduced, supporting the concept that clinicians were using the pathological fracture codes for SFs prior to having specific SF codes [38]. The third AFHSB database was that of the Military Entrance Processing Station which provided sex, height, and weight of the recruits. The AFHSC provided the investigators with a single de-identified database linking information from these three databases.

In all databases where available, age was calculated as year of entry into BCT minus birth year. BMI was calculated as weight/height^2. In the database used to develop the %BF predictive equation, non-linear regression techniques were applied, but they accounted for little additional variance in %BF compared to linear techniques so the latter was used to develop the equation. Predictive residual sums of squares (PRESS) statistics were used to cross-validate the %BF predictive equation [39]. PRESS statistics compute residual errors based on successive removal and subsequent replacement of cases. These PRESS-residuals are summed and replace the residual sum of squares for the entire model to provide a modified correlation coefficient (r-value) and standard error of estimate (SEE).

SF incidence was calculated as: recruits with one or more SFs / total number of recruits X 1000 (cases/1000 recruits). Univariate logistic regression was performed to quantify risk of SFs at deciles of estimated %BF. Simple contrasts were used, comparing the risk at a baseline (referent) decile of %BF (defined with a risk ratio of 1. 00) to other deciles of that variable. The baseline decile of %BF was selected such that it included the mean BF value. A multivariate logistic regression model was constructed with SF incidence as the dependent variable and race/ethnicity and %BF as independent variables to see if race/ethnicity modified the relationship between

Table 1 Physical Characteristics of Men and Women in Databases

Database	Variable	Men (Mean ± SD)	Women (Mean ± SD)
Body Composition	Age (yr)	22 ± 4	21 ± 3
	Height (cm)	176.5 ± 7.1	163.1 ± 6.2
	Weight (kg)	78.9 ± 12.7	62.6 ± 9.8
	BMI (kg/m2)	25.3 ± 3.7	23.5 ± 3.0
	Body Fat (%)	16.7 ± 6.3	28.8 ± 6.5
Recruit Population 1997–2007	Age (yr)	21 ± 3	21 ± 4
	Height (cm)	175.6 ± 6.9	162.7 ± 6.4
	Weight (kg)	76.1 ± 13.3	61.8 ± 9.5
	BMI (kg/m2)	24.6 ± 3.8	23.3 ± 3.0
	Body Fat (%)	15.7 ± 5.6	28.5 ± 4.3

%BF and SF incidence. In both regression models, odds ratios (OR) and 95% confidence intervals (95%CI) were calculated comparing each decile to the referent decile. Statistical Software for the Social Sciences (SPSS, version 24.0) was used to analyze all data.

Results

The addition of BMI, age, and sex to the regression model accounted for significant portions of the variance in DXA %BF ($p < 0.05$) but race/ethnicity did not ($p = 0.94$). The racial distribution of the BCD sample was 55.01% White, 28.65% Black, 12.32% Hispanic, 2.29% Asian, 1.43% American Indian, and 1 recruit without race specified. The resulting multiple linear regression equation was:

$$\%BF = -7.53 + 1.43 \bullet BMI + 0.13 \bullet age - 14.73 \bullet sex,$$

where BMI was in kg/m^2, age in years, and sex coded as either 1 (men) or 0 (women). For this equation, the $r = 0.88$ and the SEE = 4.2 %BF. The PRESS estimated r-value was 0.84 and the SEE was 4.2 %BF. Adding interaction terms (age X BMI, age X sex, BMI X sex) accounted for little additional variance ($r < 0.01$).

Table 2 Association between Stress Fracture Incidence and Body Fat

Sex	Percentile	Body Fat Range (%)	n	Injury Incidence (cases/1000)	Logistic Regression Odds Ratio (95%CI)	*p*-value
Men	1–10	< 8.90	47,545	23.7	1.27 (1.17–1.40)	< 0.01
	11–20	8.90–10.62	47,603	18.2	0.98 (0.89–1.07)	0.62
	21–30	10.63–12.08	47,382	16.6	0.87 (0.79–0.96)	0.02
	31–40	12.09–13.51	47,706	16.3	0.90 (0.82–0.99)	< 0.01
	41–50	13.52–15.05	47,431	16.8	0.89 (0.81–0.98)	0.03
	51–60	15.06–16.73	47,778	18.6	1.00	Referent
	61–70	16.74–18.60	47,579	20.0	1.07 (0.98–1.18)	0.13
	71–80	18.61–20.61	47,525	20.4	1.10 (1.00–1.20)	0.05
	81–90	20.62–23.52	47,605	21.1	1.14 (1.04–1.24)	< 0.01
	91–100	≥ 23.53	47,591	21.4	1.15 (1.05–1.26)	< 0.01
Women	1–10	< 22.90	10,779	90.1	1.20 (1.09–1.32)	< 0.01
	11–20	22.90–24.56	10,802	81.4	1.07 (0.97–1.18)	0.18
	21–30	24.57–25.97	10,805	80.2	1.05 (0.95–1.16)	0.32
	31–40	25.98–27.23	10,752	79.6	1.04 (0.95–1.16)	0.38
	41–50	27.24–28.53	10,712	76.6	1.00	Referent
	51–60	28.54–29.55	10,827	81.0	1.06 (0.96–1.18)	0.22
	61–70	29.56–30.78	10,842	80.8	1.06 (0.96–1.17)	0.24
	71–80	30.79–32.21	10,788	72.8	0.95 (0.86–1.05)	0.30
	81–90	32.22–34.20	10,793	77.3	1.01 (0.92–1.12)	0.83
	91–100	≥ 34.21	10,806	79.2	1.04 (0.94–1.15)	0.45

Age and physical characteristics of the men and women in the database used to develop the predictive equation are shown in Table 1.

The database containing all individuals in BCT between 1997 and 2007 included 614,606 recruits. Of these, 30,955 recruits (5.0%) were missing either birth year, gender, height, and/or weight and were not considered further in the analysis. The final dataset used for analysis contained 583,651 recruits, with 475,745 men and 107,906 women. Age and physical characteristics of these recruits are shown in Table 1.

The overall SF incidence was 1.9% for men and 8.0% for women as reported previously [38]. Table 2 shows the SF risk for men and women by deciles of estimated %BF. The men demonstrated a bimodal relationship with elevated SF risk in the lowest and highest %BF groups compared to the decile containing the mean %BF. The women had high SF risk at the lowest %BF decile compared to the mean %BF decile, but the SF risk at the higher BF deciles were similar to the mean decile.

Table 3 shows that the addition of race to the logistic regression model did little to modify the relationship

Table 3 Multivariate Association between Stress Fractures, Body Fat, and Race/Ethnicity

Sex	Variable	Strata	n	Injury Incidence (cases/ 1000)	Multivariate Logistic Regression Odds Ratio (95%CI)	*p*-value
Men	Body Fat	< 8.90%	47,545	23.7	1.27 (1.16–1.39)	< 0.01
		8.90–10.62%	46,603	18.2	0.98 (0.89–1.07)	0.61
		10.63–12.08%	47,382	16.6	0.89 (0.81–0.98)	0.02
		12.09–13.51%	47,706	16.5	0.89 (0.80–0.97)	0.01
		13.52–15.05%	47,431	16.6	0.89 (0.81–0.99)	0.04
		15.06–16.73%	47,778	18.7	1.00	Referent
		16.74–18.60%	47,579	20.0	1.07 (0.97–1.17)	0.17
		18.61–20.61%	47,525	20.4	1.08 (0.99–1.19)	0.09
		20.62–23.52%	47,605	21.1	1.13 (1.03–1.23)	0.01
		≥ 23.53%	47,591	21.4	1.17 (1.07–1.28)	< 0.01
	Race/Ethnicity	Black	72,155	12.2	1.00	Referent
		White	324,089	21.0	1.72 (1.60–1.85)	< 0.01
		Hispanic	52,684	19.3	1.56 (1.43–1.71)	< 0.01
		Asian	15,439	17.0	1.38 (1.20–1.59)	< 0.01
		Am Indian	4812	21.8	1.75 (1.42–2.15)	< 0.01
		Other	1393	25.8	2.12 (1.52–2.98)	< 0.01
		Unknown	5173	16.0	1.31 (1.04–1.64)	0.02
Women	Body Fat	< 22.90%	10,779	90.1	1.22 (1.11–1.35)	< 0.01
		22.90–24.56%	10,802	81.4	1.09 (0.98–1.20)	0.10
		24.57–25.97%	10,805	80.2	1.06 (0.96–1.18)	0.22
		25.98–27.23%	10,752	79.6	1.05 (0.95–1.16)	0.35
		27.24–28.53%	10,712	76.6	1.00	Referent
		28.54–29.55%	10,827	81.1	1.07 (0.97–1.18)	0.21
		29.56–30.78%	10,842	80.8	1.06 (0.96–1.17)	0.23
		30.79–32.21%	10,788	72.6	0.95 (0.86–1.06)	0.35
		32.22–34.20%	10,793	77.4	1.03 (0.93–1.13)	0.63
		≥ 34.21%	10,806	79.2	1.07 (0.97–1.18)	0.18
	Race/Ethnicity	Black	31,661	60.9	1.00	Referent
		White	55,580	90.5	1.54 (1.46–1.63)	< 0.01
		Hispanic	13,388	81.5	1.37 (1.27–1.48)	< 0.01
		Asian	3608	76.8	1.28 (1.12–1.46)	< 0.01
		Am Indian	1784	81.3	1.37 (1.15–1.64)	< 0.01
		Other	428	102.8	1.77 (1.29–2.43)	< 0.01
		Unknown	1457	74.1	1.23 (1.01–1.51)	0.04

between %BF and SF risk. Race was an independent risk factor in the multivariate model with black recruits having lower SF risk than other race/ethnic groups.

Discussion

The major finding of the study was that women and men in the lowest decile of body fatness had a 20–27% higher relative risk of developing a SF during BCT. Moreover, men in the upper most decile had a 15% greater risk of SFs compared to men in the mean BF decile. The same did not hold for women, however. Gender differences in fat mass and bioavailability of estrogens in young adults [40] may provide a partial explanation for the sex differences at the higher %BF levels. Estrogens have positive effects on bone formation [41] and adipocytes produce estrogens [42]. Thus, women with higher %BF may have similar SF risk to women with less BF because of higher estrogen levels. The increase in SF risk at the lowest BF deciles may be related to frame size. In previous studies, low BF was associated with smaller bone width, reflective of small frames size [43], and individuals with smaller tibia and femur widths were more likely to experience lower body SFs in basic training [16].

To examine the contribution of %BF to the risk of developing a SF during BCT, an equation was derived to predict %BF, as %BF is not routinely measured on recruits. Our hypothesis that there would be an acceptable strength of the association between predicted and actual %BF using BMI, age and sex was confirmed as the resulting equation had an $r = 0.88$ and a standard error of estimate of 4.2%BF, which was very similar to the strength of associations and errors of estimate derived by others [28–33] (see Table 3). Inclusion of race did little to improve the model. Initially it was assumed that race could contribute to the predictability of %BF because of known racial differences in body composition [34]. However, other investigations [29, 31] that have examined or included race/ethnicity in their %BF predictive equations also showed that this variable contributes little to the prediction of %BF when BMI, age and gender were included. The present study did find that individuals self-reporting as black had a lower risk of SFs than other racial groups, a finding that has been replicated in many other investigations [2, 9, 12–15]. The lower SF risk among blacks could be partly related to the higher bone mineral density and thicker bone cortical areas of blacks compared to other racial/ethnic groups [44–47]. The racial difference in bone mineral density between blacks and whites persists after adjustments for body composition, dietary history, sun exposure, biochemical bone markers, lifestyle characteristics, and other factors [47].

The PRESS statistic produced an r-value and SEE that were very similar to that obtained from the original data in the multiple linear regression model. This indicated that that the original model was consistent and that the equation produced an adequate prediction of %BF from BMI,

Table 4 Equations Estimating %BF from BMI, Age, and Gender

Study	Criterion Method for BF Determination	Participants	Equation for % Body Fat Prediction	r^2	SEE
Deurenberg et al. [28]	Underwater weighting	749 healthy M & W, 16–83 yr. in Netherlands	−5.4 + 1.20 • BMI + 0.23 • age - 10.8 • sex	0.79	4.1
Gallagher et al. [29]	4 compartment models using dual energy x-ray absorptiometry, doubly-labled water, & underwater weighting	706 M & W, 20–94 yr., BMI < 35 kg/m^2, residing near NY city	−10.02 + 1.46 • BMI + 0.12 • age - 11.61 • sex	0.67	5.7
Gallagher et al. [30]	4 compartment models using dual energy x-ray absorptiometry, doubly-labled water, & underwater weighting	1626 M & W, 20–97 yr., convenience sample from UK, US, and Japan	64.5–848 • (1/BMI) + 0.079 • age-16.4 • sex + 0.05 • sex • age + 39.0 • sex • (1/BMI)	0.74	5.0
Jackson et al. [31, 49, 50]	Underwater weighting	679 M & W, 18–61 yr., from 3 US locations	−13.9 + 1.61 • BMI + 0.13 • age - 12.1 • sex	0.75	5.5
Pasco et al. 2012 [32]	Dual-energy x-ray absorptiometry	1766 M & W, 20–74 yr., in Australia	37.8 + 1.62 • (BMI-mean) -16.7 • sex - 0.06 • (BMI-mean)^2 + 0.02 • age - 0.17• sex • (BMI-mean) + 0.03 • gender • (BMI-mean) + 0.04 • sex • age	0.83	4.1
Gomez-Ambrosi et al. 2012 [33]	Air displacement plethysmography	6123 Caucasians, 18–80 yr. in Spain	−44.988 + (0.503 • age) + (10.689 • sex) + (3.172 • BMI) − (0.026 • BMI^2) + (0.181 • BMI • sex) − (0.02 • BMI • age) − (0.005 • BMI^2 • sex) + (0.00021 • BMI^2 • age)	0.79	4.7
Present Study	Dual-energy x-ray absorptiometry	349 healthy men and women 18–35 yr., in US Army BCT	−7.53 + 1.43 • BMI + 0.13 • age - 14.73 • sex	0.77	4.2

In all models, BMI is in kg/m^2, age in years, and in all models except Gomez Ambrosi, sex is 0 = women, 1 = men. For Gomez Ambrosi, sex is 0 = men, 1 = female
Abbreviations: r^2 explained variance (%), *SEE* standard error of the estimate (% body fat), *US* United States, *UK* United Kingdom, *NY* New York, *BCT* Basic Combat Training, *M* men, *W* women

age, and gender in our sample of male and female recruits. Future BCT studies that collect height, weight, age and gender may be able to use this equation to predict %BF.

Although no previous study has examined associations between SF risk and body fat in BCT, three studies have prospectively examined associations between BF and overall BCT injury risk [3, 5, 48]. Jones et al. [3] found a trend for a bimodal relationship between time-loss injuries and skinfold determined %BF in male recruits ($n = 124$) but not female recruits ($n = 186$). Knapik et al. [48] found a trend toward increasing risk of injuries of any type when the lowest DXA-determined %BF tertile was compared with the highest %BF tertile among both men ($n = 169$) and women ($n = 164$). Westphal et al. [5] actually found a trend indicating lower risk of any injury and time-loss injury among groups with the highest and lowest %BF groups compared to women in a mid %BF range ($n = 156$). These equivocal results may be partially explained by the relatively low sample sizes, few injury cases, and likely low statistical power. In the present study, we included 95% of recruits who attended BCT over an 11-year period which included a very large number of SFs ($n = 17{,}811$).

At least four investigations have examined the association between %BF and SFs in athletes. One study [22] of elite female runners ($n = 19$ reporting SFs and 19 not reporting SFs) found that DXA-determined %BF was lower but not significantly different among women self-reporting a previous history of SFs (16.6% vs 17.4%, $p > 0.05$). Another study [23] of university male and female lacrosse players ($n = 5$ men with and 30 men without SFs; $n = 7$ women with and 42 without SFs) also found no relationship between %BF (determined with a Tanita MC-190 body composition analyzer) and self-reported SFs. A third study of 54 female runners ($n = 22$ with SFs) found no difference in %BF between SF cases (17.0% BF) and non-SF cases (17.7% BF) ($p > 0.05$). Finally, the fourth study [25] matched 19 athletes with diagnosed SFs (by X-ray, bone scan, or magnetic resonance imaging) with 19 healthy athletes without SFs and found no significant difference in DXA-determined %BF between the two groups ($p = 0.31$). Most studies [22–24] relied on self-reports of SFs and all [22–25] had few SF cases, likely making them underpowered to detect a significant relationship between SF and %BF. Further, these studies [22–25] compared average %BF among those with and without SFs and did not compare risk at various %BF levels as reported in the present study.

Several previous studies have examined the ability of BMI, age, gender, and/or race to predict %BF [28–33] and data on these studies and the equations developed are shown in Table 4. Compared to the present investigation, these previous studies used samples that possessed more diversity in terms of age, BMI, and %BF. Yet the equation produced here has similar level of prediction strength as these other studies.

Limitations to this study should be noted. The %BF body fat equation developed here was based on a sample of Army recruits and the predictive equation is most appropriately applied to this population. Nonetheless, men and women entering the Army come from a wide-ranging cross-section of the US and are broadly representative of individuals of similar age within this national population. The most obvious limitation is that the %BF values in this study were estimated from a predictive equation. Studies should be conducted that measure actual BF in a large group of recruits and follow those recruits through BCT to obtain SF incidence and examine if the relationships established here are confirmed.

Conclusion

In summary, we developed a useful equation to predict %BF in US Army recruits and showed that this equation (using BMI, age, and sex) was consistent and produced an adequate prediction of %BF. We applied this equation to show that SF risk was higher among male and female recruits with low %BF and among male recruits with higher body fat.

Abbreviations

%BF: Percent body fat; 95%CI: 95% Confidence interval; AFHSB: Armed Forces Health Surveillance Branch; BCT: Basic combat training; BF: Body fat; BMI: Body Mass Index; DMDC: Defense Manpower Data Center; DXA: dual-energy x-ray absorptiometry; ICD-9: International Classification of Diseases; OR: Odds ratio; PRESS: Predictive residual sums of squares; SEE: Standard error of estimate; SF: Stress fracture; US: United States

Acknowledgements

We would like to thank Dr. Angie Cost from the Armed Forces Health Surveillance Branch of the Defense Health Agency for providing us with the 11-year recruit data for analyses.

Funding

This study used internal funding from the US Army Research Institute of Environmental Medicine.

Authors' contributions

JJK conceived the study, compiled and analyzed the data, and drafted the manuscript. SJM and MAS assisted in conceiving the study, collected the data, and assisted in manuscript preparation. All authors read and approved the final manuscript.

Authors' information

The views, opinions, and/or findings contained in this report are those of the author(s) and should not be construed as an official Department of the Army position, policy, or decision, unless so designated by other official documentation. In the conduct of research involving human subjects, the investigator(s) adhered to the policies regarding the protection of human subjects as prescribed by Department of Defense Instruction 3216.02 (Protection of Human Subjects and Adherence to Ethical Standards in DoD-Supported Research) dated 8 November 2011.

Competing interests

The authors declare that they have no competing interests.

References

1. Reinker KA, Ozburne S. A comparison of male and female orthopedic pathology in basic training. Milit Med. 1979;144:532–6.
2. Brudvig TGS, Gudger TD, Obermeyer L. Stress fractures in 295 trainees: a one-year study of incidence as related to age, sex, and race. Milit Med. 1983;148:666–7.
3. Jones BH, Bovee MW, Harris JM, Cowan DN. Intrinsic risk factors for exercise-related injuries among male and female Army trainees. Am J Sports Med. 1993;21:705–10.
4. Bensel CK, Kish RN. Lower extremity disorders among men and women in Army basic training and effects of two types of boots. Natick: U.S. Army Natick Research and Development Laboratories Technical TR-83/026 TR-83/026; 1983.
5. Westphal KA, Friedl KE, Sharp MA, King N, Kramer TR, Reynolds KL, Marchitelli LJ. Health, performance and nutritional status of U.S. Army women during basic combat training. Natick: U.S. Army Research Institute of Environmental Medicine Technical Report Number T96–2; 1995.
6. Pester S, Smith PC. Stress fractures of the lower extremities of soldiers in basic training. Orthop Rev. 1992;21:297–303.
7. Knapik JJ, Montain SJ, McGraw S, Grier T, Ely M, Jones BH. Stress fracture risk factors in basic combat training. Int J Sports Med. 2012;33:940–6.
8. Hauret KG, Shippey DL, Knapik JJ. The physical training and rehabilitation program: duration of rehabilitation and final outcome of injuries in basic combat training. Milit Med. 2001;166:820–6.
9. Mattila VM, Niva M, Kiuru M, Pihlajmaki H. Risk factors for bone stress injuries: a follow-up study of 102,515 person-years. Med Sci Sports Exerc. 2007;39:1061–6.
10. Macleod MA, Houston AS, Sanders I, Anagnostopoulos C. Incidence of trauma related to stress fractures and shin splints in male and female Army recruits: retrospective case study. Br Med J. 1999;318:29.
11. Protzman RR, Griffis CC. Comparative stress fracture incidence in males and females in equal training environments. Athl Train. 1977;12:126–30.
12. Lappe JM, Stegman MR, Recker RR. The impact of lifestyle factors on stress fractures in female Army recruits. Osteopros Int. 2001;12:35–42.
13. Gardner LI, Dziados JE, Jones BH, Brundage JF, Harris JM, Sullivan R, Gill P. Prevention of lower extremity stress fractures: a controlled trial of a shock absorbent insole. Am J Public Health. 1988;78:1563–7.
14. Kelly EW, Johnson SR, Cohen ME, Shaffer R. Stress fractures of the pelvis in female navy recruits: an analysis of possible mechanisms of injury. Milit Med. 2000;165:142–6.
15. Friedl KE. Body composition and military performance: origins of the Army standards. In: Marriott BM, Grumstrup-Scott J, editors. Body composition and military performance. Washington, DC: National Academy Press; 1992. p. 31–55.
16. Beck TJ, Ruff CB, Mourtada FA, Shaffer RA, Maxwell-Williams K, Kao GL, Sartoris DJ, Brodine S. Dual energy X-ray absorptiometry derived structural geometry for stress fracture prediction in male US marine corps recruits. J Bone Mineral Res. 1996;11:645–53.
17. Giladi M, Milgrom C, Simkin A, Danon Y. Stress fractures. Identifiable risk factors. Am J Sports Med. 1991;19:647–52.
18. Finestone A, Shlamkovitch N, Eldad A, Laor A, Danon YL, Milgrom C. Risk factors for stress fractures among Israeli infantry recruits. Milit Med. 1991;156:528–30.
19. Shaffer RA, Rauh MJ, Brodine SK, Trone DW, Macera CA. Predictors of stress fractures in young female recruits. Am J Sports Med. 2006;34:108–15.
20. Valimaki W, Alfthan E, Lehmuskallio E, Loyttyniemi E, Sah T, Suominen H, Valimakii MJ. Risk factors for clinical stress fractures in male military recruits: a prospective cohort study. Bone. 2005;37:267–73.
21. Givon U, Friedman E, Reiner A, Vered I, Finestone A, Shemer J. Stress fractures in the Israeli defense forces from 1995 to 1996. Clin Orthop Relat Res. 2000;373:227–32.
22. Duckham RL, Peirce N, Meyer C, Summers GD, Cameron N, Brooke-Wavell K. Risk factors for stress fractures in female endurance athletes: a cross-sectional study. BMJ Open. 2012;2:e001920.
23. Wakamatsu K, Sakuraba K, Suzuki Y, Maruyama A, Tsuchiya Y, Shikakura J, El O. Association between stress fracture and bone metabolism/quality markers in lacrosse players. Open Access J Sports Med. 2012;3:67–71.
24. Bennell KL, Malcolm SA, Thomas SA, Ebeling PR, McCrory PR, Wark JD, Brukner PD. Risk factors for stress fractures in female track-and-field athletes: a retrospective analysis. Clin J Sports Med. 1995;5:229–35.
25. Schnackenburg KE, MacDonald HM, Ferber R, Wiley JP, Boyd SK. Bone quality and muscle strength in female athletes with lower limb stress fractures. Med Sci Sports Exerc. 2011;43:2110–9.
26. Knapik JJ, Burse RL, Vogel JA. Height, weight, percent body fat and indices of adiposity for young men and women entering the U.S. Army. Aviat Space Environ Med. 1983;54:223–31.
27. Roche AF, Siervogel RM, Chumlea WM, Webb P. Grading body fatness from limited anthropometric data. Am J Clin Nutr. 1981;34:2831–8.
28. Deurenberg P, Weststrate JA, Seidell JC. Body mass index as a measure of body fatness: age- and sex-specific prediction formulas. Brit J Nutr. 1991;65:105–14.
29. Gallagher D, Visser M, Supulveda D, Pierson RN, Harris T, Heymsfield SB. How useful is body mass index for comparison of body fat across age, sex and ethnic groups. Am J Epidemiol. 1996;143(3):228–39.
30. Gallagher D, Heymsfield SB, Heo M, Jebb SA, Murgatroyd PA, Sakamoto Y. Healthy percent body fat ranges: an approach for developing guidelines on body mass index. Am J Clin Nutr. 2000;72:694–701.
31. Jackson AS, Stanforth PR, Gagnon J, Rankinen T, Leon AS, Rao DC, Skinner JS, Bouchard C, Wilmore JH. The effect of sex, age, and race on estimating percentage of body fat from body mass inde: the heritage family study. Int J Obes. 2002;26:789–96.
32. Pasco JA, Nicholson GC, Brennan SL, Kotowicz MA. Prevalence of obesity and the relationship between the body mass index and body fat: cross-sectional, population-based data. PLoS One. 2012;7(1):e29580.
33. Gomez-Ambrosi J, Silva C, Galofre JC, Escalada J, Santos S, Millan D, Vila N, Ibanez P, Gil MJ, Valenti V, et al. Body mass index classification misses subjects with increased cardiometabolic risk factors related to elevated adiposity. Int J Obes. 2012;36:286–94.
34. Fernandez JR, Heo M, Heymsfield SB, Pierson RN, Pi-Sunyer FX, Wang ZM, Wang J, Hayes M, Allison DB, Gallagher D. Is percent body fat differentially related to body mass index in Hispanic Americans, African Americans, and European Americans? Am J Clin Nutr. 2003;77:71–5.
35. Rauh MJ, Macera CA, Trone DW, Shaffer RA, Brodine SK. Epidemiology of stress fracture and lower-extremity overuse injuries in female recruits. Med Sci Sports Exerc. 2006;38:1571–7.
36. Sharp MA, Knapik JJ, Patton JF, Smutok MA, Hauret K, Chervak M, Ito M, Mello RP, Frykman PN, Jones BH. Physical fitness of soldiers entering and leaving basic combat training. Natick: US Army Research Institute of Environmental Medicine Technical Report Number T00-13; 2000.
37. Nana A, Slater GJ, Stewart AD, Burke LM. Methodological review: using dual-energy X-ray absorptiometry (DXA) for the assessment of body composition in athletes and active people. Int J Sports Nutr Exerc Metabol. 2014;24:196–215.
38. Knapik JJ, Montain SJ, McGraw SM, Grier T, Ely MR, Jones BH. Risk factors for stress fractures in basic combat training. Int J Sports Med. 2012;33:940–6.
39. Holiday DB, Ballard JE, Mckeown BC. PRESS-related statistics: regression tools for cross-validation and case diagnostics. Med Sci Sports Exerc. 1995;27:612–20.
40. Cauley JA. Estrogen and bone health in men and women. Steroids. 2015;99:11–5.
41. Khosla S, Oursler MJ, Monroe DG. Estrogens and the skeleton. Trends Endrocriol Metab. 2012;23(11):576–81.
42. Li J, Papadopoulos V, Vihma V. Steroid biosynthesis in adipose tissue. Steroids. 2015;103:89–104.
43. Chumlea WC, Wisemandle W, Guo SS, Siervogel RM. Relations between frame size and body composition and bone mineral status. Am J Clin Nutr. 2002;75:1012–6.
44. Trotter M, Broman GE, Peterson RR. Densities on bones of white and negro skeletons. J Bone Joint Surg Am. 1960;42A:50–8.
45. Bachrach LK, Hastie T, Wang MC, Narssimhan R, Marcus R. Bone mineral acquisition in healthy Asian, hispanic, black and caucasian youth: a longitudinal study. J Clin Endocrinol Metab. 1999;84:4702–12.
46. Nelson DA, Barondess DA, Hendrix SL, Beck TJ. Cross-sectional geometry, bone strength, and bone mass in the proximal femur in black and white postmenopausal women. J Bone Mineral Metabol. 2000;15:1992–7.
47. Ettinger B, Sidney S, Cummings SR, Libanati C, Bikle DD, Tekawa IS, Tolan K, Steiger P. Racial differences in bone mineral density between young adult black and white subjects persist after adjustment for anthropometric, lifestyle, and biochemical differences. J Clin Endocrinol Metab. 1997;82:429–34.

20

Serial changes in the head-shaft angle of proximal humeral fractures treated by placing locking plates

Ji-Qi Wang†, Bing-Jie Jiang†, Wei-Jun Guo and You-Ming Zhao*

Abstract

Background: Although the proximal humeral fractures (PHFs) treated with locking plate have been well applied, there are few studies concerning on the serial HSA changes after locking plate placement. The purpose of this retrospective study was to explored the clinical significance of serial HSA changes after surgery.

Methods: We retrospectively analyzed the clinical data of 122 patients between January 2012 to December 2016 in our hospital. The serial change of the HSA and Neer's score of 122 patients were recorded and analyzed. Then, we evaluated the HSA changes affected functional recovery in conjunction with medial support (MS). Moreover, multivariable linear regression analysis was performed to identify any potential confounding factors that may influence functional recovery.

Results: Of 146 patients, 122 (50 males and 72 females) patients were finally enrolled in our study. Our preliminary data suggested that the most decrease of HSA occurred in the period of 1 to 3 months ($p < 0.001$) postoperatively, and functional recovery was significantly related with the change of HSA ($R^2 = 0.647$, $p < 0.001$). The presence of MS plays an important role in maintaining postoperative HSA and restoring function. Moreover, Neer type 4 fracture, the difference between the postoperative HSA (on the injured side) and that of the uninjured side (the ΔHSA), and the HSA change to the end of follow-up were all significantly associated with functional recovery.

Conclusions: Serial HSA changes were evident in PHF patients in whom locking plates had been inserted; it is essential to maintain reduction for 1–3 months postoperatively. MS is important in this context and surgeons must maximally restore MS. Furthermore, the functional outcome tended to improve when the HSA of the injured side was restored to a value close to that of the uninjured side.

Keywords: Proximal humeral fractures, Locking plate, Head-shaft angle, Functional outcomes, Medial support

Background

Proximal humeral fractures (PHFs) represent 5% of all fractures [1]and require surgical treatment, especially in elderly patients for whom high-level functional recovery is important [2]. Placement of a proximal humeral internal locking system (PHILOS) is the current mainstay of treatment to achieve minimal loss of function [3]. Despite the advantages of this technique, the use of locking plates to surgically treat PHF is associated with high complication rates (16–36%) [4]. The major complications are reduction loss and varus malunion [3, 5, 6]; reduction loss can be associated with screw perforation of the articular surface, triggering a need for re-operation, or even causing complete fixation failure [7]. Recent studies showed that a lack of medial support (MS) might play an important role in reduction loss [8–10].

Generally, the humeral head-shaft angle (HSA) dictates the choice of plate length [11];our understanding of the HSA is continuously improving. To the best of our knowledge, the HSA is closely associated with shoulder function and is affected by many factors. However, only a few studies focused on serial HSA changes after locking plate placement. We explored the clinical

* Correspondence: wmuorthopaedic@sina.com
†Ji-Qi Wang and Bing-Jie Jiang contributed equally to this work.
Department of Orthopaedics, The Second Affiliated Hospital and Yuying Children's Hospital of Wenzhou Medical University, 109# Xue Yuan Xi Road, Wenzhou, Zhejiang 325000, China

significance of serial HSA changes after surgery. We retrospectively evaluated the changes, i.e. how they affected functional recovery in conjunction with MS, and the relationship between HSA changes and clinical outcomes after PHILOS fixation of PHFs.

Methods

Study design

We retrospectively reviewed serial HSA changes in PHF patients treated via locking plate placement. Our institutional ethics committee approved the study and all participants provided written informed consent prior to data collection.

Patients

The inclusion criteria were as follows: an acute closed fracture < 14 days old treated via PHILOS; age ≥ 18 years; no complication such as nerve or vascular injury; no history of an upper extremity fracture; and complete follow-up. From January 2012 to December 2016, we treated 146 PHF patients using the PHILOS. Of these, 24 were excluded: 3 with open fractures, 3 with a history of upper extremity fracture, 4 with nerve injury, and 14 lost to follow-up. Thus, 122 patients (50 males and 72 females) met the inclusion criteria and were enrolled; we also measured the HSAs of the uninjured sides. According to the Neer classification [12], we treated 44 two-part, 58 three-part, and 20 four-part fracture patients.

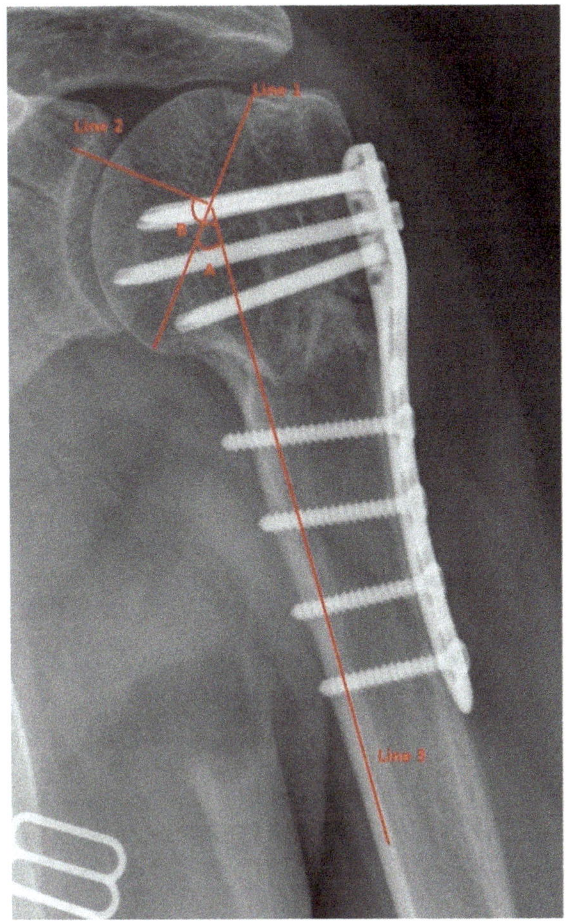

Fig. 1 The head-shaft angle (HSA) measurement method. A vertical line is drawn from the superior to the inferior border of the articular surface (Line 1) and a line perpendicular to this line is then drawn to run through the centre of the humeral head (Line 2). The angle between the latter line and a line parallel to the long axis of the humeral shaft (Line 3) is the humeral head-shaft angle. We found that this angle (angle B) was equal to the angle between the vertical and the long axes (angle A) plus 90°

Surgical technique

All patients underwent a standard procedure via a deltopectoral approach while in the beach-chair position. After confirming satisfactory reduction, fragments were temporarily fixed with K-wires. Next, appropriate locking proximal humeral plates (Proximal Humeral Inter-locking System; Synthes; Oberdorf, Switzerland) were used to fix the fractures.

All patients underwent similar postoperative rehabilitation; the shoulders were sling-immobilised for 3–6 weeks, followed by controlled passive mobilisation exercises (pendulum exercise, flexion, and external rotation) for 1–6 weeks depending on fracture type and bone healing. For all patients, stretching and resistive strengthening exercises were recommended until complete fracture healing was evident on radiographs.

Postoperative follow-up

X-rays were taken immediately after the operation; at 1, 3, 6, and 12 months; and at the last follow-up. The HSA was measured as described by Agudelo et al. [13] (Fig. 1).A vertical line was first drawn from the superior to the inferior border of the articular surface (Line 1) and a line perpendicular to this line was then drawn through the centre of the humeral head (Line 2). The angle between the latter line and a line parallel to the long axis of the humeral shaft (Line 3) was defined as the humeral HSA. We found that this angle (angle B) was identical to the angle between the vertical and long axes (angle A), plus 90°. HSAs were independently assessed (twice) by two reviewers blinded to the clinical outcomes; the average of each set of four values was used in the analysis. In addition, following the recommendation of Greiner [14], an HSA < 120° was considered indicative of varus malunion. Using the criterion of Owsley [15], loss of reduction was defined as an HSA reduction > 10°.

Functional recovery was evaluated using the Neer criteria [16] at the last follow-up.

Statistical analysis

All statistical analyses were performed using SPSS software (ver. 19.0; SPSS Inc., Chicago, IL, USA). Numerical data were compared using Student's t-test. One-factor analysis of variance (ANOVA) was employed to compare group means, and the LSD test was used to perform multiple comparisons. The Kruskal–Wallis test was employed to compare differences in Neer scores during follow-up; multiple comparisons were performed with the Tamhane T2 test. Categorical data were compared using the chi-squared ($\chi 2$) and Fisher's exact tests. We performed linear regression analysis to identify relationships between functional outcomes and HSA changes. Univariate analysis was employed to explore associations between various factors and the Neer scores; multivariable linear regression was then performed to control for confounding effects. The level of significance was set to 0.05 for all analyses.

Results

In total, 122 patients (50 males and 72 females) were included; their demographic data are listed in Table 1. The mean age was 61.1 years (range: 37–87 years). Over a mean of 16.2 months of follow-up (range: 12–24 months), all patients achieved bony union; the mean healing time was 4.4 months (range: 3–12 months). We treated 44 two-part, 58 three-part, and 20 four-part fracture patients; the mean HSA of the uninjured side was 136.5 ± 4.8°. Reduction loss was observed in 18 patients, of whom 16 experienced varus malunion, 2 subacromial impingement, 2 screw penetration requiring re-operations to remove the screws, and 4 delayed union that healed only after 12 months of follow-up.

We found that most of the HSA reduction occurred from 1 to 3 months postoperatively, and the reduction amount was 4.9 ± 3.3° ($p < 0.001$, Fig. 2). We divided the patients into two groups: with and without MS. We found no significant difference in HSA loss between the groups at 1 month postoperatively. However, after 3 months, the HSA of patients with MS was significantly greater than that of patients without MS (Table 2). Figure 3 shows the HSA trends during follow-up. The Neer score of patients with MS was significantly higher than that of patients lacking MS; the former patients enjoyed better functional recovery. Also, patients lacking MS were at a significantly increased risk of reduction loss than those with MS (Table 2, $p = 0.005$). The mean Neer score in the varus malunion group (HSA < 120°) at the last follow-up was 73.6 ± 11.6, versus 84.2 ± 9.2 in the non-varus malunion group (HSA ≥ 120°) ($p < 0.001$, Fig. 4).

Linear regression showed that the Neer score was negatively associated with HSA change (R2 = 0.647, p < 0.001; Fig. 5). On univariate analyses, Neer type 4 fracture, the difference between the postoperative HSA (on the injured side) and that of the uninjured side (the ΔHSA), healing time, and the HSA change to the end of follow-up were all significantly associated with the Neer score (Table 3). On multivariate linear regression analysis, only healing time among the above four factors was excluded from the final model (R2 = 0.692, Table 4).

Table 1 Patient's demographic information

Total patients	122
Male	50
Female	72
Age (year)	61.1 ± 12.3
Fracture type	
two-part	44
three-part	58
four-part	20
Healing time (months)	4.4 ± 1.3
Follow-up time (months)	16.2 ± 3.2
Uninjured side HSA (°)	136.5 ± 4.8
Complications	
Reduction loss	18
Varus malunion	16
Subacromial impingement	2
Delayed union	4
Reoperation	2

HSA head-shaft angle

Discussion

HSA loss was maximal from 1 to 3 months postoperatively, in agreement with the literature [8, 17]. The average healing time was 4.4 months; the HSA remained essentially unchanged after 6 months. Of fractures that did not heal within 3 months, significant differences were evident between the HSA in the immediate postoperative phase and the values measured over 1–3 months. We suspected that this might reflect early voluntary exercise. Most patients could endure residual pain 1 month after surgery and, after 2 months of functional exercise, limb function partially recovered. Hence, some patients may have commenced internal forward rotation, and even stretching and weight-bearing activities. Muscle action during such exercises might change the HSA. In addition, the biomechanical stability of the proximal humerus may be compromised by fracture-healing during this period. Primitive bone callus formation varies among

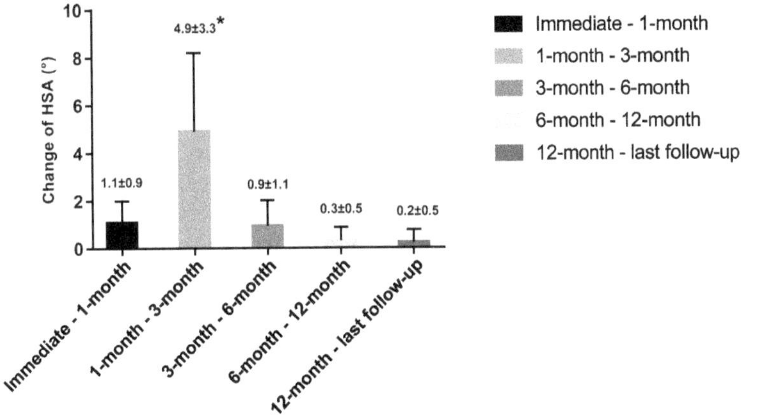

Fig. 2 The change of HSA in each follow-up period. HSA, head-shaft angle; * indicate that most decrease of HSA occurs in the period of 1 to 3 months ($p < 0.001$)

individuals; premature exercise may change the HSA but further research is required to confirm this.

The mean HSA of the with-MS group was significantly greater than that of the without-MS group at 3 months postoperatively ($p = 0.003$); MS was associated with less reduction loss. Overall, the reduction loss rate was significantly higher in the without-MS group ($p = 0.005$), consistent with other studies [18–20].Jung et al. [21] reported that inadequate MS was an independent risk factor for reduction loss after surgery to treat PHFs. In the absence of MS, the fixed-angle screws must serve as perpendicular struts aiding the humeral head to resist varus displacement. Therefore, MS is important for maintenance of reduction in patients with PHFs; surgeons must maximally restore MS.

Earlier studies on the functional and radiological outcomes of PHFs reached conflicting conclusions. Yüksel et al. [22] found no relationship between the HSA and the Constant score (which measures

Table 2 Comparison of head-shaft angle and clinical outcomes between patient with medial support and without medial support

		With MS	Without MS	*p* value
Mean HSA (°)	Immediate	135.6 ± 5.7	135.9 ± 5.0	0.752
	1-month	134.2 ± 5.8	135.0 ± 5.1	0.412
	3-month	127.9 ± 6.5	131.5 ± 6.7	0.003
	6-month	126.7 ± 6.3	130.7 ± 6.8	0.001
	12-month	126.4 ± 6.1	130.3 ± 6.7	< 0.001
	Last follow-up	126.2 ± 6.1	130.2 ± 6.9	0.001
Neer's criteria				0.056
	Excellent (> 89)	14	28	
	Satisfactory (80–89)	20	24	
	Unsatisfactory (70–79)	14	12	
	Failure (< 70)	10	0	
Neer's score		78.9 ± 11.6	86.3 ± 7.2	0.004
Complication				
	Reduction loss	14	4	0.005
	Varus malunion	10	6	0.199
	Subacromial impingement	0	2	0.175
	Delayed union	2	2	0.920
	Reoperation	2	0	0.134

HSA head-shaft angle, *MS* medial support

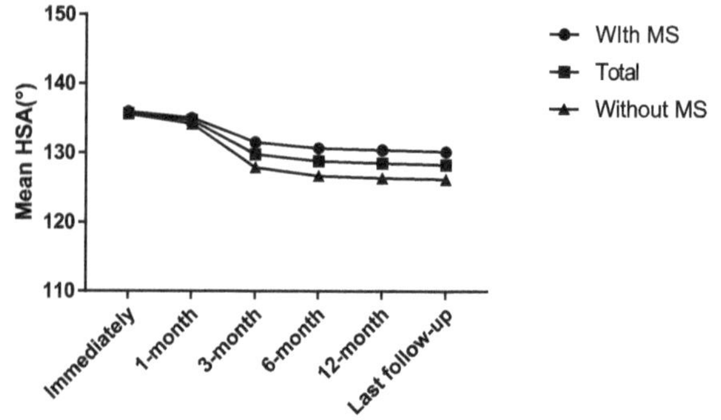

Fig. 3 The HSA trends during follow-up. HSA, head-shaft angle; MS, medial support

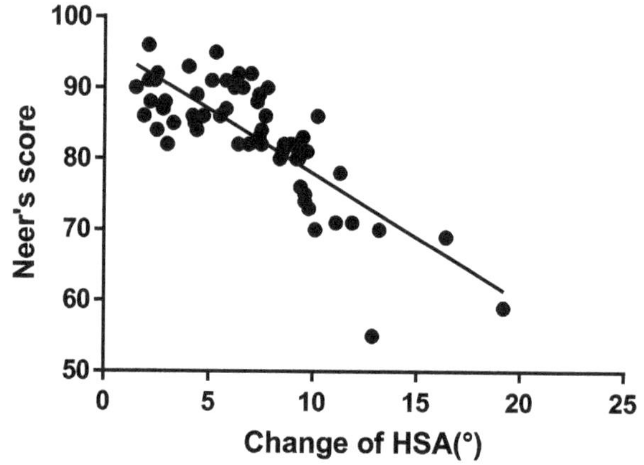

Fig. 5 Linear regression analysis of Neer's score and the HSA change to the end of follow-up. HSA, head-shaft angle

recovery); however, Bai et al. [23] reported that an HSA change > 10° significantly reduced the score. We investigated the relationship between the HSA and functional recovery in PHF patients in whom locking plates were placed and found that HSA change was negatively associated with recovery. Court-Brown et al. [24] found no association between increasing varus angulation and shoulder function; Capriccioso et al. [25] reported that the initial surgical neck displacement (varus or valgus) did not significantly affect functional outcomes. Conversely, 16 of our patients experienced varus malunion; their mean Neer score was 73.6 ± 11.6, thus lower than that of non-varus malunion patients (84.2 ± 9.2, $p < 0.001$). However, we would mention that three patients in the varus malunion group enjoyed excellent or satisfactory functional outcomes; all uninjured side HSAs were < 130°, and the Neer scores were 84, 92, and 83. A previous study found no significant between-group difference in bilateral HSAs [26].Therefore, we used multivariable linear regression to control for confounding effects; we found that Neer type 4 fracture, the postoperative HSA difference between the injured and uninjured side, and the change in HSA to completion of follow-up may influence the Neer score. Similarly, a previous study reported that, in patients with two- and three-part fractures, the overall functional results were usually satisfactory; but this was not always the case in those with four-part fractures [27, 28]. We suggest that the latter fractures usually develop in osteoporotic patients, often associated with proximal fractures and medial metaphyseal comminution [29].We found that the postoperative HSA difference between the treated and uninjured side, and the

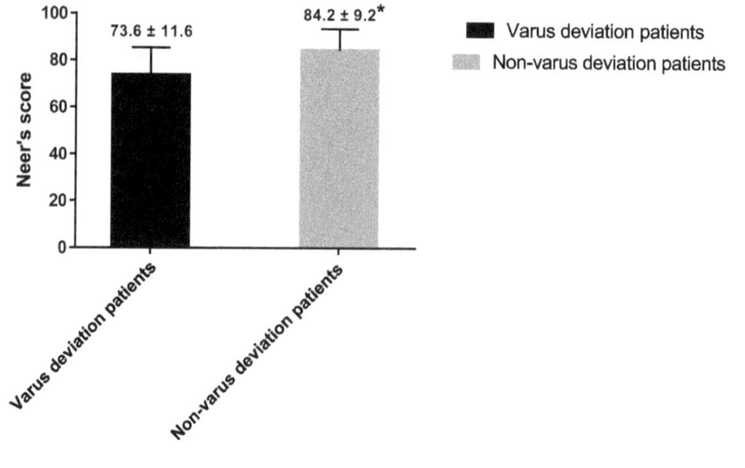

*, p<0.001.

Fig. 4 The mean Neer's score in varus malunion and non-varus malunion patients. *, $p < 0.001$

Table 3 Univariate association for each risk factor and Neer's score

Characteristics	RR (95% CI)	p value
Age (year)	0.08 (−0.04, 0.19)	0.212
Sex		
Female	Ref.	
Male	0.25 (−2.72, 3.22)	0.868
Fracture type		
2	Ref.	
3	2.42 (0.69, 5.52)	0.129
4	4.21 (2.32, 8.40)	0.041
Uninjured side HSA	0.10 (−0.21, 0.40)	0.535
Postoperative HSA	0.17 (−0.11, 0.44)	0.245
ΔHSA	−2.04 (−3.36, −0.71)	0.003
Healing time (month)	−1.54 (−2.61, −0.47)	0.005
Change of HSA	−1.80 (−2.04, −1.56)	< 0.001

HSA, head-shaft angle; ΔHSA, the difference between the postoperative HSA (on the injured side) and that of the uninjured side; Change of HSA, the HSA change to the end of follow-up

change in HSA to completion of follow-up, were negatively associated with the Neer score. Thus, restoration of the native HSA afforded better functional recovery. We identified a trend toward improved function when it was possible to restore the HSA of the injured side to a value similar to that of the uninjured side. Also, we could not rule out an effect of reduction loss in patients for whom the pre-injury HSA was < 130°.

Our study had certain limitations. First, it used a retrospective design and the sample size relatively small; we also cannot exclude potential effects of unmeasured factors. Furthermore, we prescribed a general postoperative rehabilitation protocol, but some patients may have individualised needs regarding the timing of passive range-of-motion exercises; this could affect the clinical and radiographic outcomes. A future prospective study with a larger sample size is required to validate our findings.

Table 4 Multivariable linear regression model for Neer's score

Characteristics	Coefficient	95% CI	p value
Fracture type 4	−4.31	−7.16, − 1.46	0.004
ΔHSA	−1.03	−1.84, −0.23	0.014
Healing time	0.08	−0.74, 0.89	0.857
Change of HSA	−1.70	−14.01, − 1.93	< 0.001

HSA, head-shaft angle; ΔHSA, the difference between the postoperative HSA (on the injured side) and that of the uninjured side; Change of HSA, the HSA change to the end of follow-up

Conclusions

Serial HSA changes were evident in PHF patients in whom locking plates had been inserted; it is essential to maintain reduction for 1–3 months postoperatively. MS is important in this context and surgeons must maximally restore MS. Furthermore, the functional outcome tended to improve when the HSA of the injured side was restored to a value close to that of the uninjured side.

Abbreviations

HSA: head-shaft angle; MS: medial support; PHF: Proximal humeral fracture; PHILO: The proximal humeral internal locking system; ΔHSA: the difference between the postoperative HSA (on the injured side) and that of the uninjured side

Acknowledgements

JQW and BJJ contributed equally to this work and should be considered co-first authors. We thank all the colleagues for their valuable assistance during the implementation of this study.

Funding

This study was funded by Natural Science Foundation of Zhejiang Province (LY15H060009). Natural Science Foundation of Zhejiang Province was involved in the study design, data collection, data analysis, and preparation of the manuscript.

Authors' contributions

YMZ: Study design, corresponding author; JQW: Analysis and interpretation of data, draft the manuscript; BJJ: Data collection and analysis; WJG: Supervise this study, critically revise the manuscript, and search the literature. All authors read and approved the final manuscript.

Consent for publication

Not applicable.

Competing interests

The authors declare that they have no competing interest.

References

1. Passaretti D, Candela V, Sessa P, Gumina S. Epidemiology of proximal humeral fractures: a detailed survey of 711 patients in a metropolitan area. J Shoulder Elb Surg. 2017;26(12):2117–24. https://doi.org/10.1016/j.jse.2017.05.029.
2. Hinds RM, Garner MR, Tran WH, Lazaro LE, Dines JS, Lorich DG. Geriatric proximal humeral fracture patients show similar clinical outcomes to non-geriatric patients after osteosynthesis with endosteal fibular strut allograft augmentation. J Shoulder Elb Surg. 2015;24(6):889–96. https://doi.org/10.1016/j.jse.2014.10.019.
3. Shulman BS, Egol KA. Open reduction internal fixation for proximal humerus fractures indications, techniques, and pitfalls. Bulletin of the Hospital for Joint Disease (2013). 2013;71(Suppl 2):54–9.
4. Jung WB, Moon ES, Kim SK, Kovacevic D, Kim MS. Does medial support decrease major complications of unstable proximal humerus fractures

treated with locking plate? BMC Musculoskelet Disord. 2013;14:102. https://doi.org/10.1186/1471-2474-14-102.
5. Gregory TM, Vandenbussche E, Augereau B. Surgical treatment of three and four-part proximal humeral fractures. Orthop Traumatol Surg Res. 2013;99(1 Suppl):S197–207. https://doi.org/10.1016/j.otsr.2012.12.006.
6. Clavert P, Adam P, Bevort A, Bonnomet F, Kempf JF. Pitfalls and complications with locking plate for proximal humerus fracture. J Shoulder Elb Surg. 2010;19(4):489–94. https://doi.org/10.1016/j.jse.2009.09.005.
7. Gonc U, Atabek M, Teker K, Tanriover A. Minimally invasive plate osteosynthesis with PHILOS plate for proximal humerus fractures. Acta Orthop Traumatol Turc. 2017;51(1):17–22. https://doi.org/10.1016/j.aott.2016.10.003.
8. Zhang L, Zheng J, Wang W, Lin G, Huang Y, Zheng J, Edem Prince GA, Yang G. The clinical benefit of medial support screws in locking plating of proximal humerus fractures: a prospective randomized study. Int Orthop. 2011;35(11):1655–61. https://doi.org/10.1007/s00264-011-1227-5.
9. Krappinger D, Bizzotto N, Riedmann S, Kammerlander C, Hengg C, Kralinger FS. Predicting failure after surgical fixation of proximal humerus fractures. Injury. 2011;42(11):1283–8. https://doi.org/10.1016/j.injury.2011.01.017.
10. Konigshausen M, Kubler L, Godry H, Citak M, Schildhauer TA, Seybold D. Clinical outcome and complications using a polyaxial locking plate in the treatment of displaced proximal humerus fractures. A reliable system? Injury. 2012;43(2):223–31. https://doi.org/10.1016/j.injury.2011.09.024.
11. Buchler P, Farron A. Benefits of an anatomical reconstruction of the humeral head during shoulder arthroplasty: a finite element analysis. Clinical biomechanics (Bristol, Avon). 2004;19(1):16–23.
12. Neer CS 2nd. Displaced proximal humeral fractures. I. Classification and evaluation. J Bone Joint Surg Am. 1970;52(6):1077–89.
13. Agudelo J, Schurmann M, Stahel P, Helwig P, Morgan SJ, Zechel W, Bahrs C, Parekh A, Ziran B, Williams A, Smith W. Analysis of efficacy and failure in proximal humerus fractures treated with locking plates. J Orthop Trauma. 2007;21(10):676–81. https://doi.org/10.1097/BOT.0b013e31815bb09d.
14. Greiner S, Kaab MJ, Haas NP, Bail HJ. Humeral head necrosis rate at mid-term follow-up after open reduction and angular stable plate fixation for proximal humeral fractures. Injury. 2009;40(2):186–91. https://doi.org/10.1016/j.injury.2008.05.030.
15. Owsley KC, Gorczyca JT. Fracture displacement and screw cutout after open reduction and locked plate fixation of proximal humeral fractures [corrected]. J Bone Joint Surg Am. 2008;90(2):233–40. https://doi.org/10.2106/jbjs.f.01351.
16. Neer CS 2nd. Four-segment classification of proximal humeral fractures: purpose and reliable use. J Shoulder Elb Surg. 2002;11(4):389–400. https://doi.org/10.1067/mse.2002.124346.
17. Pawaskar AC, Lee KW, Kim JM, Park JW, Aminata IW, Jung HJ, Chun JM, Jeon IH. Locking plate for proximal humeral fracture in the elderly population: serial change of neck shaft angle. Clin Orthop Surg. 2012;4(3):209–15. https://doi.org/10.4055/cios.2012.4.3.209.
18. Gardner MJ, Weil Y, Barker JU, Kelly BT, Helfet DL, Lorich DG. The importance of medial support in locked plating of proximal humerus fractures. J Orthop Trauma. 2007;21(3):185–91. https://doi.org/10.1097/BOT.0b013e3180333094.
19. Erdogan M, Desteli EE, Imren Y, Uzturk A, Kilic M, Sezgin H. The effect of inferomedial screw on postoperative shoulder function and mechanical alignment in proximal humerus fractures. Eur J Orthop Surg Traumatol. 2014;24(7):1055–9. https://doi.org/10.1007/s00590-013-1391-y.
20. Gadea F, Favard L, Boileau P, Cuny C, d'Ollone T, Saragaglia D, Sirveaux F. Fixation of 4-part fractures of the proximal humerus: can we identify radiological criteria that support locking plates or IM nailing? Comparative, retrospective study of 107 cases. Orthop Traumatol Surg Res. 2016;102(8):963–70. https://doi.org/10.1016/j.otsr.2016.09.015.
21. Jung SW, Shim SB, Kim HM, Lee JH, Lim HS. Factors that influence reduction loss in proximal Humerus fracture surgery. J Orthop Trauma. 2015;29(6):276–82. https://doi.org/10.1097/bot.0000000000000252.
22. Yuksel HY, Yilmaz S, Aksahin E, Celebi L, Muratli HH, Bicimoglu A. The results of nonoperative treatment for three- and four-part fractures of the proximal humerus in low-demand patients. J Orthop Trauma. 2011;25(10):588–95. https://doi.org/10.1097/BOT.0b013e318210ea56.
23. Bai L, Fu ZG, Wang TB, Chen JH, Zhang PX, Zhang DY, Jiang BG. Radiological evaluation of reduction loss in unstable proximal humeral fractures treated with locking plates. Orthop Traumatol Surg Res. 2014; 100(3):271–4. https://doi.org/10.1016/j.otsr.2013.12.024.
24. Court-Brown CM, McQueen MM. The impacted varus (A2.2) proximal humeral fracture: prediction of outcome and results of nonoperative treatment in 99 patients. Acta Orthop Scand. 2004;75(6):736–40.
25. Capriccioso CE, Zuckerman JD, Egol KA. Initial varus displacement of proximal humerus fractures results in similar function but higher complication rates. Injury. 2016;47(4):909–13. https://doi.org/10.1016/j.injury.2016.01.021.
26. Malavolta EA, Assuncao JH, Pagotto RA, Avelino RL, Gracitelli ME, Pereira CA, Jacomo AL, Ferreira Neto AA. The rotation of the humeral head does not alter radiographic evaluation of the head-shaft angle. J Shoulder Elb Surg. 2016;25(4):543–7. https://doi.org/10.1016/j.jse.2015.09.026.
27. Fankhauser F, Boldin C, Schippinger G, Haunschmid C, Szyszkowitz R. A new locking plate for unstable fractures of the proximal humerus. Clin Orthop Relat Res. 2005;430:176–81.
28. Thanasas C, Kontakis G, Angoules A, Limb D, Giannoudis P. Treatment of proximal humerus fractures with locking plates: a systematic review. J Shoulder Elb Surg. 2009;18(6):837–44. https://doi.org/10.1016/j.jse.2009.06.004.
29. Sohn HS, Shin SJ. Minimally invasive plate osteosynthesis for proximal humeral fractures: clinical and radiologic outcomes according to fracture type. J Shoulder Elb Surg. 2014;23(9):1334–40. https://doi.org/10.1016/j.jse.2013.12.018.

21

Polyaxial locking plates in treating distal humeral fractures

Moritz Crönlein[1], Martin Lucke[3], Marc Beirer[1], Dominik Pförringer[1], Chlodwig Kirchhoff[1], Peter Biberthaler[1], Karl F. Braun[1] and Sebastian Siebenlist[1,2*]

Abstract

Background: Management of distal humeral fractures remains to be one of the most challenging aspects in trauma surgery. Low profile plating systems with variable angle screw fixation represent a crucial advancement to the established angular stable locking plates with considerable attention in current research. The aim of the prospective randomized trial was to review the preliminary results and patients' outcome following treatment with these newly developed implants and to rule out potential differences in fracture treatment of two different plating systems.

Methods: Twenty patients with distal humeral fractures (AO 13-A1 – AO 13-C3) were included in the current study since 2014. After completing the randomization plan, patients were distributed into two groups for different variable angle locking plates (DePuy Synthes® VA-LCP vs. Medartis® Aptus Elbow). Functional elbow scoring (ROM, MEPS, QuickDASH) served as primary outcome parameter, while radiological fracture consolidation served as secondary outcome parameter. Follow-ups were conducted 6 weeks, 12 weeks, 6 months and 12 months after the operation.

Results: Seventeen of 20 patients (85%) concluded all follow-up examinations. Postoperative elbow extension deficiencies showed significant differences between the two groups in all follow-up examinations with a mean of Ø 18 +/− 7.4 degrees in the DePuy Synthes® VA-LCP group compared to a mean of Ø 6.5 +/− 7.5 degrees in the Medartis® Aptus Elbow group ($p = 0.002$) 12 months postoperatively. Functional scoring showed a disparate pattern. The Medartis® Aptus Elbow group achieved significantly better MEP scores during follow-up. However, the analysis of the QuickDash revealed better results of the DePuy Synthes® VA-LCP group in the first half and better results of the Medartis® Aptus Elbow group in the second half of the follow-up examination instead.

Conclusions: Considering the complexity of distal humeral fractures, the usage of anatomically preshaped low profile variable angle locking plates for operative treatment leads to good clinical results. Even though there might be some advances of the Medartis® Aptus Elbow plating system concerning postoperative ROM and elbow function, a consistent difference in the overall clinical outcome between the two plating systems could not be detected.

Keywords: Distal humeral fracture, Locking plate, Anatomical preshaped, Polyaxial, Outcome

* Correspondence: Sebastian.siebenlist@mri.tum.de
[1]Department of Trauma Surgery, Klinikum rechts der Isar, Technical University of Munich, Ismaninger Strasse 22, 81675 Munich, Germany
[2]Department of Orthopaedic Sports Medicine, Klinikum rechts der Isar, Technical University of Munich, Ismaninger Strasse 22, 81675 Munich, Germany
Full list of author information is available at the end of the article

Background

Distal humeral fractures are still very rare accounting for only 1–2% of all fractures [1]. Concerning the complex fracture pattern of these fractures together with the growing age of the patients, management remains to be one of the most challenging aspects in modern trauma surgery [2]. Dealing with these challenges, a large variety of different treatment options can be found in current literature, ranging from conservative treatment [3, 4] to different operative fixation techniques [5–8] up to total joint replacements [9].

The essential goal to achieve best results for patients suffering from distal humeral fractures is to restore joint congruency irrespective of patient's age. Considering that, conservative treatment frequently leads to a painful limited range of motion (ROM) quite often. Over the last decades, therefore, open reduction and internal fixation (ORIF) is known to be the treatment of choice [10]. Due to the importance of the distal humerus for elbow function and stability, new specific angular stable implant systems and innovative fixation techniques have been developed in the recent past [11]. Biomechanical analysis of angle stable locking plates already show promising results for fracture treatment especially in the osteoporotic bone [12]. As an advancement to the known angle stable locking plates where screws can only be placed in the predetermined direction, low profile plating systems with a variable angle for screw fixation gain considerable attention in current research. The usage of anatomically preshaped plates with variable possibilities for angular stable screw fixation already showed promising results in dealing with various complex fracture types like distal femur fractures [13], distal tibial fractures [14], distal radial fractures [15], clavicle fractures [16] or radial head fractures [15, 17]. However, little about these modern implants is known in terms of dealing with distal humeral fractures.

With the Medartis® Aptus Elbow distal Humerus Plates 2.8 (Medartis®, Basel, Switzerland) and the DePuy Synthes® VA-LCP distal Humerus Plates 2.7/3.5 (DePuy Synthes®, Umkirch, Germany), two modern plating systems have recently been introduced. Both plating systems consist of an anatomically preshaped low-profile design with variable angle for locking screw fixation and especially designed for fracture treatment of the distal humerus. Therefore, the aim of the present prospective randomized trial was to review the preliminary functional outcomes following treatment with these anatomically preshaped low-profile plating implants in the short-term and to rule out potential differences between both plating systems.

Methods

Patients

Before study initiation the approval of the local ethics committee of (Trial Number 253/14) was obtained. The comparative prospective randomized clinical trial included 20 patients with fractures of the distal humerus recruited from a level-one university trauma centre. Patient recruitment was conducted between 03/2014 and 12/2015. Fractures of the distal humerus, as defined by the AO classification system (AO 13-A1 – AO 13-C3), were included in this study as they were identified by the treating surgeon being applicable for locking plate treatment and after written informed consent of the patients was obtained. All patients were randomized following a randomization plan (Randlist®, DatInf GmbH, Tübingen, Germany) for either being treated with the DePuy Synthes® VA-LCP 2.7/3.5 mm (DePuy Synthes®, Umkirch, Germany) or with the Medartis® Aptus Elbow system 2.0/3.8 mm (Medartis®, Basel, Switzerland). Both include anatomically preshaped, polyaxial angular stable locking plates in various sizes. Angle stable screw positioning with the freedom of +/– 15° off-axis screw placement gives the surgeon a large variety in both systems.

The inclusion criteria involve all patients from the age of 18 to 95 years who suffered from a distal humeral fracture (AO 13-A1 – AO 13-C3) that had to undergo operative treatment. The exclusion criteria involve all under-aged patients (< 18 years), pregnant patients and patients with a mental disorder as well as patients under comprehensive legal support. In addition, pathological fractures had been excluded from the study.

Surgical technique

All patients were operated by consultant orthopaedic and trauma surgeons, experienced in upper extremity surgery. The mean interval between injury and operation was 2.4 days (range 0–12 days). General anaesthesia was used in all cases and a single dose of 1.5 mg cephalosporin was given preoperatively for prophylaxis. Patients were positioned in prone position with the injured arm on a radiolucent, small padded arm holder. Under tourniquet control, the posterior approach (Bryan-Morrey) to the distal humerus was performed in all cases. Additional olecranon osteotomy was performed in 7 cases (3× DePuy Synthes® vs. 4× Medartis® Aptus Elbow) presenting with AO type 13 C2 and AO type 13 C3 fractures. Postoperatively, physiotherapy was initiated using the same rehabilitation protocol for both groups. Passive and active assisted ROM was permitted immediately without limitations, while weight bearing was restricted for 6 weeks.

Follow-up evaluation

All patients were initially followed-up 6 weeks after operation. Additional follow-ups were performed 3, 6 and 12 months postoperatively. The follow-up examinations were carried out by an independent investigator not involved in patient's initial surgical treatment (MC) in the outpatient clinic of our level-one university trauma centre.

For the assessment of pain, the visual analogue scale (VAS), ranging from 0 "no pain" to 10 "worst imaginable pain" was documented. ROM and collateral ligament stability were registered on standardized scoring sheets. For subjective evaluation, patients rated their satisfaction for elbow use on a scale of 1 to 6 (1–highly satisfied; 2–satisfied; 3–moderate; 4–sufficient; 5–unsatisfied; 6-very unsatisfied). Moreover, sensomotoric disturbances and postoperative complications were recorded. Minor complications had been defined as complications that could be treated conservatively (e.g. superficial wound infections, delayed union etc.), whereas major complications needed operative revision (e.g. secondary loss of reduction, non-unions, severe wound infections etc.). For functional upper extremity and elbow scoring the shortened Disabilities of the Arm, Shoulder and Hand Score (QuickDASH) and the Mayo Elbow Performance Score (MEPS) were comprised. Postoperative x-rays were evaluated with special respect to bony healing, secondary loss of reduction and heterotopic ossifications.

Statistics

Statistical analyses were performed using the statistical software SigmaStat (version 3.5; Systat Software, San Jose, CA, USA). The scores at certain time points were compared with an independent t test after a normality check had been passed and equal variances had been detected. Normal distributed data with unequal variances would have been compared with Welch's t test. Arbitrarily data was tested with Mann-Whitney U test. The significance level was set at $p = 0.05$.

Results

Epidemiological data

Seventeen of 20 patients (85%) were able to conclude all follow up examinations (see Fig. 1). Three patients were lost to follow-up. One patient died 6 months postoperatively of unrelated cause to the surgery, the other two patients never returned for postoperative clinical and radiological control of unknown cause. These both patients also couldn't be found for follow-up survey. The remaining 17 patients presented with a mean age of 79 years (range 31–91 years) at the time of injury with no statistically differences between groups. Most common injury types were falls from less than three meters. Gender distribution showed differences with only 1 male patient compared to 16 female patients (see Table 1).

Clinical outcome

Clinical follow-up included documentation of swelling, redness, joint effusion, delay of wound healing, crepitation and muscular atrophy. At no timepoint during the follow-up survey any differences could be determined between the two groups concerning these clinical parameters. Even though pain levels of the DePuy Synthes® VA-LCP group turned out to be higher in all of the follow-up examinations, significant

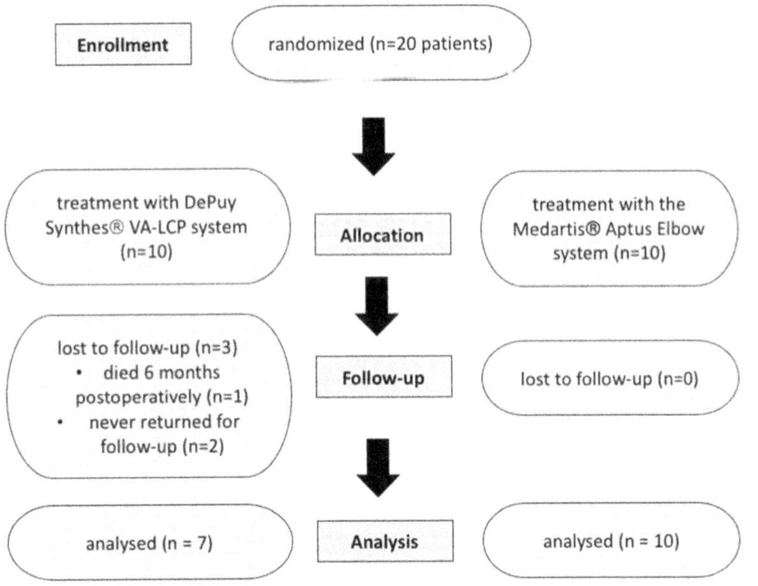

Fig. 1 Flow diagram of the progress through the phase of the prospective randomized trial

Table 1 A total of 17 patients, presenting with a distal humeral fracture (AO-type 13 A-C), were recruited to this prospective randomized trial, either being treated with DePuy Synthes® VA-LCP or Medartis® Aptus Elbow plating systems. There were no statistically significant differences in patients` demographics or injury characteristics between the groups

Characteristics	DePuy Synthes® VA-LCP	Medartis® Aptus Elbow
Mean age (years)	81	76
Sex (male: female)	0:7	1:9
AO classification		
13-A	2	1
13-B	0	0
13-C	5	9

differences could only be observed in the 6 weeks and 12 months follow-ups compared to the Medartis® Aptus Elbow group (see Table 2). Nerve injury had been detected in one patient with a partial sensomotoric palsy of the ulnar nerve, following ORIF of a comminuted AO type 13-C3 fracture using the DePuy Synthes® VA-LCP plating system (see Table 3). After neurolysis of the ulnar nerve the motoric palsy fully recovered whereas sensory ulnar nerve palsy remained.

Compared to the uninjured arm postoperative elbow extension deficiencies showed significant differences between both groups at every follow-up examination with a mean value of Ø 18 +/− 7.4 degrees in the DePuy Synthes® VA-LCP group compared to a mean value of Ø 6.5 +/− 7.5 degrees in the Medartis® Aptus Elbow group ($p = 0.002$) at 12 months postoperatively (see Fig. 2). For flexion and pronosupination no differences were seen between groups. Likewise, there were no signs of collateral ligament instability in both groups.

For subjective evaluation, patients rated their satisfaction for elbow use. Overall, 14 patients rated their satisfaction from very satisfied to sufficient (3× very satisfied, 6× satisfied, 4× moderate, 1× sufficient) and would undergo surgery again. The remaining three patients were not satisfied at time of last survey (2× Medartis® Aptus Elbow, 1× DePuy Synthes®). Differences between the two plating systems could not be detected for this subgroup analysis.

The elbow scoring showed a different result pattern for the QuickDash. In the first two clinical follow-ups (after 6 and 12 weeks) the DePuy Synthes® VA-LCP group showed better results than the Medartis® Aptus Elbow group, however not statistically significant. After 6 and 12 months on the other hand statistically significant better results were determined in the Medartis® Aptus Elbow group (see Table 2). The Medartis® Aptus Elbow group achieved significantly better MEP Scores in all of the postoperative follow-up examinations with good results 6 weeks postoperatively and excellent results 12 weeks, 6 months and 12 months

Table 2 Functional elbow scoring was assessed using MEPs and QuickDash Scores for each plating system (DePuy Synthes® vs. Medartis® Aptus Elbow) separately, 6 weeks, 12 weeks, 6 months and 12 months postoperatively.

Scoring System	Plating System	6 weeks	12 weeks	6 months	12 months
VAS	DePuy Synthes® VA-LCP	Ø 4.7 +/− 1.1	Ø 1.4 +/−0.8	Ø 3.5 +/− 1.7	Ø 2.3 +/− 1.8
	Medartis® Aptus Elbow	Ø 2,3 +/− 2.2	Ø 0.8 +/− 0.9	Ø 1.1 +/− 1.5	Ø 1 +/− 0.9
	p value	0.006	0.163	0.630	0.074
Quick Dash	DePuy Synthes® VA-LCP	Ø 69.5 +/− 13.1	Ø 19.5 +/− 10.5	Ø 56.4 +/− 15.6	Ø 57.2 +/− 16
	Medartis® Aptus Elbow	Ø 74.1 +/− 21.1	Ø 52.3 +/− 4.8	Ø 25.5 +/− 21.2	Ø 25.5 +/− 10.1
	p value	0.634	0.092	0.002	0.002
MEPS	DePuy Synthes® VA-LCP	Ø 53 +/− 5.2	Ø 80 +/− 10	Ø 74 +/− 12.1	Ø 75.7 +/− 12.1
	Medartis® Aptus Elbow	Ø 75 +/− 10	Ø 91.4 +/− 12.1	Ø 90.6 +/− 10.7	Ø 90.9 +/− 10.7
	p value	0.001	0.009	0.004	0.007

Results are given as Ø mean +/− standard deviation

Table 3 Overview of the complications following fracture treatment for each plating system (DePuy Synthes® vs. Medartis® Aptus Elbow)

Complication	DePuy Synthes® VA-LCP	Medartis® Aptus Elbow
Non-union	0	2
Secondary fracture dislocation	1	0
Nerve injuries	1	0
Infections	0	0
Heterotopic ossifications	1	1

postoperatively compared to the DePuy Synthes® VA-LCP group (see Table 2).

Radiological follow-up

Eleven fractures showed a fracture healing without complications at final follow-up of 12 months (4× DePuy Synthes® vs. 7 x Medartis® Aptus Elbow) (see Figs. 3 and 4). Non-unions were detected in two patients, both following treatment of an AO type 13 C3 fracture with the Medartis® Aptus Elbow system. One of them, a 74-year-old female suffering from multiple comorbidities (i.e. diabetes type 2, obesity, COPD), presented with a non-union which resulted in secondary plate loosening. The other patient, 68-year-old female, presented as a heavy smoker (>25 pack years) and a history of recurrent falls of unknown cause, following initial distal humeral plating. Both patients have been revised using allogenic bone grafts with subsequent osseous healing. A secondary loss of reduction was seen in one 80-year-old female patient following treatment with the DePuy Synthes®, VA-LCP system. Due to her age and comorbidities, elbow replacement after plate removal was performed 5 months after index operation. Heterotopic ossifications were seen in two patients, one of each treatment group (see Table 3). One of them, a 55-years-old female (Medartis® Aptus Elbow), had to be revised due to ROM deficiencies based on massive heterotopic ossifications 13 months following plate osteosynthesis. In the sequel, an open arthrolysis and implant removal was performed after fracture consolidation. According to medical records, this patient was satisfied with the postoperative result 6 months after implant removal and arthrolysis.

Discussion

A recent advance in the treatment of complex distal humeral fractures has been the introduction of anatomically preshaped, polyaxial angular stable locking plates [18–20]. Besides acting as internal fixators due to their locking fixation, screw positioning within a total range of up to 30° can be chosen, giving the surgeon a larger variety of screw placement [15]. The purpose of the present study therefore was to review the short-term results following treatment with these novel implants.

The most important finding was that usage of polyaxial angular stable plating systems leads to reliable results with good functional outcome in the majority of patients. Substantial differences between both evaluated plating systems could neither be detected for subjective evaluation nor for functional elbow scoring. Patients' satisfaction is directly constrained to elbow mobility. The postoperative ROM showed significant better results with decreased extension deficits in the Medartis® Aptus Elbow group compared to the DePuy Synthes® group (see Fig. 2). However, an overall extension deficit of 12.3° (see Fig. 2) 12 months after osteosynthesis was found for both groups which is sufficient to fulfil most of the personal daily routine activities (functional arc of elbow

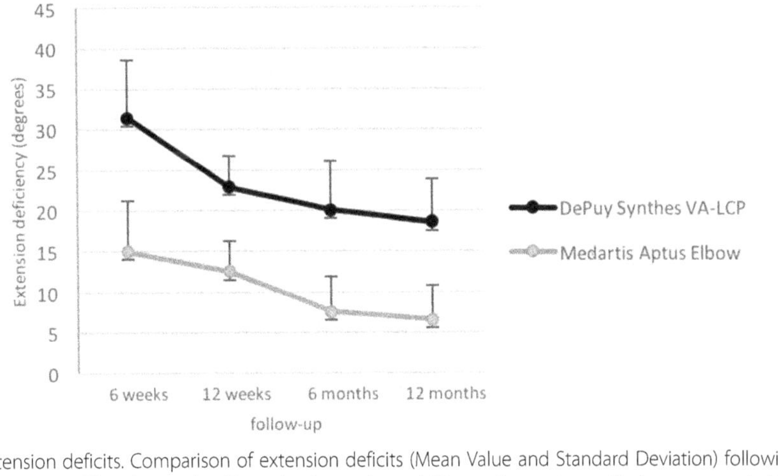

Fig. 2 Illustration of the extension deficits. Comparison of extension deficits (Mean Value and Standard Deviation) following distal humeral plating (DePuy Synthes® vs. Medartis® Aptus Elbow) 6 weeks, 12 weeks, 6 months and 12 months postoperatively are presented in this figure. At all times of follow-up evaluation, the extension deficits showed significant differences between the two groups ($p < 0.05$)

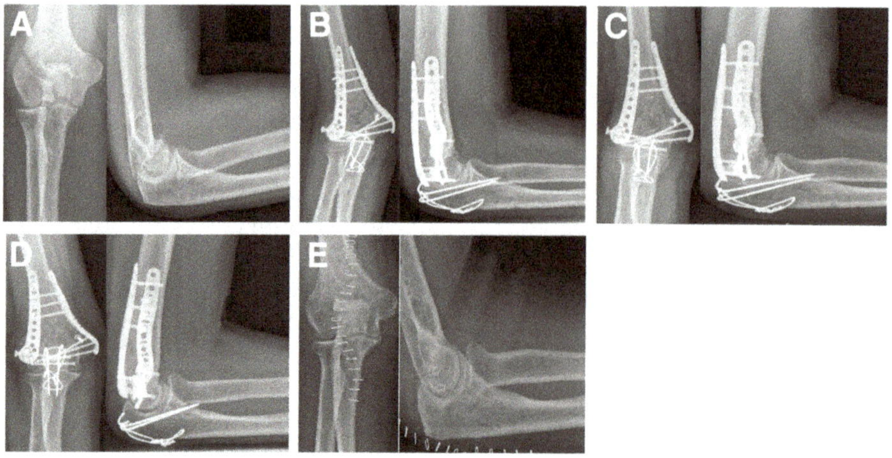

Fig. 3 ORIF of a distal humerus fracture (AO 13-C3) with the Medartis® Aptus Elbow System. Radiographs of a 55-year-old female patient with a AO type 13-C3 fracture resulting from a bicycle accident: preoperative x-rays (**a**), postoperative results, 6 weeks (**b**), 12 weeks (**c**) and 6 months (**d**) following Medartis® Aptus Elbow plating. Implant removal could be obtained after fracture consolidation (**e**)

motion according to BF Morrey) [10]. While both plating systems provide comparable implants in terms of diameter, length and material, there might be advantages in the plate design of the lateral Medartis® Aptus Elbow plates, which are twisted from distal lateral to proximal posterior for parallel plating in order to reduce soft tissue detachment during the operation and postoperative soft tissue irritation as well. This design feature might at least explain parts of the slightly higher postoperative ROM, even though not proven based on the present data. Obvious restrictions in the postoperative ROM or postoperative stiffness, however, defy explanation by implant size or configuration. Rather reasonable for postoperative stiffness in general, is the prolonged postoperative immobilization, often used to compensate inadequate fixation [21]. As another reason for postoperative stiffness, heterotopic ossifications or capsule adhesions are described with rates up to 8.6% in the current literature [22]. Two patients with extension deficiencies due to heterotopic ossifications were determined in our trial (see Table 3), with only one of them needing revision after fracture consolidation. In cases of major extension deficiencies open arthrolysis and implant removal is recommended [22], as we performed in

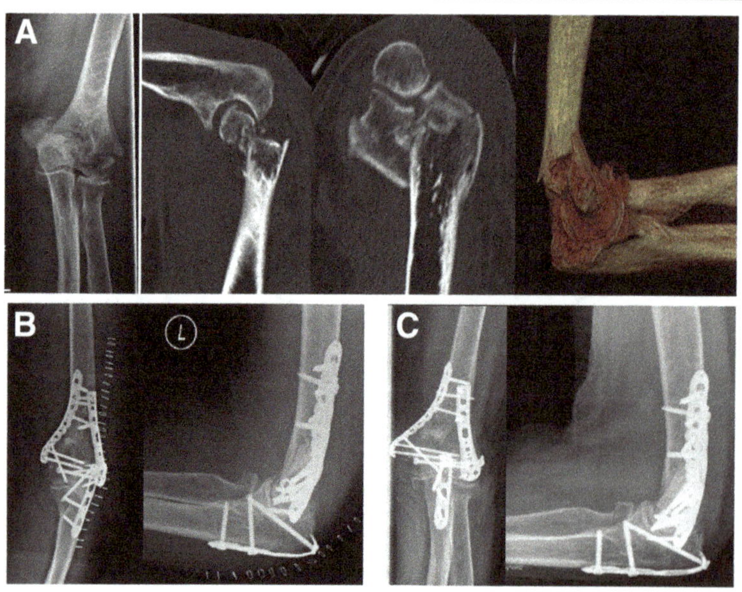

Fig. 4 ORIF of a distal humerus fracture (AO 13-C3) with the DePuy Synthes® VA-LCP System. Radiographs and CT Scans of a 82-year-old female patient with a AO type 13-C3 fracture resulting from a fall. Preoperative x-rays and CT Scans (**a**), postoperative results, 6 weeks (**b**) and 12 months (**c**) following DePuy Synthes® VA-LCP plating

our case with good clinical outcome. Postoperative Indomethacin therapy seems promising to prevent from heterotopic ossifications following ORIF of distal humeral fractures, though significant advantages are still missing in current literature [22]. In this survey no postoperative prophylaxis for heterotopic ossifications was performed. However, different plate configurations are not known to have an impact on postoperative heterotopic ossifications. Known risk factures are rather associated brain injury or delayed surgical treatment [22].

Knowing that bicolumnar plating is an effective and reliable method in treating complex distal humeral fractures [6, 23], there is little evidence of the ideal plate positioning [24, 25]. Especially the differences of orthogonal plating vs. parallel plating are discussed controversially in current literature. While few authors showed higher biomechanical stability following orthogonal (90°-90°) plating, especially in the osteoporotic bone [23, 26], other authors refer to higher stability rates following parallel plaiting [21, 27, 28]. Current biomechanical examinations of Kudo et al. [29], using the DePuy Synthes® VA-LCP system showed a higher rate of secondary displacement in the orthogonal plating orientation than in the parallel orientation. In matters of theses controversial studies we believe, according to the latest publication of Govindasamy et al. [25], that plate orientation should be chosen according to the fracture pattern, as both variants seem to provide enough stability to fix distal humerus fractures.

Besides the previously discussed plate positioning, screw orientation is known to influence fracture stability, with conventional angle stable locking systems providing higher stability especially against rotational failure than variable locking systems [30]. Highest stability in variable angle locking systems can be achieved inserting the screws perpendicular to the plate [30]. So, a higher variability in fragment fixation using variable plating systems, seems to be at the expense of stability. However, statistically significant differences in postoperative stability due to the used two different implant systems, with only one patient showing a secondary loss of reduction following treatment with the DePuy Synthes® VA-LCP and orthogonal plating position could not be detected in our study.

The complication rates in our study (see Table 3) are consistent with the rates described in the current literature, accounting up to 35% [19]. These high rates can be explained due to numerous reasons, such as the complexity of distal humerus fractures, the low amount of cancellous bone in the distal fragments and the tendency of the elbow joint to develop joint stiffness [10, 19, 31].

This study has several limitations, including the small number of only 17 examined patients at last follow-up survey and the disparity of both groups (7 patients DePuy Synthes® VA-LCP vs. 10 patients Medartis® Aptus Elbow). Due to the small number of patients, a differentiation between the treated fracture types and the used plate positioning (parallel plating vs. perpendicular plating) was not reasonable with respect to functional outcomes. Also, the influence of implant removal was not analysed. However, the presented follow-up rate of 85%, the wide assessment of functional parameters and the prospective randomized character certainly present the strengths of the present survey. To the best of our knowledge, moreover, this is the first randomized controlled trial to compare two modern polyaxial plating systems in distal humeral fracture treatment.

Conclusion

The usage of anatomically preshaped low profile locking plates in fracture treatment of distal humeral fractures leads to good clinical results. Even though there might be a trend of some advances of the Medartis® Aptus Elbow plating system concerning postoperative ROM and elbow scoring, a crucial difference in the overall clinical outcome between the two plating systems could not be detected in the short-term follow-up. Further trials with higher sample sizes are needed to prove the advantages of these novel implant systems in the treatment of these challenging fractures.

To sum up, successful management of distal humerus fractures is essentially constrained to a correct fracture reduction, a sufficient reconstruction of the articular surface and a high primary stability for early functional rehabilitation.

Abbreviations

MEPS: Mayo elbow performance score; ORIF: Open reduction internal fixation; QuickDASH: Disabilities of the arm, shoulder and hand score; ROM: Range of motion; VAS: Visual analogue scale

Acknowledgments

We thank Fritz Seidl, M.A. Interpreting and Translating, for professional language editing.

Funding

No funding was obtained for this study.

Authors' contributions

MC, ML and SS were substantially involved in conception and design of the study. MC and DP carried out patients evaluation and drafted the manuscript. KFB and MB assisted in the literature research and performed the statistical analysis. PB, SS and CK participated in the design of the study, helped to draft the manuscript and noted critical revisions of the manuscript for important intellectual content. All authors read and approved the final manuscript.

Consent for publication
Written informed consent for publication was obtained from all participants.

Competing interests
Marc Beirer, MD, is a member of the Editorial Board of BMC Musculoskeletal Disorders.
The authors declare that there are no financial or personal conflicts of interests that could have influenced this work.

Author details
[1]Department of Trauma Surgery, Klinikum rechts der Isar, Technical University of Munich, Ismaninger Strasse 22, 81675 Munich, Germany. [2]Department of Orthopaedic Sports Medicine, Klinikum rechts der Isar, Technical University of Munich, Ismaninger Strasse 22, 81675 Munich, Germany. [3]Department of Trauma Surgery, Chirurgisches Klinikum München Süd, Am Isarkanal 30, 81379 Munich, Germany.

References

1. Bonnaire F, Bula P. Distale Humerusfrakturen. Trauma Berufskr. 2010;12(S2): 96–103.
2. Charissoux JL, Vergnenegre G, Pelissier M, Fabre T, Mansat P. Sofcot: epidemiology of distal humerus fractures in the elderly. Orthop Traumatol Surg Res. 2013;99(7):765–9.
3. Pidhorz L, Alligand-Perrin P, De Keating E, Fabre T, Mansat P. Societe francaise de chirurgie orthopedique et t: distal humerus fracture in the elderly: does conservative treatment still have a role? Orthop Traumatol Surg Res. 2013;99(8):903–7.
4. Ring D, Waters P. Operative fixation of Monteggia fractures in children. J Bone Joint Surg Br. 1996;78(5):734–9.
5. Zogbi DR, Terrivel AM, Mouraria GG, Mongon ML, Kikuta FK, Filho AZ. Fracture of distal humerus: MIPO technique with visualization of the radial nerve. Acta Ortop Bras. 2014;22(6):300–3.
6. Jung SW, Kang SH, Jeong M, Lim HS. Triangular fixation technique for Bicolumn restoration in treatment of distal Humerus Intercondylar fracture. Clin Orthop Surg. 2016;8(1):9–18.
7. Munde SL, Bhatti MJ, Siwach RC, Gulia A, Kundu ZS, Bansal S, Middha S, Kamra HT. Double tension band Osteosynthesis in inter-Condylar humeral fractures. J Clin Diagn Res. 2015;9(12):RC08–11.
8. Park JS, Kim YT, Choi SJ. Crisscross-type screw fixation for transcondylar fractures of distal humerus in elderly patients. Arch Orthop Trauma Surg. 2015;135(1):1–7.
9. Pooley J, Salvador Carreno J. Total elbow joint replacement for fractures in the elderly-functional and radiological outcomes. Injury. 2015; 46(Suppl 5):S37–42.
10. Schmidt-Horlohe K, Siebenlist S, Stockle U, Hoffmann R. Distal humeri fractures. Z Orthop Unfall. 2011;149(1):95–108. quiz 109-110
11. Amir S, Jannis S, Daniel R. Distal humerus fractures: a review of current therapy concepts. Curr Rev Musculoskelet Med. 2016;9(2):199–206.
12. Korner J, Diederichs G, Arzdorf M, Lill H, Josten C, Schneider E, Linke B. A biomechanical evaluation of methods of distal humerus fracture fixation using locking compression plates versus conventional reconstruction plates. J Orthop Trauma. 2004;18(5):286–93.
13. El-Zayat BF, Efe T, Ruchholtz S, Khatib S, Timmesfeld N, Krüger A, Zettl R. Mono- versus polyaxial locking plates in distal femur fractures – a biomechanical comparison of the non-contact-bridging- (NCB) and the PERILOC-plate. BMC Musculoskelet Disord. 2014;15(369):369-76.
14. Yenna ZC, Bhadra AK, Ojike NI, Burden RL, Voor MJ, Roberts CS. Polyaxial screws in locked plating of Tibial Pilon fractures. Orthopedics. 2015;38(8):e663–7.
15. Mehling I, Scheifl R, Mehler D, Klitscher D, Hely H, Rommens PM. Are there any differences in various polyaxial locking systems? A mechanical study of different locking screws in multidirectional angular stable distal radius plates. Biomed Tech (Berl). 2013;58(2):187–94.
16. van Olden GDJ. VA-LCP anterior clavicle plate: the anatomically precontoured fixation system with angular stability for clavicle shaft. Musculoskelet Surg. 2014;98(3):217–23.
17. Crönlein M, Zyskowski M, Beirer M, Imhoff FB, Pforringer D, Sandmann GH, Kirchhoff C, Biberthaler P, Siebenlist S. Using an anatomically preshaped low-profile locking plate system leads to reliable results in comminuted radial head fractures. Arch Orthop Trauma Surg. 2017;137(6):789-95.
18. Hanschen M, Aschenbrenner IM, Fehske K, Kirchhoff S, Keil L, Holzapfel BM, Winkler S, Fuechtmeier B, Neugebauer R, Luehrs S, et al. Mono- versus polyaxial locking plates in distal femur fractures: a prospective randomized multicentre clinical trial. Int Orthop. 2014;38(4):857–63.
19. Greiner S, Haas NP, Bail HJ. Outcome after open reduction and angular stable internal fixation for supra-intercondylar fractures of the distal humerus: preliminary results with the LCP distal humerus system. Arch Orthop Trauma Surg. 2008;128(7):723–9.
20. Chen H, Li D, Zhang J, Xiong X. Comparison of treatments in patients with distal humerus intercondylar fracture: a systematic review and meta-analysis. Ann Med. 2017;49(7):1–13.
21. O'Driscoll SW. Optimizing stability in distal humeral fracture fixation. J Shoulder Elb Surg. 2005;14(1 Suppl S):186S–94S.
22. Begue T. Articular fractures of the distal humerus. Orthop Traumatol Surg Res. 2014;100(1 Suppl):S55–63.
23. Leigey DF, Farrell DJ, Siska PA, Tarkin IS. Bicolumnar 90-90 plating of low-energy distal humeral fractures in the elderly patient. Geriatr Orthop Surg Rehabil. 2014;5(3):122–6.
24. Abzug JM, Dantuluri PK. Use of orthogonal or parallel plating techniques to treat distal humerus fractures. Hand Clin. 2010;26(3):411–21. vii
25. Govindasamy R, Shekhawat V, Banshiwal RC, Verma RK. Clinico-radiological outcome analysis of parallel plating with perpendicular plating in distal humeral intra-articular fractures: prospective randomised study. J Clin Diagn Res. 2017;11(2):RC13–6.
26. Gerich TG. Intra-articular fractures of the distal humerus : aspects of fracture treatment in geriatric patients. Orthopade. 2014;43(4):347–52.
27. Stoffel K, Cunneen S, Morgan R, Nicholls R, Stachowiak G. Comparative stability of perpendicular versus parallel double-locking plating systems in osteoporotic comminuted distal humerus fractures. J Orthop Res. 2008;26(6):778–84.
28. Arnander M, Reeves A, MacLeod IA, Pinto T, Khaleel A. A biomechanical comparison of plate configuration in distal humerus fractures. J Orthop Trauma. 2008;22(5):332–6.
29. Kudo T, Hara A, Iwase H, Ichihara S, Nagao M, Maruyama Y, Kaneko K. Biomechanical properties of orthogonal plate configuration versus parallel plate configuration using the same locking plate system for intra-articular distal humeral fractures under radial or ulnar column axial load. Injury. 2016; 47(10):2071-6.
30. Tidwell JE, Roush EP, Ondeck CL, Kunselman AR, Reid JS, Lewis GS. The biomechanical cost of variable angle locking screws. Injury. 2016; 47(8):1624–30.
31. Fan D, Wang W, Hildebrand KA, Fan CY. Open arthrolysis for elbow stiffness increases carrying angle but has no impact on functional recovery. BMC Musculoskelet Disord. 2016;17(1):388.

Above-versus below-elbow casting for conservative treatment of distal radius fractures

Aldo Okamura[1*], Gabriel Maciel de Mendonça[1], Jorge Raduan Neto[2], Vinicius Ynoe de Moraes[2], Flavio Faloppa[2] and João Carlos Belloti[2]

Abstract

Background: A variety of cast options are available for the non-surgical treatment of distal radius fractures (DRF) in adults. However, the literature is inconclusive regarding the need to immobilize the elbow joint after reduction in order to prevent rotation of the forearm in order to maintain the reduction of DRF. This study aimed to evaluate the best method of immobilization between above-elbow (AE) and below-elbow (BE) cast groups at the end of six-month follow-up.

Methods: This is a randomized clinical trial with parallel groups and a blinded evaluator. There are two non-surgical interventions: AE and BE. Patients will be randomly assigned. A hundred twenty eight consecutive adult patients with acute (up to 7 days) displaced DRF of type A2, A3, C1, C2 or C3 by the Arbeitsgemeinschaft für Osteosynthesefragen (AO) classification will be included. The primary outcome will be the maintenance of reduction by evaluation of radiographic parameters and Disabilities of the Arm, Shoulder and Hand Questionnaire (DASH). Secondary outcomes include function measured by Patient Rated Wrist Evaluation (PRWE), pain measured by the Visual Analogue Scale (VAS), objective functional evaluation (goniometry and dynamometry) and rate of complications. Evaluations will be performed at 1, 2, 3, 4, 6, 8, 12 and 24 weeks. For the Student's t-test, a difference of 10 points in DASH score, with 95% confidence interval, a statistical power of 95%, and 20% sampling error. We consider an extra 10% for balancing follow up losses results in 64 patients per group.

Discussion: Results from this study protocol will help to define the need for elbow immobilization in maintenance of reduction, as well as functional performance of below elbow cast versus above elbow cast immobilization during the immobilization period.

Keywords: Distal radius fracture, Conservative treatment, Treatment outcome, Randomized, Prospective

* Correspondence: aldookamura@gmail.com
[1]Hospital Municipal do Campo Limpo Dr. Fernando Mauro Pires da Rocha, Estrada de Itapecerica, 1661 - Campo Limpo, São Paulo, SP 05835-005, Brazil
Full list of author information is available at the end of the article

Background

Although distal radius fractures (DRF) are among the most frequent of the upper limb [1], the best method of treatment and outcome of these fractures has not yet been fully defined [2, 3]. Regarding non-surgical treatment, Cochrane review based on randomized controlled trials has concluded there are controversial in terms of the type of casting to be applied after the initial fracture reduction and there is no conclusive evidence of difference in outcome between different positions and methods of plaster and brace management for the common types of DRF [4–6].

Below-elbow (BE) splinting is easier to apply, is lower in cost, lighter, provides greater comfort, better function for daily life activities and less articular stiffness of the elbow [7–9]. Casts that include the elbow joint, which prevents the rotation of the forearm, may result in greater stability of the fracture and less risk of loss of reduction and need for re-reduction [10–12]. Other studies found similar results between immobilization methods in maintaining the initial fracture reduction [13, 14].

This study is based on the hypothesis that above-elbow (AE) splint immobilization in patients with DRF will present better results for loss of reduction and radiographic parameters, but more complication rate and worse functional outcomes when compared to below-elbow (BE) immobilization methods at the end of a six-month follow-up.

Methods/design

Aim

To determine the best method of immobilization in patients with distal radius fractures at the end of a six-months: below-elbow versus above-elbow cast.

Design and setting

Randomized controlled trial developed at Federal University of São Paulo - UNIFESP and Hospital Municipal Dr. Fernando Mauro Pires da Rocha - SP.

Participant characteristics

Adults with growth plate closure, both genders, with unilateral and closed acute displaced DRF (up to 1 week), associated or not with the ulnar styloid fractures with no other fractures, which may be closed reduced and meet inclusion criteria (Fig. 1).

Inclusion criteria

Displaced and reducible fractures classified by AO as type A2, A3, C1, C2 and C3 will be included if one of these conditions is present.

- Radial height – loss >2 mm [15–19].
- Radial Inclination - loss >4° [17, 20, 21].
- Dorsal angulation >10° [5, 18, 20].
- Positive ulnar variance – loss >3 mm [19–21].
- Intra-articular step off or gap – >2 mm [5, 19, 22].
- Carpal malalignment [19, 23].

The contralateral side is used as a reference.

Exclusion criteria

Patients presenting one or more of the following criteria will be excluded from this study:

- Open fractures, bilateral fracture or associated with tendon or neurovascular lesions.
- Associated carpal fractures.
- Marginal fractures or fractures from shearing mechanism.
- Fractures with palmar deviation (Smith's fracture).
- Irreducible fractures (closed method).
- Prior history of a degenerative or traumatic disorder of the affected or contralateral wrist joint.
- Systemic diseases or traumatic lesions associated with fracture that restrict the application of methods or the evaluation of results.
- Cognitive deficit that does not allow the patient to understand the elements of the functional evaluation.
- Consent Form Refusal.

Radiological measurements

The volar tilt, the radial inclination, the radial height, the ulnar variance and the intra-articular step off or gap were determined on posteroanterior (PA) and lateral (L) radiographs views obtained using a standardised procedure [24].

The standard method of obtaining a PA radiograph is with the shoulder in 90° of abduction, the elbow in 90° of flexion and the wrist in a neutral position. For the lateral view, the shoulder is adducted and the elbow is in 90° of flexion with the hand positioned in the same plane as the humerus [19].

The volar tilt, also called palmar tilt is measured on the lateral view and refers to the distance between a line through the dorsal and palmar boundary points of the radial joint surface and the perpendicular to the longitudinal axis of the radial shaft.

The radial inclination, also know as radial deviation is measured on the PA view and refers to the distance between a line through the radial and ulnar boundaries of the radial joint surface and the perpendicular to the longitudinal axis of the radial shaft.

The radial height, also called radial lenght is measured on the PA view and refers to the difference in axial direction of the radius between the distal tip of the radial styloid and the most distal aspect of the ulnar articular surface.

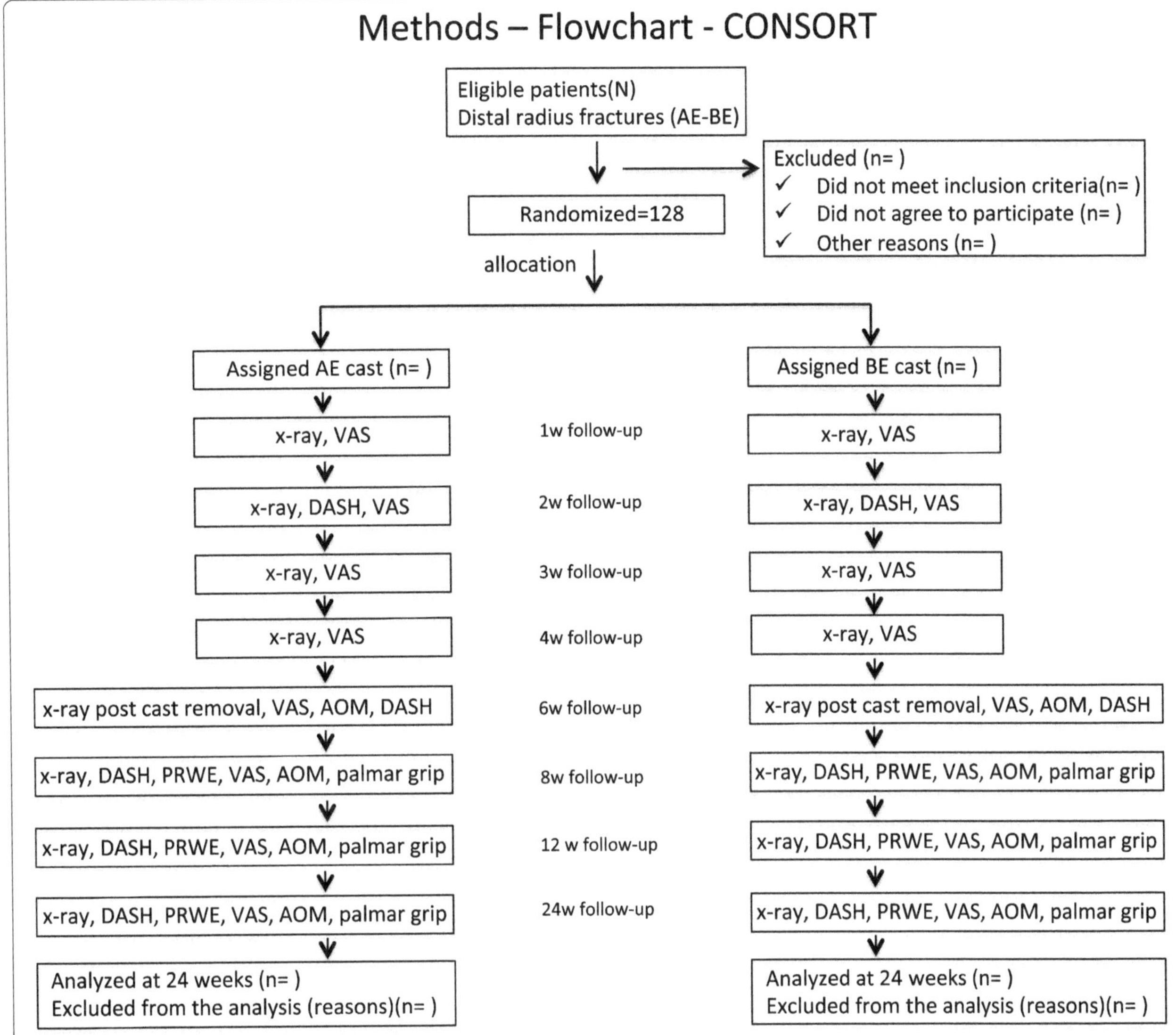

Fig. 1 Flowchart of patients included in this study

The ulnar variance, also called the radioulnar index is measured on the PA view and refers to the vertical distance between a line parallel to the medial corner of the articular surface of the radius and a line parallel to the most distal point of the articular surface of the ulnar head, both of which are perpendicular to the long axis of the radius.

The intra-articular step off or gap is measured on PA or lateral view and refers articular incongruity.

The carpal alignment is measured on lateral view. Two lines are drawn, one along the long axis of the capitate and other along the long axis of the radius. The lines do intersect within the carpus.

Initial treatment

All the patients with a distal radius fracture who arrive at the emergency room will undergo a standard protocol with clinical and radiographic examination (bilateral x-rays of the wrist in PA and lateral views). After applying the inclusion and exclusion criteria, eligible individuals will be informed about the nature and purpose of the study, by reading the "Consent Form" and after signing it they will be included. On a pre-scheduled date (up to 7 days), the study participant will be referred to the main operating room to be anesthezied before closed reduction of the fracture under radioscopy control. The reducibility criteria will be evaluated and patients that have reducible fracture will be randomized and treated by one of the two methods of the study (Fig. 2). Patients that do not have closed reducible fracture will be excluded from the study and will receive surgical treatment (open reduction and internal fixation) on a date to be scheduled.

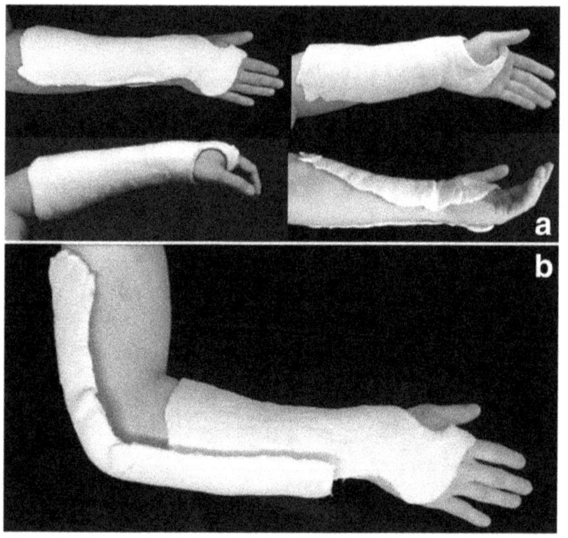

Fig. 2 Types of immobilization. Below-elbow cast (**a**). Above-elbow cast (**b**)

Anesthesia

Intravenous anesthesia will be performed by aseptic technique. A simple bolus injection with Propofol (infusion rate 180 mcg.kg^{-1}.min^{-1}) in combination with opioid (fentanyl 5–10 mcg.kg^{-1}) adjusted to the individual needs of each patient and repeated as many times as necessary according to the anesthesiologist's criteria [25, 26].

Method for closed reduction and immobilization

The patient will be submitted to the closed reduction of the fracture through a traction and counter-traction technique. Materials needed for application of the two splinting techniques will be available in the operating room. Initially, all patients will receive a short radial splint that will be performed with a 20 cm wide gypsum cut to fit the thumb (Fig. 2a). The splint will be applied to the radial aspect of the wrist covering the volar and dorsal portion of the radius to the elbow. The splint will be moulded with three point fixation as described by Charnley [27]. The three points will be defined after a metal pointer will be placed beside the limb to identify the site of fracture by using the image intensification. Patients randomized to the above-elbow splint will receive a complementation of immobilization with a 15 cm width splint on the ulnar aspect of the forearm that begins at the middle of the forearm and extends into the armpit. The elbow will be immobilized at 90 degrees, and in a neutral position to block pronosupination (Fig. 2b). Cotton tubular mesh, cotton stripes and crepe bandage will be used in both bindings. Regardless of the immobilization adopted, all wrists will be positioned with slight flexion and ulnar deviation. Patients will be encouraged to actively move their fingers and the ipsilateral shoulder.

Patients with above-elbow immobilization will remain for 4 weeks with the splint followed by 2 weeks of below-elbow immobilization. The immobilization will be removed after 6 weeks.

Clinical outcomes

The self-reported functional evaluation DASH and PRWE, visual analogue pain scale (VAS), radiographic measures, objective functional evaluation will be performed by independent evaluators at intervals provided in Table 1. For the outcomes at 8,12 and 24 weeks the evaluators will be blinded to the patient assignment groups. The minimum clinical follow-up will be 24 weeks, with the following parameters being considered to evaluate the results:

Primary outcomes

Radiographic parameters

Maintenance of reduction by evaluation wrist radiographs in PA and lateral x-rays at the following intervals: one, two, three, four, six, eight, twelve and twenty-four weeks after fracture reduction.

The radial height, radial inclination, volar tilt, ulnar variance, intra-articular step off or gap and carpal alignment will be used to determine maintenance of reduction at every follow-up visit. Measurements will be made on the radiographs with a marker, straight edge, and protractor by two researchers independently on different occasions.

We will consider maintenance of reduction if:

- loss of reduction ≤2 mm in radial height
- loss of reduction ≤4 degrees in radial inclination
- dorsal angulation ≤10°
- ≤ 2 mm intra-articular step off
- positive ulnar variance ≤3 mm
- any carpal malalignment.

The contralateral side is used as a reference.

Patient-reported functional outcomes

Functional status will be evaluated by means of DASH questionnaire (validated for the Portuguese language) at the following intervals: two, six, eight, twelve and twenty-four weeks after fracture reduction [28]. The

Table 1 Outcomes and measurement time

	1 W	2 W	3 W	4 W	6 W	8 W	12 W	24 W
X rays	x	x	x	x	x	x	x	x
DASH		x			x	x	x	x
PRWE						x	x	x
VAS	x	x	x	x	x	x	x	x
AOM					x	x	x	x
Palmar Grip						x	x	x

DASH was developed as an instrument for patients with upper-extremity injuries. The survey contains 30 questions related to the function of the hand, wrist, elbow, and shoulder based on the conditions to do certain activities in the past week, so the evaluations refer only after the beginning of the immobilization.

Secondary outcomes

Patient Rated Wrist Evaluation – PRWE; [29] Pain (VAS - Visual Analogue Pain Scale); [30, 31] Objective functional evaluation (goniometry and dynamometry); and rate of complications and failures.

The PRWE score (validated for the Portuguese language) will be obtained at eight, twelve and twenty-four weeks. The PRWE contains 15 items that are specific to determining the degree of musculoskeletal disability related to the wrist [29].

Pain in the wrist, elbow and shoulder will be measured separately in all visits at one, two, three, four, six, eight, twelve and twenty-four weeks after fracture reduction by the Visual Analogue Pain Scale (VAS). This is a unidimensional measure of pain intensity, which has been widely used in diverse adult populations [30]. Pain in VAS is a continuous scale comprised of a horizontal line of 10 cm (100 mm) in length, anchored by two verbal descriptors, one for each symptom extreme by "no pain" (score of 0) and "pain as bad as it could be" or "worst imaginable pain" (score of 100). Participants are asked to report pain intensity in the last 24 h. The respondent is asked to place a line perpendicular to the VAS line at the point that represents their pain intensity. Using a ruler, the score is determined by measuring the distance (mm) on the 100 mm line between the "no pain" anchor and the patient's mark, providing a range of scores from 0 to 100 [31].

Objective functional evaluation

Arcs of motion will be measurement for the wrist, and a goniometer will be employed to measure wrist flexion, extension, ulnar deviation, radial deviation and pronosupination at the six, eight, twelve and twenty-four week follow up visit. The flexion–extension of the elbow will be measurement at six, eight, twelve and twenty-four week follow-up visit.

Palmar grip strength with a digital dynamometer (Jamar Plus - Hand Dynamometer), at the following moments of treatment evolution: eight, twelve and twenty-four week follow-up visit.

Complications

Any clinical situation requiring treatment (clinical or surgical procedure) not provided in the protocol will be considered as a complication. All complications will be recorded for further stratification into major and minor complications.

In cases where there is loss of reduction, patients will be informed and surgical treatment indicated.

Statistical methods

Descriptive data will be exposed as means or proportions followed by standard deviations or 95% confidence intervals. As a method to confirm the effectiveness of the randomization, baseline data will be compared in the two groups of comparison. To ensure the normal distribution of data, we will use visual analysis and Shapiro-wilk test.

For comparison between proportions, we will consider Pearson's chi-square test. For continuous data, we will use Student T test. Intra-group comparison (1, 2, 3, 4, 6, 8, 12 and 24 weeks) will be analyzed by paired Student T test or Wilcoxon (if data is not normally distributed). We will consider as significant when alpha $< 0{,}05$. To analyze the occurrence of complication after treatment, we intend to perform survival analysis associated with Kaplan-Meier curves, if we find greater than 20% complication in any of the comparison groups. All statistical analysis will be performed following intention to treat principle. Statistical advisors will be blinded to the treatment groups as an effort to decrease bias.

Randomization and masking

Patients will be randomly assigned using randomization software (available at: http://www.randomizer.org). The allocation of patients in the AE or BE groups will be performed using opaque envelopes numbered on their outer face with consecutive numbers (concealment). Additionally, the envelope will be opened only in the operating room after verification of fracture reducibility and the procedure will be delegated to a person who is not directly connected to the study.

Sample size calculation

Based on data derived from one recent randomized clinical trial on the subject [32]. We considered as relevant differences on DASH scores (clinically relevant) when scores are greater than 10 points and standard deviation 15 points [33]. To detect this difference (Student T-test) and statistical power of 95% resulted in a 58 patient sample size per group. We considered an extra 10% for balancing follow up losses. Thus, our inclusion target will be 64 patients per group. We considered the test as bicaudal.

Discussion

This publication presents a randomized clinical trial of the non-operative treatment of DRF. Casts may be applied either "above elbow" or "below elbow", depending on the particular type of injury and physician preference. Often, the plaster may extend above the elbow to help provide additional stability and neutralize the extensive forces that can be generated by natural movements of the arm and forearm. Above-elbow immobilization is the conservative treatment used by most of the Brazilian orthopedic surgeons (74%) [34].

Short arm immobilization has been used by many orthopedic surgeons around the world, who claimed equally beneficial results [8, 13]. Hence, controversy still persists regarding the length of the immobilization for the treatment of DRF [4, 5].

The value of the study includes all participants will be reduced in the main operating room under general intravenous anesthesia and with the aid of radioscopy which will allow better control of the pain and maximum quality in the reduction. All reductions and immobilizations will be performed by a single researcher, specialist in hand surgery. The follow up during the immobilization period will be weekly, with radiographic documentation, which allows the early identification of the reduction loss. This is the only trial to apply DASH questionnaire at the beginning and end of immobilization period (2 and 6 weeks) to compare the groups. Pain in the wrist, elbow and shoulder will be measured separately in all visits to verify the influence of immobilization on the elbow and shoulder joints. Adults of all ages will be evaluated, it is known that the DRF in the elderly has different behavior and prognosis when compared to the young [35–38]. Randomization will equalize the distribution homogeneously between the groups, allowing the sample to be faithful to the population.

Our study has several strengths and limitations. Weekly assessments increase the chance of follow-up loss, however a strict control will be adopted. The study presents limitations because the database was constructed based on measurements of X-ray films calculated manually with goniometer and pen, which may imply in unmeasured tolerance limits. To minimize this, the measurements were performed by two senior researchers independently at different times. All patients in this study will be users of the public health system, many of them may have difficulty responding to self-reported questionnaires. A trained assistant will be available in these cases. Another important point to consider is the work compensation in some patients who want secondary gains, which can influence the information collected.

The results from this randomized clinical trial study are expected to be published in december of 2019. We hope that the study results will provide an answer as to which is the best conservative treatment method for DRF.

Abbreviations

AE: Above-elbow; AO: Arbeitsgemeinschaft für osteosynthesefragen; BE: Below-elbow; DASH: Disabilities of the arm, shoulder and hand; DRF: Distal radius fractures; Kg: Kilograms; L: Lateral; mcg: Micrograms; min: minutes; PA: Posteroanterior; PRWE: Patient rated wrist evaluation; UNIFESP: Federal University of São Paulo; VAS: Visual analogue scale

Acknowledgements

This study was conducted in the Hand, Arm and Shoulder Surgery Unit (Head: Prof. Dr. Carlos Henrique Fernandes) of the Universidade Federal de São Paulo – UNIFESP/EPM, with substantial contribution from Hospital Dr. Fernando Mauro Pires da Rocha (Head of orthopaedic unit: Dr. Jonas Aparecido Borracini).

Funding

No external funding.

Authors' contributions

AO and JCB designed the project, reviewed the literature and drafted the text. GMM assisted with manuscript writing, editing and helped to revise the manuscript. JR conceptualized the study methods. VYM performed the sample size calculations and defined the types of statistical analyzes. FF gave their expertise in the field of musculoskeletal disorders and critically revised the manuscript for important intellectual content. All authors reviewed and approved the final manuscript.

Consent for publication

Not applicable.

Competing interests

The authors declare that there are no conflicts of interest.

Author details

[1]Hospital Municipal do Campo Limpo Dr. Fernando Mauro Pires da Rocha, Estrada de Itapecerica, 1661 - Campo Limpo, São Paulo, SP 05835-005, Brazil. [2]Hand, Arm and Shoulder Surgery Unit, Department of Orthopedics and Traumatology, Universidade Federal de São Paulo, UNIFESP/EPM, Rua Borges Lagoa, 778 Vila Clementino, São Paulo, SP, Brazil.

References

1. Chung KC, Spilson SV. The frequency and epidemiology of hand and forearm fractures in the United States. J Hand Surg Am. 2001;26(5):908–15.
2. Cui Z, Pan J, Yu B, Zhang K, Xiong X. Internal versus external fixation for unstable distal radius fractures: an up-to-date meta-analysis. Int Orthop. 2011 Sep;35(9):1333–41.
3. Diaz-Garcia RJ, Oda T, Shauver MJ, Chung KC. A systematic review of outcomes and complications of treating unstable distal radius fractures in the elderly. J Hand Surg Am. 2011;36(5):824–35.
4. Handoll H, Madhok R. Conservative interventions for treating distal radial fractures in adults. Cochrane Database Syst Rev. 2003;2(2):CD000314.
5. Lichtman DM, Bindra RR, Boyer MI, Putnam MD, Ring D, Slutsky DJ, et al. Treatment of distal radius fracture. J Am Acad Orthop Surg. 2010;18:180–9.
6. Raittio L, Launonen A, Hevonkorpi T, Luokkala T, Kukkonen J, Reito A, Sumrein B, Laitinen M, Mattila VM. Comparison of volar-flexion, ulnar-deviation and functional position cast immobilization in the non-operative treatment of distal radius fracture in elderly patients: a pragmatic randomized controlled trial study protocol. BMC Musculoskelet Disord. 2017;18:401.
7. Pool C. Colles's fracture. A prospective study of treatment. J Bone Joint Surg Br. 1973 Aug;55(3):540–4.
8. Stewart HD, Innes AR, Burke FD. Functional cast-bracing for Colles' fractures a comparison between cast-bracing and conventional plaster casts. J Bone Joint Surg Br. 1984 Nov;66(5):749–53.
9. Webb GR, Galpin RD, Armstrongs DG. Comparison of short and long arm plaster casts for displaced fractures in the distal third of the forearm in children. J Bone Joint Surg Am. 2006;88:9–17.
10. Wahlstrom O. Treatment of Colles' fracture a prospective comparison of three different positions of immobilization. Acta Orthop Scand. 1982;53:225–8.
11. Sarmiento A, Pratt GW, Berry NC, Sinclair WF. Colles' fractures. Functional bracing in supination. J Bone Joint Surg Am. 1975;57(3):311–7.

12. Bunger C, Solund K, Rasmussen P. Early results after Colles' fracture: functional bracing in supination vs dorsal plaster immobilization. Arch Orthop Trauma Surg. 1984;103:251–6.
13. Bong MR, Egol KA, Leibman M, Koval KJ. A comparison of immediate postreduction splinting constructs for controlling initial displacement of fractures of the distal radius: a prospective randomized study of long- arm versus short-arm splinting. J Hand Surg Am. 2006;31:766–70.
14. Grafstein E, Stenstrom R, Christenson J, Innes G, MacCormack R, Jackson C, Stothers K, Goetz T. A prospective randomized controlled trial comparing circumferential casting and splinting in displaced Colles fractures. CJEM. 2010;12(3):192–200.
15. McQueen M, Caspers J. Colles fracture: does the anatomical result affect the final function? J Bone Joint Surg Br. 1988;70:649–51.
16. Jenkins NH, Mintowt-Czyz WJ. Mal-union and dysfunction in Colles' fracture. J Hand Surg Br. 1988;13:291–3.
17. Tumia N, Wardlaw D, Hallett J, Deutman R, Mattsson SA, Sandin B. Aberdeen Colles brace as a treatment for Colles fracture. A multicenter, prospective, randomized, controlled trial. J Bone Joint Surg Br. 2003;85(1):78–82.
18. Wilcke MK, Abbaszadegan H, Adolphson PY. Patient-perceived outcome after displaced distal radius fractures: a comparison between radiological parameters, objective physical variables, and the DASH score. J Hand Ther. 2007;20:290–8.
19. Ng CY, McQueen MM. What are the radiological predictors of functional outcome following fractures of the distal radius? J Bone Joint Surg Br. 2011;93:145–50.
20. Altissimi M, Antenucci R, Fiacca C, Mancini GB. Long-term results of conservative treatment of fractures of the distal radius. Clin Orthop Relat Res. 1986;206:202–10.
21. Grewal R, MacDermid JC. The risk of adverse outcomes in extra-articular distal radius fractures is increased with malalignment in patients of all ages but mitigated in older patients. J Hand Surg Am. 2007;32:962–70.
22. Knirk JL, Jupiter JB. Intra-articular fractures of the distal end of the radius in young adults. J Bone Joint Surg Am. 1986;68(5):647–59.
23. Batra S, Gupta A. The effect of fracture-related factors on the functional out- come at 1 year in distal radius fractures. Injury. 2002;33:499–502.
24. Mann FA, Wilson AJ, Gilula LA. Radiographic evaluation of the wrist: what does the hand surgeon want to know? Radiology. 1992;184(1):15–24.
25. Bailey PL, Stanley TH. Intravenous opioid anesthetics in: Miller DM - anesthesia. 4th ed. New York: Churchill Livingstone; 1994. p. 291–387.
26. Shafer SL. Towards optimal intravenous dosing strategies. Semin Anesth. 1993;12:222–34.
27. Charnley J. The Cooles' fracture. In: The John Charnley trust editor(s). The treatment of closed fractures. 4th ed. Cambridge: Colt Book Ltd; 1999. p. 146–70.
28. Orfale AG, Araújo PM, Ferraz MB, Natour J. Translation into Brazilian Portuguese, cultural adaptation and evaluation of the reliability of the disabilities of the arm, shoulder and hand questionnaire. Braz J Med Biol Res. 2005;38(2):293–302.
29. Rodrigues EKS, Fonseca MCR, MacDermid JC. Brazilian version of yhe patient rated wrist evaluation (PRWE-Br): cross- cultural adaptation, internal consistency, test- retest reliability, and construct validity. J Hand Ther. 2015;28(1):69–76.
30. Revill SI, Robinson JO, Rosen M, Hogg MIJ. The reliability of a linear analogue for evaluating pain. Anaesthesia. 1976;31(9):1191–8.
31. Hawker GA, Mian S, Kendzerska T, French M. Measures of adult pain: visual analog scale for pain (VAS pain), numeric rating scale for pain (NRS pain), McGill pain questionnaire (MPQ), short-form McGill pain questionnaire (SF-MPQ), chronic pain grade scale (CPGS), short Form-36 bodily pain scale (SF-36 BPS), and measure of intermittent and constant osteoarthritis pain (ICOAP). Arthritis Care Res. 2011;63:S240–52.
32. Park MJ, Kim JP, Lee HI, Lim TK, Jung HS, Lee JS. Is a short arm cast appropriate for a stable distal radius fractures in patients older than 55 years? A randomized prospective multicentre study. J Hand Surg Eur. 2017;42(5):487–92.
33. Gummersson C, Atroshi I, Ekdahl C. The disabilities of arm, shoulder and hand (DASH) outcome questionnaire: longitudinal construct validity and measuring self-rated health change after surgery. BMC Musculoskelet Disord. 2003;4:11.
34. Belloti JC, Santos JB, Atallah AN, Albertoni WM, Faloppa F. Fractures of the distal radius (Colles' fracture). Sao Paulo Med J. 2007;125(3):132–8.
35. Arora R, Gabl M, Gschwentner M, Deml C, Krappinger D, Lutz M. A comparative study of clinical and radiologic outcomes of unstable colles type distal radius fractures in patients older than 70 years: nonoperative treatment versus volar locking plating. J Orthop Trauma. 2009;23:237–42.
36. Egol KA, Walsh M, Romo-Cardoso S, Dorsky S, Paksima N. Distal radial fractures in the elderly: operative compared with non-operative treatment. J Bone Joint Surg Am. 2010;92:1851–7.
37. Wong TC, Chiu Y, Tsang WL, Leung WY, Yam SK, Yeung SH. Casting versus percutaneous pinning for extra-articular fractures of the distal radius in an elderly Chinese population: a prospective randomised controlled trial. J Hand Surg Eur. 2010;35:202–8.
38. Arora R, Lutz M, Deml C, Krappinger D, Haug L, Gabl M. A prospective randomized trial comparing nonoperative treatment with volar locking plate fixation for displaced and unstable distal radial fractures in patients sixty-five years of age and older. J Bone Joint Surg Am. 2011;93:2146–53.

Epidemiology and time trends of distal forearm fractures in adults - a study of 11.2 million person-years in Sweden

Daniel Jerrhag[1*], Martin Englund[2,3], Magnus K. Karlsson[1] and Bjorn E. Rosengren[1]

Abstract

Background: A distal forearm fracture is a very common injury causing both suffering and substantial health care costs. The incidence of this fracture type seemed to increase worldwide until the middle 1980's, but thereafter most reports have shown stable or decreasing rates. As few large studies have been presented lately we aimed to describe recent epidemiology and time trends of distal forearm fractures in adults. We paid special attention to fractures in working ages as they present challenges in terms of treatment and costs for sick-leave, and have not previously been thoroughly investigated.

Methods: By use of population data from Statistics Sweden and official in- and out-patient register data of men and women (≥17 years) in Sweden (Skåne region), we ascertained distal forearm fractures and estimated age- and sex-specific rates and time-trends from year 1999 to 2010 (11.2 million person-years (py)).

Results: The total incidence rate was 278 per 100,000 py (31,233 fractures) with 23% higher annual numbers 2010 compared with 1999. An increase in the annual age standardized incidence was found in men, +0.7% per annum (95% confidence interval (CI) 0.1, 1.4), and women, +0.9% (95% CI 0.5, 1.3), driven mainly by an increasing incidence in working ages (17–64 years). Also, expected demographic changes including a 25% population increase may result in 38% more fractures until 2050, compared to 2017.

Conclusions: The incidence of distal forearm fractures in adults in southern Sweden is increasing, mainly driven by an increase in working ages. In combination with expected demographic changes these findings may present substantial challenges for the future.

Keywords: Epidemiology, Time-trends, Wrist fracture, Distal radius fracture, Forecast

Background

The distal forearm fracture is a common orthopedic injury. The consequences for the individual patient depend on factors such as age, fracture pattern and occupation. In epidemiological studies the age rate curve has been found to be bimodal, with highest incidences found in children and elderly [1, 2].

In young adulthood and middle age the distal forearm fracture is less common than in childhood and in the elderly, but fracture patterns can be severe with consequent loss of function or absence from work. The higher incidence rates of this fracture type in the elderly result in substantial suffering as well as health care costs.

We have earlier found that the incidence of distal forearm fractures among children is increasing in the Skåne region, Sweden [3]. In adults, however, few larger studies of distal forearm fracture epidemiology have been presented recently [4, 5] and none with focus on working-age individuals. To provide politicians and public health planners with current data, we aimed to, in the Skåne region, Sweden (i) describe present epidemiology of distal forearm fractures in the adult population, specifically also in the working-age population, (ii) estimate time-trends during the most recent decade, and (iii) make a forecast to estimate the number of fractures the decades to come.

* Correspondence: Daniel.Jerrhag@med.lu.se
[1]Clinical and Molecular Osteoporosis Research Unit, Departments of Clinical Sciences and Orthopedics Malmö, Skåne University Hospital, Lund University, SE 20502 Malmo, Sweden

Methods

The *Skåne Healthcare Register (SHR)* is a register covering in- and outpatient health care provided to residents of Skåne, the southernmost region of Sweden from year 1998. The region includes both urban and rural areas and had in year 2010 a total adult (≥17 years) population of about 1.0 million. From year 1999 to 2010 we used the SHR to ascertain distal forearm fractures in adults (≥17 years) residing in the region (11.2 million py) by using physician-set diagnostic codes according to the Swedish version of the International Classification of Diseases (ICD) 10 system (S52.50, S52.51, S52.60, S52.61). Bilateral fractures were counted as only one fracture as the database does not include information about side. The washout period was set to 1 year (365 days) for each fracture and unique individual and we consequently also included year 1998 data to create a reference for washouts year 1999. From the complete data set we estimated sex-specific incidence rates per 100,000 py using the cumulative annual adult population, in one year age classes from Statistics Sweden as denominator (population at risk) [6]. For estimation of temporal trends, we tabulated data by year and used Poisson regression of annual direct age-standardized incidence rates (with the average population during the examined years as the standard population) and included 95% confidence intervals (95% CI) to describe uncertainty. The validity of the register, in terms of distal forearm fractures, has previously been examined with a sensitivity of 90% and positive predictive value of 94% for the register data compared to gold standard [7].

To estimate the number of distal forearm fractures in the whole of Sweden the forthcoming decades, the overall incidence in 1-year age groups during the examination period from 1999 to 2010 from the Skåne region was applied to demographic forecasts from Statistics Sweden for the years 2017–2050 [8].

We used SAS system v 9.2, SPSS v17.0, and Microsoft Excel 2003 for data management and statistical calculations. All tests were two-tailed and we considered a p-value lower than 0.05 to be statistically significant. The study has been approved by the Ethical Review Board (ERB) at Lund University (2011/432).

Results

From year 1999 to 2010 we identified 31,233 distal forearm fractures (male to female ratio 1:3) during 11.2 million py. This represents an overall incidence of 278 per 100,000 py (Table 1).

Adults in working ages (17–64 years) contributed to 15,052 fractures (48% of all fractures, male to female ratio 1:1.5). Correspondingly, those older than 64 years contributed to 16,181 fractures (52% of all, male to female ratio 1:6.5). From 1999 to 2010 the overall annual number of distal forearm fractures increased from 2368 to 3089, with underlying increases in both men (from 589 to 766) and women (from 1779 to 2323). An additional file shows the number of persons at risk, and the number of fractures more in detail (additional file 1).

There was also a significant increase in the annual age-standardized incidence in both men (+0.7% per annum, 95% CI 0.1, 1.4), and women (+0.9%, 95% CI 0.5,

Table 1 Population at risk, number of fractures and overall wrist fracture incidence

Age stratum (years)	Men			Women		
	At risk	Fractures	Incidence	At risk	Fractures	Incidence
≥ 17	5,478,970	8217	150	5,762,155	23,016	399
17–64	4,412,748	6045	137	4,342,588	9007	207
≥ 65	1,066,222	2172	204	1,419,567	14,009	987
17–49	3,081,881	4106	133	3,016,896	3425	114
≥ 50	2,397,089	4111	171	2,745,259	19,591	714
17–19	264,337	781	295	255,140	343	134
20–29	897,345	1152	128	889,840	835	94
30–39	983,138	946	96	951,017	954	100
40–49	937,061	1227	131	915,592	1293	141
50–59	920,560	1287	140	916,685	3201	349
60–69	734,078	1117	152	757,112	4699	621
70–79	476,240	843	177	588,380	5269	896
80–89	235,815	717	304	399,501	4989	1249
≥90	30,398	147	484	88,891	1433	1612

Different age-strata (years) and incidence per 100,000 py during 1999–2010 in the Skåne region, Sweden

1.3). For adults in working ages (17–64 years) the incidence increased significantly for both men (+0.8%, 95% CI 0.02, 1.5) and women (+2.1%, 95% CI 1.5, 2.8) while it was stable in their counterparts ≥65 years. Detailed data including other relevant age groups are presented in Table 2.

Even though the Swedish population ≥ 17 years is estimated to increase by only 25% from 8,110,000 (year 2017) to 10,100,000 (year 2050) we project an increase in number of forearm fractures by 38% from 22,600 (year 2017) to 31,000 (year 2050) due to shifts in age structure (Fig. 1). In working ages (17–64 years) the total number of fractures is projected to increase from 10,400 to 12,500, representing an increase by 20%. In the age-group ≥65 years the number of fractures is projected to increase from 12,200 to 18,600, an increase by 52% (Fig. 2).

Discussion

In our study of 11.2 million py in a well-defined Swedish population we found that the age-standardized incidence in both adult (≥17 years) men and women increased significantly from year 1999 to 2010. This was driven mainly by an increase in working ages (17–64 years). With an increasing population and the expected demographic changes until year 2050 we project the number of distal forearm fractures to increase by 38% in Sweden from 2017 to year 2050, even though the actual number of citizens is only estimated to increase by 25%.

Table 2 Annual change in age standardized rates in different age-strata in the Skåne County 1999–2010

	Annual percent change (95% CI)	
Age stratum (years)	Men	Women
Primary analyses		
≥ 17	**+0.7 (0.1, 1.4)**	**+0.9 (0.5, 1.3)**
17–64	**+0.8 (+0.0, 1.5)**	**+2.1 (1.5, 2.8)**
≥ 65	+0.5 (−0.7, 1.8)	+0.1 (−0.3, 0.6)
Secondary analyses		
17–49	+0.7 (−0.2, 1.6)	+1.0 (−0.0, 1.9)
≥ 50	+0.8 (−0.1, 1.7)	**+0.5 (0.1, 0.9)**
Tertiary analyses		
17–19	+1.7 (−0.4, 3.8)	+2.3 (−0.8, 5.5)
20–29	+1.3 (−0.4, 3.0)	+0.0 (−1.9, 2.0)
30–39	+0.4 (−1.4, 2.3)	−0.5 (−2.3, 1.3)
40–49	−0.2 (−1.8, 1.4)	**+2.3 (0.7, 4.0)**
50–59	**+2.0 (0.4, 3.7)**	**+3.4 (2.3, 4.4)**
60–69	−0.7 (−2.4, 1.0)	**+1.7 (0.9, 2.6)**
70–79	+0.0 (−1.9, 2.0)	**+2.0 (1.2, 2.9)**
80–89	+2.1 (−0.1, 4.3)	+0.2 (−0.6, 1.0)
≥ 90	−0.8 (−5.4, 4.0)	+0.6 (−0.9, 2.1)

For clarity rather than for precision one decimal is given. Statistically significant changes are bolded

Distal forearm fracture rates have been superintended episodically and most studies agree on an increase from the 1950's to the 1980's [2, 9–12]. After the 1980's some studies have reported decreasing or stable adult distal forearm fracture rates [5, 13–20], whilst some recent reports, from Denmark and Taiwan, infer an increasing incidence [4, 21] (Fig. 3a, b).

A new large British study [20] during years 1988–2012 however reports a lower incidence in the entity radius/ulnar fractures (not only distal forearm fractures) than that we found for only distal forearm fractures. Since definition of fracture, ascertainment method, geographical regions and age stratification differ substantially between studies, direct comparisons are difficult (Tables 3 and 4).

We therefore primarily compared our results to earlier reports from the Skåne region, Sweden [2, 9, 13] (Fig. 3a, b). Jonsson et al. [13] reported a lower incidence in both genders in the adult population in Malmö (the largest city in the Skåne region) 1991–1992 compared to 1980–1981. In our data from the period 1999–2010, the incidence in men ≥17 years (150 per 100,000 py) were at the level of those for Malmö 1980–1981 but higher than those from 1991 to 1992. In contrast, for women, the incidence was lower during 1999–2010 (339 per 100,000 py), than in Jonsson et al. 1991–1992 [13]. In the north-eastern part of the Skåne region, Brogren et al. [22] reported an incidence in men ≥19 years of 120 per 100,000 py and in women of 390 per 100,000 py in year 2001. In Finland, Flinkkilä et al. reported an incidence for men and women ≥16 years, of 147 and 363 per 100,000 py, respectively, in year 2008. Both Brogren et al. and Flinkkilä et al. base their results on fracture ascertainment through radiographs and medical charts and their results are similar to ours.

In our study we found a significant annual increase in the age standardized distal forearm fracture rate in adult men and women. As a distal forearm fracture has been found to be an indicator of osteoporosis [23] and also forecast subsequent fractures, [24, 25] these results may have implication for the future fracture burden. Our results are in some contrast to Wilcke et al. [5] who in Stockholm, Sweden, found a decreasing forearm fracture rate from year 2004 to 2010 in individuals ≥65 years of age. However, their findings must be interpreted with care as they included only one fracture per individual, rendering a decreasing population at risk with successive years without a corresponding decrease in the denominator and without adjustment for lower risks in those who remained eligible. On the other hand Abrahamsen et al. [4] in a recent large register based study in Denmark, found a higher incidence compared to earlier. Their reported incidence for men (153 per 100,000 py)

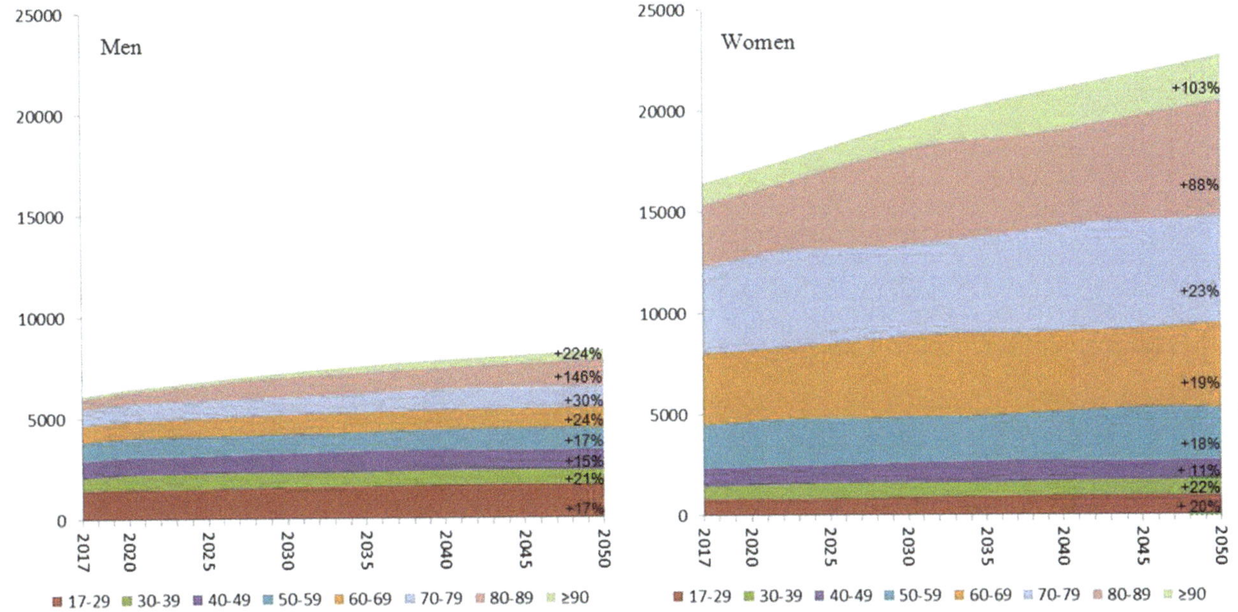

Fig. 1 Projection of numbers of distal forearm fractures in Sweden the forthcoming decades (2017–2050). Age strata in years. Change in % from 2017 to 2050. Over all incidence in 1-year age groups in Skåne region, Sweden 1999–2010 used for calculation (see methods)

was nearly the same as we found, but for women (530 per 100,000 py) somewhat higher (Fig. 3a, b).

The reasons behind the increase in incidence we found during 1999–2010 are not examined in this study but several factors may have contributed including an increased prevalence of osteoporosis. Trend data available for osteoporosis in the Skåne region, Sweden [26–28], do however not indicate this. More recent studies from other countries including Finland and USA, actually point in the opposite direction with an increasing time trend in bone mineral density (BMD) [29, 30]. A more strict postmenopausal estrogen prescription compared to earlier may have contributed to an increased fracture incidence but this effect is likely small as the incidence is increasing in both men and women. In Sweden, as in many other countries, body mass index (BMI) is

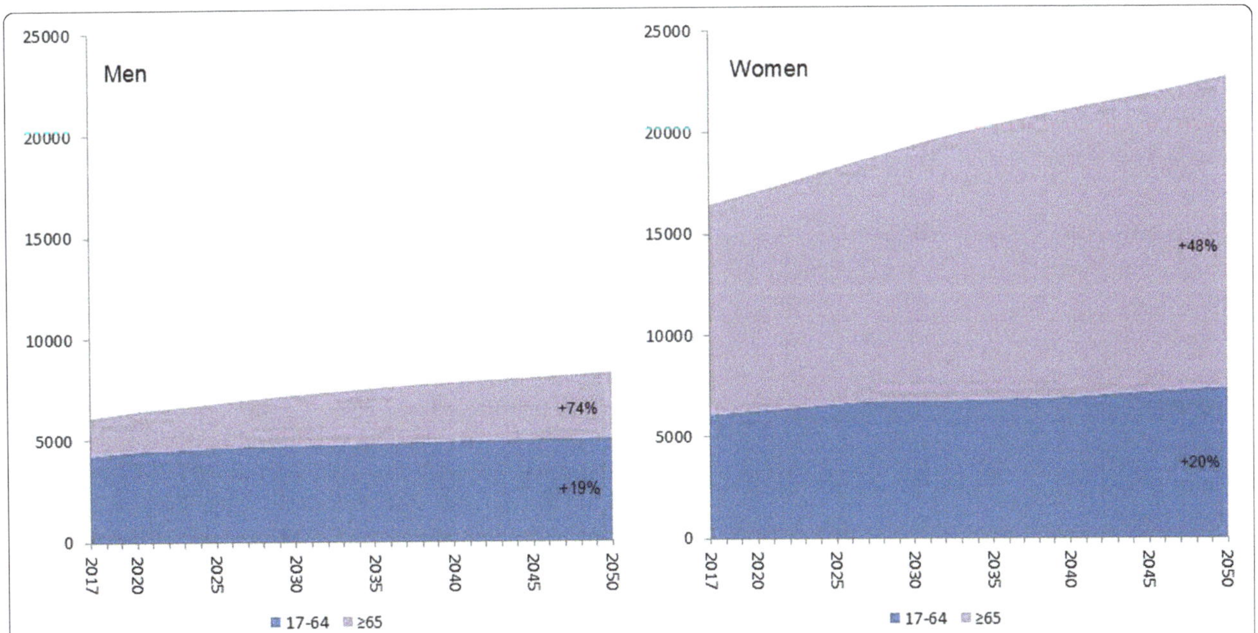

Fig. 2 Projection of numbers of distal forearm fractures in Sweden in working and non-working ages. Age strata in years. Change in % from 2017 to 2050. Over all incidence in 1-year age groups in Skåne region, Sweden 1999–2010 used for calculation (see methods)

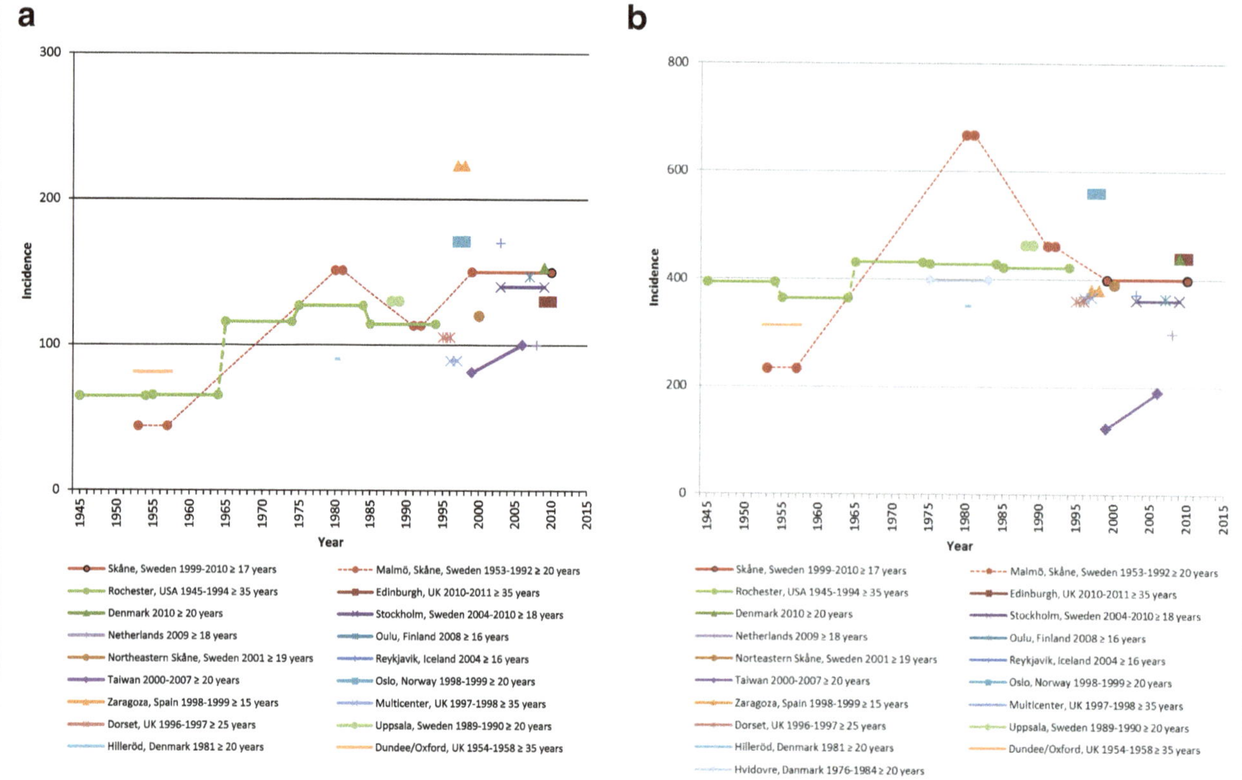

Fig. 3 a. Reported incidence of distal forearm fractures in men per 100,000 py during the last 6 decades. **b**. Reported incidence of distal forearm fractures in women per 100,000 py during the last 6 decades. [2, 4, 5, 9, 11, 13–18, 21, 22, 39–45]

Table 3 Reported incidence of distal forearm fractures in adults (≥ 50 years) during 7 decades

Population at risk	Year	Incidence	
		Men	Women
Skåne, Sweden[a]	1999–2010	171	712
Denmark[a] [4]	2010	203	926
Austria[b] [46]	2010	162	607
Oulu, Finland[a] [16]	2008	223	710
Netherlands[a] [44]	2009	147	612
Kristiansand, Norway[b] [47]	2004–2005	189	751
Northeastern Skåne, Sweden[a] [22]	2001	152	677
Austria[b] [46]	1999	171	709
Oslo, Norway[a] [14]	1998–1999	254	1098
Malmö, Sweden[a] [13]	1991–1992	157	827
Uppsala, Sweden[a] [42]	1989–1990	217	970
Malmö, Sweden[ac] [9]	1980–1981	158	462
Hvidovre, Danmark[a] [45]	1976–1984	-	695
Hilleröd, Denmark[a] [11]	1981	116	824
Oslo, Norway[a] [40]	1979	234	1137
Malmö, Sweden[a] [2]	1953–1957	53	510

Incidence per 100,000 py
[a]Crude incidence
[b]Age standardized incidence
[c]Numbers derived from Jónsson et al. [13]

increasing [31]. The importance of BMI for fracture risk has been known since long but recent insights have inferred that a higher BMI, apart from giving a lower risk for hip fracture, also confers a higher risk for upper extremity fracture [32].

Apart from consequences for the individual there are other implications of fractures. As the distal forearm fracture is the most common of fractures, even a minor increase in occurrence could substantially impact health care resource demands and public health costs. This would be especially true if the increase occurs in working ages where patients need sick-leave, depending on occupation, for 5–12 weeks or more. Any permanent loss of function may also result in inability to work with loss of competence for both employer, and society. The mean fracture-related cost of a distal forearm fracture in Sweden, in patients ≥50 years, during the year following the diagnosis, has been estimated to € 2147 in 2005 [33]. This was however just before the volar locking plate became the dominating surgical treatment [19] and therefore cost per treated patient is supposedly higher now.

As the volar locking plate is a more expensive treatment than other alternatives like casting, wire fixation and external fixation a question needed to put forward is whether it should be the gold standard procedure or not

Table 4 Reported incidence of distal forearm fractures in adults in different countries or areas

Population at risk	Year	Age (Years)	Incidence	
			Men	Women
Skåne, Sweden[a]	1999–2010	≥ 17	150	399
Edinburgh, UK[a] [41]	2010–2011	≥ 35	130	440
Denmark[a] [4]	2010	≥ 20	153	530
Stockholm, Sweden[a] [5]	2004–2010	≥ 18	140	360
Oulu, Finland[a] [16]	2008	≥ 16	147	363
Netherlands[a] [44]	2009	≥ 18	100	298
Taiwan[a] [21]	2007	≥ 20	100	189
Reykjavik, Iceland[a] [17]	2004	≥ 16	170	370
Northeastern Skåne, Sweden[a] [22]	2001	≥ 19	120	390
Taiwan[a] [21]	2000	≥ 20	81	123
Oslo, Norway[a] [14]	1998–1999	≥ 20	171	560
Dorset, UK[a] [18]	1996–1997	≥ 25	105	359
Zaragoza, Spain[a] [39]	1998–1999	≥ 15	223	380
Multicenter, UK[a] [43]	1997–1998	≥ 35	90	368
Malmö, Sweden[a] [13]	1991–1992	≥ 20	113	461
Rochester, Minnesota[b] [15]	1985–1994	≥ 35	114	421
Uppsala, Sweden[a] [24]	1989–1990	≥ 20	130	463
Rochester, Minnesota[b] [15]	1975–1984	≥ 35	127	428
Hvidovre, Danmark[a] [45]	1976–1984	≥ 20	c	397
Malmö, Sweden[ad] [9]	1980–1981	≥ 20	140	667
Hilleröd, Denmark[a] [11]	1981	≥ 20	90	350
Oslo, Norway[a] [40]	1979	≥ 20	169	673
Rochester, Minnesota[b] [15]	1965–1974	≥ 35	116	432
Rochester, Minnesota[b] [15]	1955–1964	≥ 35	65	364
Dundee/Oxford, UK[af] [41]	1954–1958	≥ 35	81	313
Rochester, Minnesota[b] [15]	1945–1954	≥ 35	65	393
Malmö, Sweden[ad] [2]	1953–1957	≥ 20	44	233

Incidence per 100,000 py
[a]Crude incidence
[b]Age standardized incidence
[c]No male figures given
[d]Numbers derived from Jónsson et al. [13]
[f]Numbers derived from Court-Brown et al. [41]

and this has been debated lately. Cost-benefit analyses have revealed small or no gains measured in Quality Adjusted Life Years (QALY) comparing volar plating procedures with other treatment options [34, 35].

With the expected demographic changes with a growing proportion of elderly citizens the number of fractures is likely to increase even if the fracture incidence, despite the findings in this study, should remain stable (Figs. 1 and 2). We have earlier found an increasing incidence also in distal forearm fractures in children [3]. As there are data supporting the idea that childhood fractures are forecasters of future fracture risk [36–38], our projections for the future may underestimate the future number of fractures especially as an incidence increase was also found in working ages in the current study. Interestingly, Mellstrand-Navarro et al. [19] reported that the rate of patients treated operatively with plating increased most (3–4 fold) from 2005 to 2010 in the age group ≥50 years. As our findings suggest an over 50% increase in fractures in the population ≥ 65 years until year 2050 it is of even more interest to make the treatment both evidence-based and as cost-effective as possible (Fig. 2). Therefore further studies are needed.

The strengths of our study include the coverage of a large adult population including all individuals in a well-defined geographical area during 12 years (11.2 million py) with validated data on distal forearm fractures [7]. However, the examination of registers rather than individual patients, charts or X-rays makes selection bias, random or systematic, possible. A previous validation of the register for this particular fracture type has however shown a very high accuracy [7]. Furthermore our results are very similar to those of Brogren et al. from Skåne region [22] and Flinkkilä et al. [16] from Finland who both utilized the gold standard of chart and X-ray review. Even though our case-finding strategy appears valid, estimations of absolute numbers from registers are always difficult. Relative changes (such as time trends) are however more easily subjected to examination and results more robust. We chose a wash-out period of one year, because the vast majority of all distal forearm fractures are then healed and thus, will not appear in the medical records again as a result of that fracture. If an individual appears in the register again, after more than a year with the same diagnosis, the most likely reason is a new fracture and the individual would then be included once more. Bilateral simultaneous fractures will however be counted only as one fracture, as the register does not include information about side. It would have been preferable with in-detail patient level data to identify possible explanatory factors.

Conclusion

The incidence of distal forearm fractures is increasing in both adult men and women in the Skåne region, Sweden. It is especially worrying that this seems driven by an increase in working ages (17–64 years) as this may present special challenges to both the healthcare system and loss of resources in society during time of sick-leave. The reasons for the increase in incidence are unknown and need further exploration but may include increasing prevalence of osteoporosis and overweight. We suggest similar examinations in other settings with uniform data collection and presentation to verify our results and to enable comparisons and merger of data. Collection and analysis of patient specific risk factors may provide additional insights to the origin of the changes. Cost analysis (including societal costs) and cost-benefit analyses of different treatments in both younger adults and elderly are scarce. Such data would contribute to understanding the effects of our findings and help decision makers to plan best use of resources in the future.

Abbreviations

BMD: Bone mineral density; BMI: Body mass index; CI: Confidence interval; Py: Person-years; QALY: Quality adjusted life years; SHR: Skåne health care register

Acknowledgements

Not applicable.

Funding

Funding was received from the Swedish Research Council, from Government Funding of Clinical Research within the National Health Service (ALF), from FoU Skåne, from the Herman Järnhardt Foundation, from the Johan and Greta Kock Foundation, and from the Faculty of Medicine, Lund University, Sweden.

Authors' contributions

BR, ME and MK designed the study. BR and ME extracted the original data. BR and DJ made all calculations. DJ wrote the first draft and edited the manuscript first together with BR and then together with all authors. All authors have read and revised the final manuscript. All authors read and approved the final manuscript.

Competing interests

The authors declare that they have no competing interests.

Consent for publication

Not applicable.

Author details

[1]Clinical and Molecular Osteoporosis Research Unit, Departments of Clinical Sciences and Orthopedics Malmö, Skåne University Hospital, Lund University, SE 20502 Malmo, Sweden. [2]Department of Clinical Sciences Lund, Orthopedics, Clinical Epidemiology Unit, Lund University, Faculty of Medicine, Lund, Sweden. [3]Clinical Epidemiology Research and Training Unit, Boston University School of Medicine, Boston, MA, USA.

References

1. Buhr AJ, Cooke AM. Fracture patterns. Lancet. 1959;1:531–6.
2. Alffram PA, Bauer GC. Epidemiology of fractures of the forearm. A biomechanical investigation of bone strength. J Bone Joint Surg Am. 1962;44-A:105–14.
3. Jerrhag D, Englund M, Petersson I, Lempesis V, Landin L, Karlsson MK, et al. Increasing wrist fracture rates in children may have major implications for future adult fracture burden. Acta Orthop. 2016;87:296–300.
4. Abrahamsen B, Jorgensen NR, Schwarz P. Epidemiology of forearm fractures in adults in Denmark: national age- and gender-specific incidence rates, ratio of forearm to hip fractures, and extent of surgical fracture repair in inpatients and outpatients. Osteoporos Int. 2015;26:67–76.
5. Wilcke MK, Hammarberg H, Adolphson PY. Epidemiology and changed surgical treatment methods for fractures of the distal radius: a registry analysis of 42,583 patients in Stockholm County, Sweden, 2004-2010. Acta Orthop. 2013;84:292–6.
6. Statistics Sweden. 1 May 2013 edition.
7. Rosengren BE, Karlsson M, Petersson I, Englund M. The 21st-century landscape of adult fractures: cohort study of a complete adult regional population. J Bone Miner Res. 2015;30:535–42.
8. Statistics Swedens. 13 Feb 2017 edition.
9. Bengner U, Johnell O. Increasing incidence of forearm fractures. A comparison of epidemiologic patterns 25 years apart. Acta Orthop Scand. 1985;56:158–60.
10. Miller SW, Evans JG. Fractures of the distal forearm in Newcastle: an epidemiological survey. Age Ageing. 1985;14:155–8.
11. Solgaard S, Petersen VS. Epidemiology of distal radius fractures. Acta Orthop Scand. 1985;56:391–3.
12. Owen RA, Melton LJ 3rd, Johnson KA, Ilstrup DM, Riggs BL. Incidence of Colles' fracture in a North American community. Am J Public Health. 1982;72:605–7.
13. Jonsson B, Bengner U, Redlund-Johnell I, Johnell O. Forearm fractures in Malmo, Sweden. Changes in the incidence occurring during the 1950s, 1980s and 1990s. Acta Orthop Scand. 1999;70:129–32.
14. Lofthus CM, Frihagen F, Meyer HE, Nordsletten L, Melhuus K, Falch JA. Epidemiology of distal forearm fractures in Oslo, Norway. Osteoporos Int. 2008;19:781–6.
15. Melton LJ 3rd, Amadio PC, Crowson CS, O'Fallon WM. Long-term trends in the incidence of distal forearm fractures. Osteoporos Int. 1998;8:341–8.
16. Flinkkila T, Sirnio K, Hippi M, Hartonen S, Ruuhela R, Ohtonen P, et al. Epidemiology and seasonal variation of distal radius fractures in Oulu, Finland. Osteoporos Int. 2011;22:2307–12.

17. Sigurdardottir K, Halldorsson S, Robertsson J. Epidemiology and treatment of distal radius fractures in Reykjavik, Iceland, in 2004. Comparison with an Icelandic study from 1985. Acta Orthop. 2011;82:494–8.
18. Thompson PW, Taylor J, Dawson A. The annual incidence and seasonal variation of fractures of the distal radius in men and women over 25 years in Dorset, UK. Injury. 2004;35:462–6.
19. Mellstrand-Navarro C, Pettersson HJ, Tornqvist H, Ponzer S. The operative treatment of fractures of the distal radius is increasing: results from a nationwide Swedish study. Bone Joint J. 2014;96-B:963–9.
20. Curtis EM, van der Velde R, Moon RJ, van den Bergh JP, Geusens P, de Vries F, et al. Epidemiology of fractures in the United Kingdom 1988-2012: Variation with age, sex, geography, ethnicity and socioeconomic status. Bone. 2016;87:19–26.
21. Tsai CH, Muo CH, Fong YC, Lo WY, Chen YJ, Hsu HC, et al. A population-based study on trend in incidence of distal radial fractures in adults in Taiwan in 2000-2007. Osteoporos Int. 2011;22:2809–15.
22. Brogren E, Petranek M, Atroshi I. Incidence and characteristics of distal radius fractures in a southern Swedish region. BMC Musculoskelet Disord. 2007;8:48.
23. Cummings SR, Kelsey JL, Nevitt MC, O'Dowd KJ. Epidemiology of osteoporosis and osteoporotic fractures. Epidemiol Rev. 1985;7:178–208.
24. Mallmin H, Ljunghall S, Persson I, Naessen T, Krusemo UB, Bergstrom R. Fracture of the distal forearm as a forecaster of subsequent hip fracture: a population-based cohort study with 24 years of follow-up. Calcif Tissue Int. 1993;52:269–72.
25. Kanis JA, Johnell O, De Laet C, Johansson H, Oden A, Delmas P, et al. A meta-analysis of previous fracture and subsequent fracture risk. Bone. 2004;35:375–82.
26. Rosengren BE, Ahlborg HG, Gardsell P, Sernbo I, Daly RM, Nilsson JA, et al. Bone mineral density and incidence of hip fracture in Swedish urban and rural women 1987-2002. Acta Orthop. 2010;81:453–9.
27. Rosengren BE, Ahlborg HG, Gardsell P, Sernbo I, Nilsson JA, Daly RM, et al. Forearm bone mineral density and incidence of hip fractures in Swedish urban and rural men 1987-2002. Scand J Public Health. 2012;40:102–8.
28. Ahlborg HG, Rosengren BE, Jarvinen TL, Rogmark C, Nilsson JA, Sernbo I, et al. Prevalence of osteoporosis and incidence of hip fracture in women–secular trends over 30 years. BMC Musculoskelet Disord. 2010;11:48.
29. Uusi-Rasi K, Karinkanta S, Heinonen A, Sievanen H. Improved femoral neck BMD in older Finnish women between 2002 and 2010. Maturitas. 2013;75:241–5.
30. Looker AC, Melton LJ 3rd, Borrud LG, Shepherd JA. Changes in femur neck bone density in US adults between 1988-1994 and 2005-2008: demographic patterns and possible determinants. Osteoporos Int. 2012;23:771–80.
31. Johansson S, Wilhelmsen L, Welin C, Eriksson H, Welin L, Rosengren A. Obesity, smoking and secular trends in cardiovascular risk factors in middle-aged women: data from population studies in Goteborg from 1980 to 2003. J Intern Med. 2010;268:594–603.
32. Prieto-Alhambra D, Premaor MO, Fina Aviles F, Hermosilla E, Martinez-Laguna D, Carbonell-Abella C, et al. The association between fracture and obesity is site-dependent: a population-based study in postmenopausal women. J Bone Miner Res. 2012;27:294–300.
33. Borgstrom F, Zethraeus N, Johnell O, Lidgren L, Ponzer S, Svensson O, et al. Costs and quality of life associated with osteoporosis-related fractures in Sweden. Osteoporos Int. 2006;17:637–50.
34. Shauver MJ, Clapham PJ, Chung KC. An economic analysis of outcomes and complications of treating distal radius fractures in the elderly. J Hand Surg Am. 2011;36:1912–8. e1911-1913
35. Tubeuf S, Yu G, Achten J, Parsons NR, Rangan A, Lamb SE, et al. Cost effectiveness of treatment with percutaneous Kirschner wires versus volar locking plate for adult patients with a dorsally displaced fracture of the distal radius: analysis from the DRAFFT trial. Bone Joint J. 2015;97-B:1082–9.
36. Amin S, Melton LJ 3rd, Achenbach SJ, Atkinson EJ, Dekutoski MB, Kirmani S, et al. A distal forearm fracture in childhood is associated with an increased risk for future fragility fractures in adult men, but not women. J Bone Miner Res. 2013;28:1751–9.
37. Buttazzoni C, Rosengren BE, Tveit M, Landin L, Nilsson JA, Karlsson MK. Does a childhood fracture predict low bone mass in young adulthood? A 27-year prospective controlled study. J Bone Miner Res. 2013;28:351–9.
38. Farr JN, Khosla S, Achenbach SJ, Atkinson EJ, Kirmani S, McCready LK, et al. Diminished bone strength is observed in adult women and men who sustained a mild trauma distal forearm fracture during childhood. J Bone Miner Res. 2014;29:2193–202.
39. Cuenca J, Martinez AA, Herrera A, Domingo J. The incidence of distal forearm fractures in Zaragoza (Spain). Chir Main. 2003;22:211–5.
40. Falch JA. Epidemiology of fractures of the distal forearm in Oslo, Norway. Acta Orthop Scand. 1983;54:291–5.
41. Court-Brown CM, Biant L, Bugler KE, McQueen MM. Changing epidemiology of adult fractures in Scotland. Scott Med J. 2014;59:30–4.
42. Mallmin H, Ljunghall S. Incidence of Colles' fracture in Uppsala. A prospective study of a quarter-million population. Acta Orthop Scand. 1992;63:213–5.
43. O'Neill TW, Cooper C, Finn JD, Lunt M, Purdie D, Reid DM, et al. Incidence of distal forearm fracture in British men and women. Osteoporos Int. 2001;12:555–8.
44. Bentohami A, Bosma J, Akkersdijk GJ, van Dijkman B, Goslings JC, Schep NW. Incidence and characteristics of distal radial fractures in an urban population in The Netherlands. Eur J Trauma Emerg Surg. 2014;40:357–61.
45. Lauritzen JB, Schwarz P, Lund B, McNair P, Transbol I. Changing incidence and residual lifetime risk of common osteoporosis-related fractures. Osteoporos Int. 1993;3:127–32.
46. Dimai HP, Svedbom A, Fahrleitner-Pammer A, Resch H, Muschitz C, Thaler H, et al. Epidemiology of distal forearm fractures in Austria between 1989 and 2010. Osteoporos Int. 2014;25:2297–306.
47. Diamantopoulos AP, Rohde G, Johnsrud I, Skoie IM, Hochberg M, Haugeberg G. The epidemiology of low- and high-energy distal radius fracture in middle-aged and elderly men and women in Southern Norway. PLoS One. 2012;7:e43367.

24

Clinical and radiological outcomes of arthroscopically assisted cannulated screw fixation for tibial eminence fracture in children and adolescents

Chang Ho Shin, Doo Jae Lee, In Ho Choi, Tae-Joon Cho and Won Joon Yoo*

Abstract

Background: The purpose of this study was to determine the efficacy and complications of arthroscopically assisted reduction and fixation with cannulated screws for tibial eminence fracture in skeletally immature patients.

Methods: This was a retrospective case series study. Forty-eight patients who were skeletally immature at the time of tibial eminence fracture were treated in a tertiary children's hospital between May 2004 and August 2015. Twenty-one patients were excluded due to non-operative treatment ($n = 10$), other surgical treatments ($n = 9$), multiple fracture (n = 1), and follow-up < 1 year (n = 1). Twenty-seven knees of 27 patients were analyzed. Avulsed fragment was reduced arthroscopically. One to three cannulated screws (4.0 mm or 5.0 mm in diameter) were used for fixation. Passive knee motion was started in 3–4 weeks. Clinical outcomes were evaluated by Lysholm score, instability of the knee, and complications. Radiological outcomes including nonunion and malunion of the avulsed fragment and physeal growth disturbance were evaluated.

Results: Mean age at the time of surgery was 10.1 years (range, 6.2 to 13.8 years). Patients were followed up for a mean of 3.9 years (range, 1.0 to 7.6 years). Fracture types included type III ($n = 13$), type II ($n = 12$), and type IV ($n = 2$) according to Zaricznyj modification of Meyers and McKeever classification. Meniscus was entrapped in five patients. Six patients showed concomitant meniscal tear. Mean Lysholm score at the latest follow-up was 95 (range, 78 to 100). Joint instability was not observed in any patient except one (instability of 5–10 mm). All patients showed full range of knee motion except one (10 degrees of flexion contracture). Screw head impingement against intercondylar notch of the femur was observed in two patients during screw removal procedure. Five knees showed prominent tibial eminence without symptoms. The injured lower limb was longer than the contralateral normal side by a mean of 6.2 mm (range, − 4 to 18 mm).

Conclusions: Arthroscopically assisted reduction and fixation with cannulated screws is an effective and safe surgical option for treating tibial eminence fracture with few complications.

Keywords: Tibial eminence fracture, Cannulated screw, Arthroscopically assisted reduction, Skeletally immature patient

* Correspondence: yoowj@snu.ac.kr
Department of Orthopaedic Surgery, Seoul National University College of Medicine, 101 Daehak-ro Jongno-gu, Seoul, 03080, Republic of Korea

Background

Tibial eminence fracture is a relatively rare injury, with an incidence of approximately 3 per 100,000 per year, which mainly occurs in children and adolescents [1]. It is thought to be a pediatric equivalent of anterior cruciate ligament (ACL) tears in adults [1–3]. Meyers and Mckeever classified this fracture into three types initially in 1959 while Zaricznyj added type IV fracture in 1977 [2, 4]. Non-displaced type I fracture and slightly displaced type II fracture can be managed conservatively with successful closed reduction, while displaced fracture requires surgical treatment [5, 6].

Various surgical fixation methods are available. Cortical screw, headless screw, suture using absorbable or non-absorbable material, suture anchor, or Kirschner wire can be used to fix the fracture [7–12]. As joint stiffness associated with delayed knee mobilization after surgery is the main complication in treatment of tibial eminence fracture [13–16], the ideal fixation device should provide sufficient initial fixation strength to allow a more aggressive rehabilitation protocol. In addition, the fixation device should not traverse the proximal tibial growth plate in skeletally immature patients because of the possibility of partial physeal arrest [17, 18]. Some biomechanical studies have investigated fixation power of several internal fixation devices with different results [19–24]. Some clinical studies have reported outcomes of various fixation devices and surgical techniques with pros and cons [9, 10, 25–29]. Cannulated screw fixation has been used widely in the treatment of the tibial eminence fracture [27, 30–34]. However, only a few articles have studied this subject in skeletally immature patients who are different from adult patients in terms of knee size, screw length, and number of screws implanted [27, 33, 34].

The purpose of this study was to determine the efficacy and complications of arthroscopically assisted reduction and fixation with cannulated screws for tibial eminence fracture in skeletally immature patients.

Methods

This retrospective study was approved by our Institutional Review Board (H-1611-007-803). A total of 48 patients who sustained tibial eminence fracture before skeletal maturity and were treated in a tertiary children's hospital between May 2004 and August 2015 were reviewed. Twenty-one patients were excluded because of non-operative treatment ($n = 10$), other surgical treatments ($n = 9$, arthroscopic suture fixation in six patients, open reduction and fixation with cannulated screws in one patient, arthroscopic partial excision of tibial eminence and femoral intercondylar notchplasty in one patient, and arthroscopic exploration in one patient), multiple fractures in other body parts ($n = 1$), and follow-up of less than 1 year (n = 1). After excluding these patients, 27 knees of 27 patients remained eligible for inclusion.

Surgical technique

All operations were performed by a single surgeon (W.J.Y.). In a fresh case of fracture, the hematoma was removed first and the avulsed fragment was pushed using a guide pin to achieve reduction while extracting the interposed meniscus or intermeniscal ligament using an arthroscopic probe. And then other guide pins were inserted before inserting a screw to prevent posterior displacement or rotation of the avulsed fragment. Guide pins were driven at a 30–50 degree sagittal plane angle to the growth plate of the proximal tibia. One to three ASNIS III cannulated screws (4.0 or 5.0 mm diameter; Stryker Corporation, Kalamazoo, MI, USA) were used with or without washers. Diameter and length of screws, number of screws implanted, and usage of washers were determined intraoperatively considering fracture pattern and the size of the avulsed osteochondral fragment and the knee. Intraoperative fluoroscopy was used to avoid iatrogenic physeal penetration by screws. In a delayed case of fracture, an arthroscopic burr and curette were used to remove the organized hematoma and fibrocartilaginous tissues on the old fracture surfaces before reduction and fixation of the avulsed fragment. In some delayed cases in which reduction was difficult to achieve, a temporary suture that had been passed through ACL was pulled out under meniscus to reduce the fragment, and a guide pin was inserted.

Post-operative management/rehabilitation protocol

Postoperatively, a long leg splint was applied for 3–4 weeks with the knee in 30 degrees of flexion. Passive knee motion was then started. Weight bearing was permitted at 6 weeks after the surgery. Patients were allowed to return to sports at 3 to 4 months after the surgery.

Clinical evaluations

Clinical outcomes were evaluated with regard to the presence or absence of arthrofibrosis, instability of the knee, Lysholm knee score [35], and complications including screw head impingement at the latest follow-up. Arthrofibrosis was defined as lack of 10 degrees or more of extension, or 15 degrees or more of flexion compared to the uninjured side at 3 months after treatment [13, 14]. Instability was evaluated using the side-to-side difference of Lachman and anterior drawer tests, and anterior tibial translation at 30 degrees of flexion in a KT-1000 arthrometer (MEDmetric, San Diego, CA, USA). Instability tests were performed by a single investigator (W.J.Y.). Lysholm knee score was obtained for 22 (81%) patients. KT-1000 measurements were obtained for 17 (63%) patients.

Radiological evaluations

Radiological outcomes were evaluated with regard to penetration of proximal tibial growth plate by screws, nonunion and malunion of the avulsed fragment, and physeal growth disturbances such as leg length discrepancy (LLD) and angular deformity. LLD was assessed in 20 (74%) patients using standing whole leg anteroposterior (AP) radiograph at the latest follow-up. A patient who had suffered a femoral shaft fracture in the ipsilateral leg 5 years before tibial eminence fracture was excluded from the evaluation of LLD. Femoral length was determined by measuring the distance from the highest point of femoral head to the lowest point of medial femoral condyle. Tibial length was determined by measuring the distance from the medial tibial plateau to the tibial plafond on whole leg AP radiograph. Magnetic resonance imaging (MRI) study was taken preoperatively for all patients except two who were under Medical Aid Program. Based on MRI and arthroscopic findings, associated injury of the knee was evaluated.

Statistical analysis

Mann-Whitney U test was used to compare means between two groups. To assess the relationship between the degree of laxity measured by KT-1000 or Lachman test and the Lysholm score, Spearman's rank correlation test was used. *P* values of less than 0.05 were considered statistically significant.

Results

Descriptive data of the 27 patients are summarized in Table 1. There were 19 boys and 8 girls. Their age at the time of surgery (mean ± standard deviation) was 10.1 ± 2.2 years (range, 6.2 to 13.8 years). Follow-up period was 3.9 ± 2.2 years (range, 1.0 to 7.6 years). The interval from trauma to surgery was 48.9 ± 143.0 days (range, 0 to 731 days). The interval was more than 30 days in 6 (22%) patients. Fractures were caused by fall (n = 11, 41%), sports injuries (n = 10, 37%, skiing in 8 patients, sprinting in 1 patient, and soccer in 1 patient), traffic accident (n = 2, 7%), or collision with another person (n = 2, 7%). Fracture type was type III in 13 (48%) patients, type II in 12 (44%) patients, and type IV in 2 (7%) patients according to Zaricznyj modification of Meyers and McKeever classification [4, 36].

The number of screws used for fixation was one in three (11%) patients, two in 19 (70%) patients, and three in 5 (19%) patients. Washer was used in conjunction with the screw in 11 (41%) patients who had cartilaginous avulsion fragment with or without very thin bone sliver. The mean sagittal angle of the screw to the growth plate of the proximal tibia was 37.6 ° ± 8.0° (range, 20° to 53.4°). Five (19%) patients showed entrapment of the meniscus or intermeniscal ligament under a displaced tibial eminence fragment (intermeniscal ligament in 2 patients, medial meniscus in 2 patients, and lateral meniscus in 1 patient) (Fig. 1). Screw removal was routinely performed for all patients at postoperative 8.6 ± 5.9 months (range, 3.0 to 33.7 months).

Clinical outcomes

Screw head impingement against femoral notch was observed in two (7%) patients during screw removal. Of these two patients, one patient was treated with one 4.0 mm screw and one 5.0 mm screw for neglected type IV fracture at 141 days after trauma. Hypertrophy of distal femoral articular cartilage was observed during screw removal procedure. This was probably due to irritation by screws. Range of knee motion was 15° to 120° before removal of screws and – 5° to 145° at the latest follow-up. The other patient was treated with one 4.0 mm screw and one 5.0 mm screw for type III fracture at 32 days post trauma (Fig. 2). Incomplete distal femoral metaphyseal fracture occurred due to vigorous physical therapy by mother at postoperative 2.5 months. This interrupted physical therapy for 3 weeks. Range of knee motion was 20° to 115° at postoperative 6 months when screws were removed. The head of 5.0 mm screw impinged against the lateral portion of medial femoral condyle and caused extension deficit of the knee. Range of motion of 10° to 120° could be easily obtained after screw removal. On post-removal radiograph, radiolucent gap between avulsed fragment and host bone was observed. This was thought to be a fibrocartilaginous union to lead to bony union which was expected. However, this patient was lost to follow-up at 3 months after screw removal. When he returned to the clinic at post-removal 18 months, he showed a 25° of flexion contracture. Plain radiographs revealed re-displaced avulsion fragment. Open reduction and internal fixation with two 5.0 mm cannulated screws with two washers were performed. At the latest follow-up, he showed a 10° of flexion contracture with further flexion of 130°. Bony union of avulsed fragment was achieved. There were no signs of knee instability. This patient was the only one who showed arthrofibrosis. All other 26 patients had full range of knee motion at the latest follow-up.

Side-to-side difference in Lachman test was less than 3 mm in 23 (85%) patients, 3 to 5 mm in 2 (7%) patients, and 5 to 10 mm in 1 (4%) patient. Side-to-side difference in anterior drawer test was less than 3 mm in 24 (89%) patients, 3 to 5 mm in 2 (7%) patients, and 5 to 10 mm in 1 (4%) patient. Of 17 patients who were examined with KT-1000 arthrometer, manual maximum side-to-side difference was less than 3 mm in 14 (82%) patients, 3 to 5 mm in 2 (12%) patients, and 5 mm in 1 (6%) patient. The patient who had 5 to 10 mm of side-to-side difference in physical examinations was the patient who showed 5 mm of side-to-side difference in the KT-1000 arthrometer measurement. He had been treated with one 4.0 mm screw and two 5.0 mm screws in conjunction with three washers for type II fracture at 36 days after trauma. Continuity of his ACL was maintained on preoperative MRI and arthroscopy. At the day of screw removal, however, the diameter of ACL decreased up to 50% of normal diameter, although the

Table 1 Descriptive Data and Results of 27 Patients

Patient	Age at surgery (years)	Age at the latest follow-up (years)	Interval from trauma to surgery (days)	Gender	Side	Type[a]	Cause of Injury	Anterior drawer/ Lachman S-to-S diff (mm)	KT-1000 S-to-S diff (mm)	FC/FF at the latest follow-up (°)	Impingement	Lysholm score	Latest X-ray	LLD ICH[b] (mm)	LLD FHH[b] (mm)
1	11–12	18–19	12	F	Rt.	III	Fall	1/0		0/135	–	100	–		
2	3–4	14–15	7	F	Lt.	II	Fall	2/0		0/135	–	100	–		
3	8–9	16–17	141	M	Rt.	IV	RTA	0/0	4	−5/145	+	80	Ossicle	11	4
4	9–10	10–11	4	F	Lt.	III	Fall	0/0		−5/135	–		–		
5	8–9	13–14	4	F	Lt.	III	Collision with another person	0/0		0/135	–	100	–		
6	7–8	10–11	8	M	Lt.	II	Fall	0/0	1	−15/135	–	100	–	3	3
7	7–8	11–12	32	M	Lt.	III	Fall	0/0	1	10/130	+	85	Ossicle	−2	2
8	6–7	8–9	11	M	Lt.	II	Fall	0/1	2	−10/145	–	95	–	7	8
9	9–10	16–17	6	M	Lt.	II	Skiing	1/2		0/145	–	100	–	17	16
10	9–10	12–13	9	M	Rt.	III	Collision with another person	5/3	0	−5/150	–	100	–	13	7
11	6–7	11–12	731	M	Rt.	III	Running	3/0	0	0/140	–	93	Ledging	4	2
12	9–10	10–11	36	M	Rt.	II	Bicycling	5/9	5	0/140	–	78	–	10	7
13	10–11	15–16	3	F	Lt.	II	Skiing	3/0	1	−5/145	–	97	–	18	8
14	8–9	12–13	75	M	Rt.	IV	Fall	2/2		0/145	–	100	Ledging	11	9
15	10–11	11–12	5	M	Rt.	II	Fall	1/2	2	0/140	–	100	–	11	10
16	12–13	13–14	3	M	Rt.	II	Skiing	0/0		0/135	–		–		
17	11–12	18–19	0	M	Rt.	II	Fall	2/2	1	−10/135	–	91	Ledging	3	1
18	9–10	14–15	182	M	Rt.	III	Soccer	0/0	2	−5/135	–	100	Ledging	−4	−3
19	8–9	11–12	5	F	Lt.	III	Skiing	0/0		5/135	–		–	0	0
20	9–10	15–16	22	M	Rt.	III	Skiing	1/4	3	−5/135	–	95	–	8	8
21	12–13	16–17	1	F	Lt.	II	Skiing	0/0	2	0/135	–		–	−1	−3
22	9–10	13–14	3	M	Rt.	II	Bicycling	3/3	1	−10/150	–	100	–	5	4
23	13–14	14–15	4	M	Rt.	III	Fall	0/0	2	−5/135	–	84	–	7	5
24	13–14	17–18	3	M	Rt.	III	Fall	2/0	2	−5/150	–	94	–		
25	13–14	15–16	2	M	Rt.	II	RTA	0/0		0/135	–	99	–	3.5	4.5
26	8–9	15–16	5	F	Lt.	III	Skiing	0/0		5/135	–		–		
27	10–11	14–15	5	M	Rt.	III	Skiing	0/2	2	−10/135	–	94	Ledging	0	−4

S-to-S diff Side-to-side difference; *FC* Flexion contracture; *FF* Further flexion; *LLD* Leg length discrepancy; *ICH* Iliac crest height; FHH, femoral head height; *RTA* Road traffic accident
[a]Zaricznyj modification of Meyers and McKeever classification, [b]Positive value means that an affected leg is longer than a contralateral leg; Negative value means that a contralateral leg is longer than an affected leg

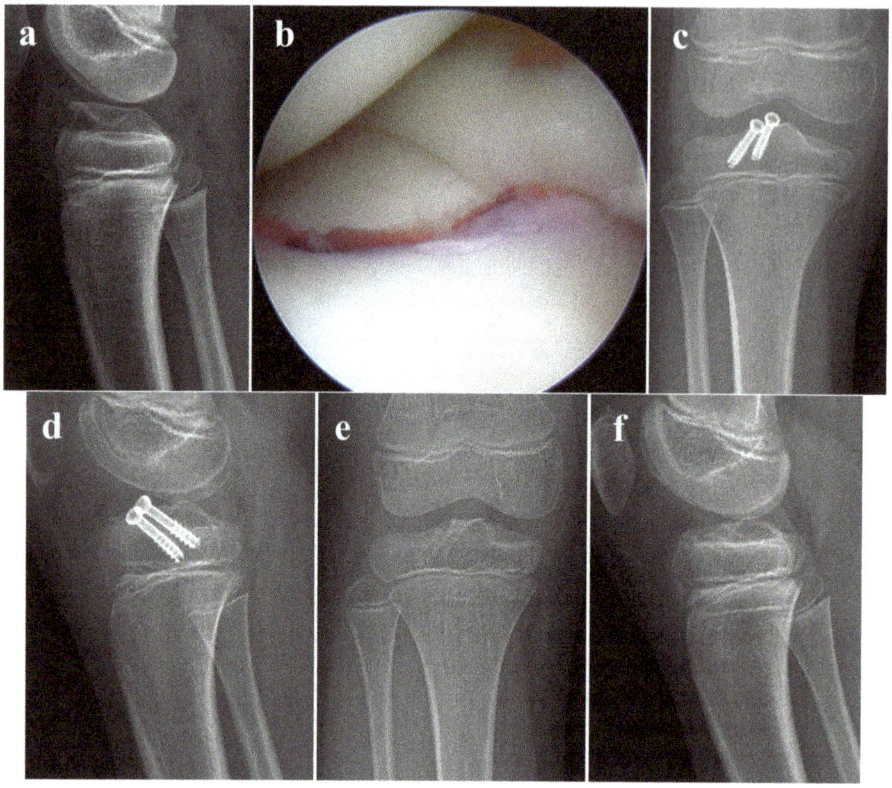

Fig. 1 a A radiograph of a 10–11 year-old girl with tibial eminence fracture. **b** Anterior horn of medial meniscus entrapped under the avulsed fragment. **c, d** Radiographs taken at postoperative one month. The avulsed fragment was fixed with two 5.0 mm cannulated screws. **e, f** Radiographs taken at postoperative one year. Screws were removed. Her Lysholm knee screw was 100. She did not have instability of the knee

tension of the ligament was acceptable. He complained intermittent pain and swelling of the knee after sports activity, although he had no pain during daily life activities.

The mean Lysholm knee score was 94.8 ± 6.8 (range, 78 to 100) at the latest follow-up. The score was more than 90 in 18 (82%) patients, 80 to 90 in 3 (14%) patients, and 78 in 1 (5%) patient who showed instability of the knee in physical examination and KT-1000 arthrometer measurement. The mean Lysholm score was 96.8 ± 4.5 (range, 84 to 100) in 16 patients whose interval from trauma to surgery was less than 30 days, and 89.3 ± 9.8 (range, 78 to 100) in 6 patients whose interval from trauma to surgery was more than 30 days (p = 0.134). The correlation between the degree of laxity measured by KT-1000 or Lachman test and the Lysholm scores was not statistically significant ($p = 0.088$ and $p = 0.910$, respectively).

Radiological outcomes

There was no case showing violation of proximal tibial physis by screws on postoperative radiographs. In 7 (26%) patients, radiologic abnormalities were found at the latest follow-up. Five (19%) had ledging which was prominent tibial eminence (Fig. 3). This might be caused by malunion and overgrowth of the avulsed fragment. Two (7%) were small ossicles above the tibial plateau (Fig. 3). Four of these 7 patients underwent operation at more than 30 days after the trauma. Extension deficit was not observed in these patients except one who underwent revision surgery due to re-displacement of avulsed fragment.

The length of the affected lower limb was 6.2 ± 5.9 mm longer (range, – 4.0 to 18.3 mm) than that of the contralateral lower limb measured against iliac crest height. It was 4.4 ± 4.7 mm longer (range, – 3.0 to 16.4 mm) measured against femoral head height. In 10 (50%) patients, the affected leg was more than 5 mm longer than the contralateral leg measured against iliac crest height. In another 10 (50%) patients, the difference in length between both legs was less than 5 mm. No patient whose contralateral leg was more than 5 mm longer than the affected leg. The mean length of femora of the affected side was 3.6 ± 4.1 mm longer (range, – 3.0 to 10.8 mm) than that of the contralateral side. The mean length of tibiae of affected side was 2.3 ± 3.4 mm longer (range, – 6.0 to 9.3 mm) than that of the contralateral side.

Associated knee injuries based on preoperative MRI and arthroscopic findings are summarized in Table 2. Six patients had lateral meniscal tear which was treated with partial meniscectomy (4 patients) or meniscal repair (2 patients). One medial meniscal tear was treated with partial meniscectomy.

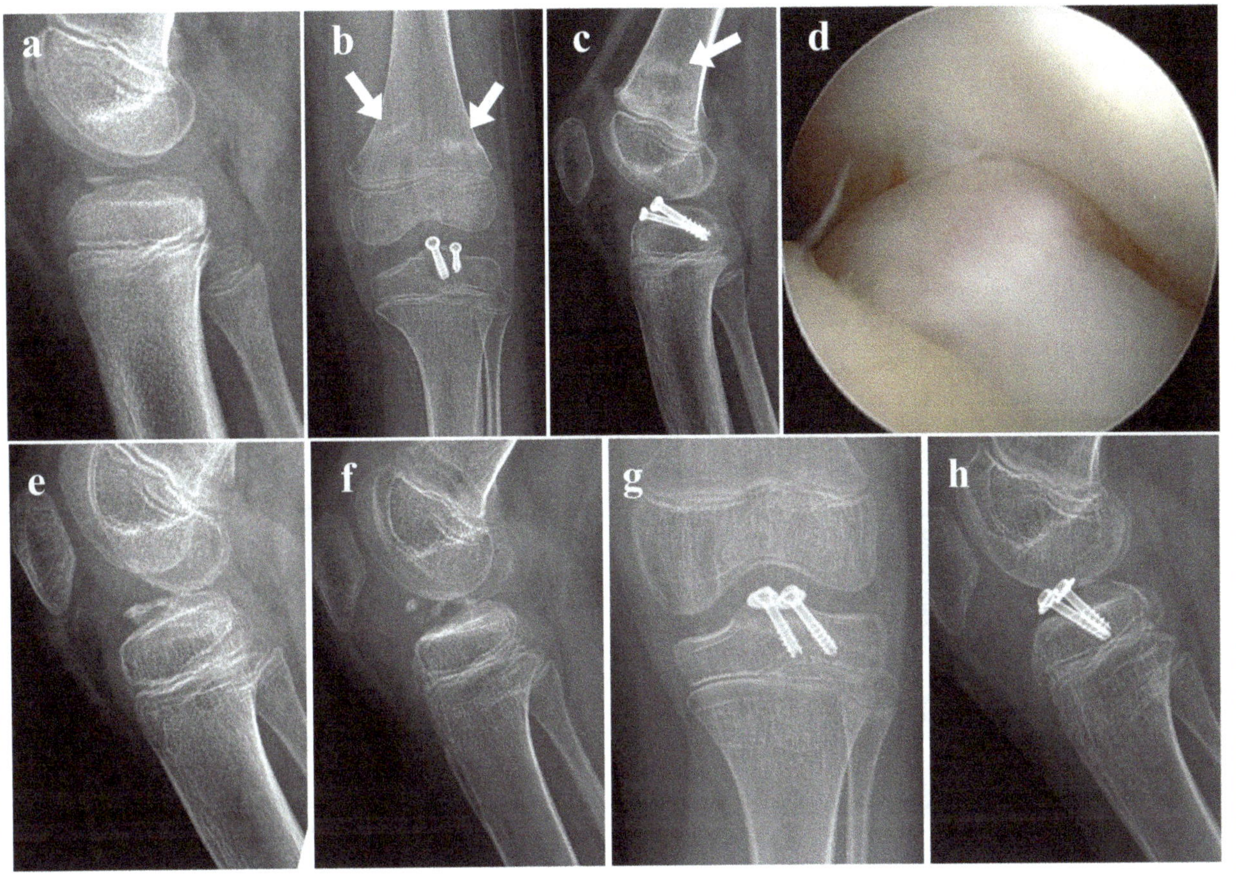

Fig. 2 **a** A 8–9 year-old boy visited the clinic at 32 days post trauma with type III tibial eminence fracture. **b, c** Radiographs taken at postoperative 2.5 months. Incomplete distal femoral metaphyseal fracture (arrow) occurred during vigorous physical therapy. **d** While removing screws, it was found that the head of 5.0 mm screw impinged against the lateral portion of the medial femoral condyle and caused extension deficit of the knee. **e** Radiolucent gap between avulsed fragment and host bone was found on the day of screw removal. **f** A radiograph taken at postoperative 18 months. He was lost to follow-up for 1 year. He returned to the clinic with flexion contracture of 25° and re-displaced avulsed fragment. **g, h** He underwent open reduction and internal fixation with two 5.0 mm screws in conjunction with two washers for re-displaced fragments

Discussion

The results show that arthroscopically assisted cannulated screw fixation is an effective and safe method for tibial eminence fracture in pediatric patients. Previous studies have described that fixation with a relatively large screw, compared to the small avulsed fragment, is technically demanding and can cause comminution of the bony fragment [28, 37, 38]. However, this complication was not found in this study. Union was achieved in almost all patients using a washer combined with a screw depending on the size of avulsed fragment and fracture pattern, consistent with prior results [32]. Other authors expressed concern that synovial leakage might occur after using a larger portal for a washer [27]. However, this complication did not occur in our series. To prevent posterior displacement of the avulsed fragment during screw insertion and consequent increased laxity, operators need to pay attention to the sagittal angle of the screw. Inserting two guide pins before screw insertion may help to prevent displacement and rotation of the fragment.

Arthrofibrosis developed in only one patient. This frequency is much less than the result of a previous multicenter study reporting an arthrofibrosis frequency of 10% in 205 patients treated with various surgical methods [14]. The authors immobilized the knee in full extension for 4 to 6 weeks in the majority of patients, which was longer than the 3 to 4 weeks in the present study. A previous systematic review reported that no patient developed arthrofibrosis in the screw fixation group compared to 6.3% of patients treated by suture fixation [39]. The data indicate that early range of motion exercise following firm fixation with cannulated screws might reduce the occurrence of arthrofibrosis.

A previous systematic review reported that 82% patients had laxity on both anterior drawer and Lachman test, while another systematic review reported abnormality on anterior drawer or Lachman test in 20% of patients [39, 40]. These rates are higher than presently observed. The discrepancy in instability might be attributable to a real difference of laxity or by heterogeneous criteria used to evaluate instability. In

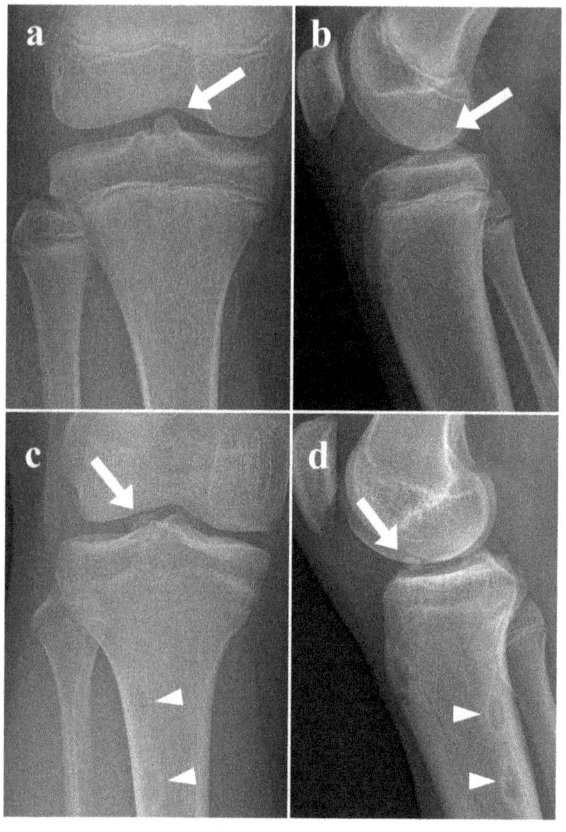

Fig. 3 a, b Radiographs showing ledging (arrow), a prominent tibial eminence, possibly caused by malunion and overgrowth of the avulsed fragment. **c, d** In two patients, ossicles (arrow) were found above the tibial plateau. One patient had well demarcated intracortical osteolytic lesions (arrowhead) in the posterolateral aspect of proximal tibia

this study, side-to-side differences on physical examinations and KT-1000 arthrometer measurement were used to determine instability for pediatric patients, who are generally suppler than adults. However, another study used the absolute value on Lachman test to judge instability [33]. Similar to the results of other studies, there was no significant relationship between laxity and subjective symptom in the current study [33, 41]. However, a patient who had 5 to 10 mm of side-to-side difference on physical examinations and KT-1000 arthrometer also had pain and swelling of the knee after strenuous exercise and recorded the lowest Lysholm score.

Table 2 Details of the associated knee injury

$N = 26$	No.
None	14 (54%)
Bone contusion in the femoral lateral condyle	5 (19%)
Lateral meniscal tear	4 (15%)
Lateral meniscal tear and bone contusion in the femoral lateral condyle	1 (4%)
Lateral and medial meniscal tear	1 (4%)
Segond fracture	1 (4%)

High Lysholm knee scores have been reported, regardless of surgical methods or fixation devices [27, 39, 42, 43]. The scores were also high in our study. Since these uniform high scores might be due to a ceiling effect of Lysholm knee score [44], caution is needed when interpreting Lysholm score as a surgical outcome. In the current study, Lysholm scores of patients who underwent surgery more than 30 days after trauma were less than those of patients who underwent surgery within 30 days after trauma. However, their differences were not statistically significant. This might be due to type-II error.

Impingement of screw head on femoral condyle or trochlea has been rarely reported. A previous study of epiphyseal or transphyseal cannulated screw fixation related no case of chondral damage from a protruded screw [45]. Another case report introduced a patient who had 15° of extension deficit and chondral damage after an epiphyseal screw fixation with a toothed washer for type II fracture [46]. The authors assumed that use of a washer might have induced bulging of the screw head, resulting in extension impingement. However, a washer was not used in the two patients who had impingement in the present study. They underwent surgery at more than 30 days after trauma and two 5.0 mm screws were used. When the period between trauma and surgery is long or diameter of a screw is large, careful inspection for impingement should be made for the whole range of motion. Intercondylar notchplasty may be considered.

Nonunion rarely occurs after a tibial eminence fracture [39, 47]. Presently, only one patient underwent additional surgery due to nonunion. On the latest radiographs, 5 (19%) patients had prominent tibial eminence, consistent with results of a previous study showing 15% patients with ledging [27]. In the latter series, one of four ledgings caused an impingement phenomenon. In the current study, however, patients with ledging did not show extension deficit except one who received revision surgery.

Some previous studies have reported physeal growth disturbance after treatment for tibial eminence fracture [32–34, 39, 47, 48]. However, LLD was rarely evaluated. Ahn and colleagues described that 2 of 5 children have LLD of 1 cm (the affected legs is longer) after arthroscopic reduction and suture fixation [48]. In our study, the mean length of the affected leg was longer than that of the contralateral leg. Interestingly, both tibiae and femora of the affected side were longer than those of the contralateral side. Because LLD was not measured preoperatively, we cannot conclusively say that tibial eminence fracture is prone to occur in a longer leg or can make the affected leg longer.

Entrapment of the meniscus or intermeniscal ligament between the avulsed fragment and host bone can obstruct the reduction of a fracture [49, 50]. A study from the United States reported this finding after tibial eminence fracture in over 50% of patients [49]. Another Western study described that 59% patients have interposition of intermeniscal ligament under the avulsed fragment [30]. In our study of Korean patients, only 19% of the patients had these findings, although distribution of fracture type was similar to that in previous studies. In contrast, associated injuries including meniscal tear were more common in our study than those in Western studies [27, 33, 49]. A Japanese study also reported associated meniscal tear in 30% of patients [51], similar to our result. More data are needed to confirm this difference between Asian and Western patients.

This study had several limitations. First, because the study design was a retrospective case series, there was no control group treated with other methods. Second, results of some examinations, such as KT-1000 arthrometer and whole leg radiograph, in some patients could not be obtained due to their circumstances. This might have caused selection bias. Third, because the number of patients with type IV fracture was small, it was difficult to assess the outcome of cannulated screw fixation for type IV fracture. Fourth, Lachman and anterior drawer tests were performed manually without taking special landmarks, which may lead to low accuracy and reliability of these tests. And the result of pivot shift test which is also commonly performed in the patients with ACL insufficiency was not presented. Fifth, although we showed Lysholm score as a functional outcome scale, it would be better if we obtained Tegner or Marx activity scale together. Lastly, the sample size was not large, in some analyses, to verify the statistical significance.

Conclusions

Arthroscopically assisted cannulated screw fixation for tibial eminence fracture in children and adolescents shows satisfactory clinical and radiological outcomes. Union can be achieved in almost every patient, and postoperative function of the knee is excellent. The occurrences of arthrofibrosis, instability, and screw head impingement are low, and the risk of violation of proximal tibial physis by screws are minimal.

Acknowledgements
Not applicable.

Abbreviations
ACL: Anterior cruciate ligament; AP: Anteroposterior; FC: Flexion contracture; FF: Further flexion; FHH: Femoral head height; ICH: Iliac crest height; LLD: Leg length discrepancy; S-to-S diff: Sde-to-side difference; RTA: road traffic accident

Funding
No funding was obtained for this study.

Authors' contributions
CHS and DJL drafted the manuscript and performed data collection and data analysis. IHC, TJC, and WJY conceived of the study, participated in the design of the study, performed data interpretation, and participated in coordination. All authors read and approved the final manuscript.

Consent for publication
Not applicable.

Competing interests
The authors declare that they have no competing interests.

References

1. Molander ML, Wallin G, Wikstad I. Fracture of the intercondylar eminence of the tibia: a review of 35 patients. J Bone Joint Surg Br. 1981;63-B(1):89–91.
2. Meyers MH, M. MF. Fracture of the intercondylar eminence of the tibia. J Bone Joint Surg Am. 1959;41-A(2):209–20. discussion 20-2
3. Skak SV, Jensen TT, Poulsen TD, Sturup J. Epidemiology of knee injuries in children. Acta Orthop Scand. 1987;58(1):78–81.
4. Zaricznyj B. Avulsion fracture of the tibial eminence: treatment by open reduction and pinning. J Bone Joint Surg Am. 1977;59(8):1111–4.
5. Lafrance RM, Giordano B, Goldblatt J, Voloshin I, Maloney M. Pediatric tibial eminence fractures: evaluation and management. J Am Acad Orthop Surg. 2010;18(7):395–405.
6. Meyers MH, McKeever FM. Fracture of the intercondylar eminence of the tibia. J Bone Joint Surg Am. 1970;52(8):1677–84.
7. Berg EE. Pediatric tibial eminence fractures: arthroscopic cannulated screw fixation. Arthroscopy. 1995;11(3):328–31.
8. Keshet D, Zaidman M, Eidelman M. Treatment of avulsion fractures of the intercondylar eminence by medial parapatellar approach, open reduction and cross wire fixation. J Pediatr Orthop B. 2015;24(4):321–5.
9. Johnson DL, Durbin TC. Physeal-sparing tibial eminence fracture fixation with a headless compression screw. Orthopedics. 2012;35(7):604–8.
10. Sawyer GA, Hulstyn MJ, Anderson BC, Schiller J. Arthroscopic suture bridge fixation of tibial intercondylar eminence fractures. Arthrosc Tech. 2013;2(4): e315–8.
11. Su WR, Wang PH, Wang HN, Lin CJ. A simple, modified arthroscopic suture fixation of avulsion fracture of the tibial intercondylar eminence in children. J Pediatr Orthop B. 2011;20(1):17–21.
12. Brunner S, Vavken P, Kilger R, Vavken J, Rutz E, Brunner R, Camathias C. Absorbable and non-absorbable suture fixation results in similar outcomes for tibial eminence fractures in children and adolescents. Knee Surg Sports Traumatol Arthrosc. 2016;24(3):723–9.
13. Nwachukwu BU, McFeely ED, Nasreddine A, Udall JH, Finlayson C, Shearer DW, Micheli LJ, Kocher MS. Arthrofibrosis after anterior cruciate ligament reconstruction in children and adolescents. J Pediatr Orthop. 2011;31(8): 811–7.
14. Vander Have KL, Ganley TJ, Kocher MS, Price CT, Herrera-Soto JA. Arthrofibrosis after surgical fixation of tibial eminence fractures in children and adolescents. Am J Sports Med. 2010;38(2):298–301.
15. Gholve PA, Voellmicke KV, Guven M, Potter HG, Rodeo SA, Widmann RF. Arthrofibrosis of the knee after tibial spine fracture in children: a report of two complicated cases. HSS J. 2008;4(1):14–9.
16. Petsche TS, Hutchinson MR. Loss of extension after reconstruction of the anterior cruciate ligament. J Am Acad Orthop Surg. 1999;7(2):119–27.
17. Larsen MW, Garrett WE, Jr., Delee JC, Moorman CT, 3rd. Surgical management of anterior cruciate ligament injuries in patients with open physes. J Am Acad Orthop Surg 2006;14(13):736–744.
18. Yoo WJ, Kocher MS, Micheli LJ. Growth plate disturbance after transphyseal reconstruction of the anterior cruciate ligament in skeletally immature adolescent patients: an MR imaging study. J Pediatr Orthop. 2011;31(6):691–6.
19. Sawyer GA, Anderson BC, Paller D, Schiller J, Eberson CP, Hulstyn M. Biomechanical analysis of suture bridge fixation for tibial eminence fractures. Arthroscopy. 2012;28(10):1533–9.
20. Mahar AT, Duncan D, Oka R, Lowry A, Gillingham B, Chambers H. Biomechanical comparison of four different fixation techniques for pediatric tibial eminence avulsion fractures. J Pediatr Orthop. 2008;28(2):159–62.
21. In Y, Kwak DS, Moon CW, Han SH, Choi NY. Biomechanical comparison of three techniques for fixation of tibial avulsion fractures of the anterior cruciate ligament. Knee Surg Sports Traumatol Arthrosc. 2012;20(8):1470–8.
22. Hapa O, Barber FA, Suner G, Ozden R, Davul S, Bozdag E, Sunbuloglu E. Biomechanical comparison of tibial eminence fracture fixation with high-strength suture, EndoButton, and suture anchor. Arthroscopy. 2012;28(5):681–7.

23. Anderson CN, Nyman JS, McCullough KA, Song Y, Uppuganti S, O'Neill KR, Anderson AF, Dunn WR. Biomechanical evaluation of physeal-sparing fixation methods in tibial eminence fractures. Am J Sports Med. 2013;41(7):1586–94.
24. Senekovic V, Balazic M. Bioabsorbable sutures versus screw fixation of displaced tibial eminence fractures: a biomechanical study. Eur J Orthop Surg Traumatol. 2014;24(2):209–16.
25. Ahn JH, Lee YS, Lee DH, Ha HC. Arthroscopic physeal sparing all inside repair of the tibial avulsion fracture in the anterior cruciate ligament: technical note. Arch Orthop Trauma Surg. 2008;128(11):1309–12.
26. Huang TW, Hsu KY, Cheng CY, Chen LH, Wang CJ, Chan YS, Chen WJ. Arthroscopic suture fixation of tibial eminence avulsion fractures. Arthroscopy. 2008;24(11):1232–8.
27. Reynders P, Reynders K, Broos P. Pediatric and adolescent tibial eminence fractures: arthroscopic cannulated screw fixation. J Trauma. 2002;53(1):49–54.
28. Wouters DB, de Graaf JS, Hemmer PH, Burgerhof JG, Kramer WL. The arthroscopic treatment of displaced tibial spine fractures in children and adolescents using meniscus arrows(R). Knee Surg Sports Traumatol Arthrosc. 2011;19(5):736–9.
29. Furlan D, Pogorelic Z, Biocic M, Juric I, Mestrovic J. Pediatric tibial eminence fractures: arthroscopic treatment using K-wire. Scand J Surg. 2010;99(1):38–44.
30. Hunter RE, Willis JA. Arthroscopic fixation of avulsion fractures of the tibial eminence: technique and outcome. Arthroscopy. 2004;20(2):113–21.
31. Pan RY, Yang JJ, Chang JH, Shen HC, Lin LC, Lian YT. Clinical outcome of arthroscopic fixation of anterior tibial eminence avulsion fractures in skeletally mature patients: a comparison of suture and screw fixation technique. J Trauma Acute Care Surg. 2012;72(2):E88–93.
32. Senekovic V, Veselko M. Anterograde arthroscopic fixation of avulsion fractures of the tibial eminence with a cannulated screw. five-year results Arthroscopy. 2003;19(1):54–61.
33. Kocher MS, Foreman ES, Micheli LJ. Laxity and functional outcome after arthroscopic reduction and internal fixation of displaced tibial spine fractures in children. Arthroscopy. 2003;19(10):1085–90.
34. Najdi H, Thevenin-Lemoine C, Sales de Gauzy J, Accadbled F. Arthroscopic treatment of intercondylar eminence fractures with intraepiphyseal screws in children and adolescents. Orthop Traumatol Surg Res. 2016;102(4):447–51.
35. Lysholm J, Gillquist J. Evaluation of knee ligament surgery results with special emphasis on use of a scoring scale. Am J Sports Med. 1982;10(3):150–4.
36. Meyers MHMF. Fractures of the intercondylar eminence of the tibia. J Bone Joint Surg Am. 1959;41:209–22.
37. EE B. Pediatric Tibia1 eminence fractures: arthroscopic cannulated screw fixation. Arthroscopy. 1995;11(3):328–31.
38. Tudisco C, Giovarruscio R, Febo A, Savarese E, Bisicchia S. Intercondylar eminence avulsion fracture in children: long-term follow-up of 14 cases at the end of skeletal growth. J Pediatr Orthop B. 2010;19(5):403–8.
39. Gans I, Baldwin KD, Ganley TJ. Treatment and management outcomes of Tibial eminence fractures in pediatric patients: a systematic review. Am J Sports Med. 2014;42(7):1743–50.
40. Bogunovic L, Tarabichi M, Harris D, Wright R. Treatment of tibial eminence fractures: a systematic review. J Knee Surg. 2015;28(3):255–62.
41. Baxter MP, Fractures WJJ. Of the tibial spine in children. An evaluation of knee stability. J Bone Joint Surg Br. 1988;70(2):228–30.
42. Janarv PM, Westblad P, Johansson C, Hirsch G. Long-term follow-up of anterior tibial spine fractures in children. J Pediatr Orthop. 1995;15(1): 63–8.
43. Perugia D, Basiglini L, Vadala A, Ferretti A. Clinical and radiological results of arthroscopically treated tibial spine fractures in childhood. Int Orthop. 2009;33(1):243–8.
44. Ra HJ, Kim HS, Choi JY, Ha JK, Kim JY, Kim JG. Comparison of the ceiling effect in the Lysholm score and the IKDC subjective score for assessing functional outcome after ACL reconstruction. Knee. 2014;21(5):906–10.
45. Parikh SN, Myer D, Eismann EA. Prevention of Arthrofibrosis after arthroscopic screw fixation of Tibial spine fracture in children and adolescents. Orthopedics. 2014;37(1):e58-e65.
46. Tsai T-Y, Chan J-H, Yeh Y-K, Chuang F-K, Liu C-W, Wang S-J. Malpractice of epiphyseal cannulated screw fixation in a child with avulsion fracture of the tibial eminence complicating with lack of knee extension and distal femoral fracture. J Med Sci. 2009;29(5):289–92.
47. Coyle C, Jagernauth S, Ramachandran M. Tibial eminence fractures in the paediatric population: a systematic review. J Child Orthop. 2014;8(2):149–59.
48. Ahn JH, Yoo JC. Clinical outcome of arthroscopic reduction and suture for displaced acute and chronic tibial spine fractures. Knee Surg Sports Traumatol Arthrosc. 2005;13(2):116–21.
49. Kocher MS, Micheli LJ, Gerbino P, Hresko MT. Tibial eminence fractures in children: prevalence of meniscal entrapment. Am J Sports Med. 2003;31(3):404–7.
50. Burstein DB, Viola A, Fulkerson JP. Entrapment of the medial meniscus in a fracture of the tibial eminence. Arthroscopy. 1988;4(1):47–50.
51. Park HJ, Urabe K, Naruse K, Aikawa J, Fujita M, Itoman M. Arthroscopic evaluation after surgical repair of intercondylar eminence fractures. Arch Orthop Trauma Surg. 2007;127(9):753–7.

25

Influence of age on results following surgery for displaced acetabular fractures in the elderly

Guo-Chun Zha[1*†], Xue-Mei Yang[2†], Shuo Feng[1], Xiang-Yang Chen[1], Kai-Jin Guo[1*] and Jun-Ying Sun[3*]

Abstract

Background: Elderly patients have more special medical needs when compared with young ones; thus, the results of open reduction and internal fixation (ORIF) for acetabular fractures should be stratified by age in these patients. This study seeks to determine whether the age of the patient influences the results of the ORIF for acetabular fractures.

Methods: We performed a retrospective analysis of prospectively collected data on 53 elderly patients with displaced acetabular fractures who underwent ORIF between May 2004 and May 2011. Patients were divided into two groups by age: young–old group (60–74 years) and old–old group (75–90 years). The number of patients in each group was 28 and 25. The reduction quality and clinical function was evaluated using the Matta criteria and modified Postel Merle D'Aubigne Score, respectively. Operative time, bleeding amount, and complications were recorded.

Results: Patients in old–old group had significantly lower anatomical reduction rate ($p = 0.024$), less operative time ($p = 0.021$), and less bleeding amount ($p = 0.016$) than those in the young–old group. The reduction quality in the young–old group was strongly associated with clinical function ($p < 0.05$). However, no difference in clinical function was detected among the different reduction qualities in the old–old group ($p > 0.05$). Moreover, no significant difference in clinical functions ($p = 0.787$) and complications ($p = 0.728$) was detected between the two groups.

Conclusions: Old–old patients may expect comparable clinical functions and complications with young–old patients. The reduction quality in old–old patients may be not significantly associated with clinical function. Different treatment strategies may be applied for acetabular fractures with ORIF in different age groups.

Keywords: Acetabular fracture, Elderly patients, Age, Outcomes

Background

The incidence of acetabular fractures in the elderly has increased [1]. However, the optimal management of displaced acetabular fractures in elderly patients remains controversial. Some surgeons prefer advocated conservative treatment for elderly patients with limited physiological reserves and medical comorbidity that may increase the risk of surgery [2, 3]. Other surgeons advise total hip arthroplasty (THA) for elderly patients with poor bone quality that may increase the risk of poor reduction and loss of reduction or failure of fixation or both [4–6]. Considering the limited life expectancy, low activity level, and low functional requirements of elderly patients, some authors believe that open reduction and internal fixation (ORIF) is suitable for these patients [1, 7, 8].

The inconsistent clinical results can be attributed in part to the following reasons: (1) previous studies included patients of a wide age variety, i.e., greater than 40 [9], 50 [10], 55 [11] to 60 [1] and 70 years old [8]; and

* Correspondence: 41049015@qq.com; xzgkj@sina.com; cgc85012@126.com
†Equal contributors
[1]Department of Orthopedic Surgery, the Affiliated Hospital of Xuzhou Medical University, No. 99 Huaihai West Road, Xuzhou, Jiangsu 221002, People's Republic of China
[3]Orthopaedic Department, the First Affiliated Hospital of Soochow University, 188 Shizi Street, Suzhou, Jiangsu 215006, People's Republic of China

(2) the results of studies that classified elderly patients as a single population were not stratified by age. Elderly patients have more special medical needs when compared with young ones; thus, different age groups of elderly patients may present different physiological reserves, lifestyle qualities, and osteoporosis degrees. Accordingly, the results of acetabular fractures in the elderly should be stratified by age. Extracting practical conclusions about the relationship of age, reduction quality, and clinical function after ORIF is difficult without a comparator group.

To the best of our knowledge, none of studies have focused exclusively on the relationship of the age to clinical function, reduction quality, and complication of ORIF for acetabular fracture in elderly patients. Therefore, this study seeks to determine whether the age of the patient influences the results of the ORIF for acetabular fractures.

Methods

Patient source

We performed a retrospective analysis of prospectively collected data on 66 consecutive elderly patients with displaced acetabular fractures between May 2004 and May 2011. Four patients were conservative therapy, and 62 patients underwent ORIF. The 62 patients were divided into two groups by age: young–old group (60–74 years) and old–old group (75–90 years). This study received approval from the institutional review board. Informed consent was obtained from all patients included in the study.

Surgical technique

All surgeries were performed by the senior author (J.Y.S) at an average of 5.8 ± 2.5 days (range, 2–14 days) from the initial injury. Skeletal traction was selectively employed through the distal femoral pin. The medical conditions of the patients were optimized through a preoperative multidisciplinary approach. Despite the absence of specific intraoperative management criteria, the surgeon closely followed the principles that accurate reduction is attempted for young–old patients with an active and good physical state. Limited operative procedure was used for old–old patients with low activity and functional requirements to achieve the stable internal fixation of fractures and prevent anatomical reduction.

All patients were placed in floppy lateral position and then operated under general anesthesia. The approach (Kocher–Langenbeck, Ilioinguinal, or Kocher–Langenbeck + Ilioinguinal) was decided according to the nature of the acetabular fracture and the preference of orthopedic surgeon (J.Y.S).

Perioperative regimen

All patients received adequate pain control during the perioperative period. The drain was removed after 48 h, and three standard plain radiographs were obtained after 3 days. On the day after surgery, the patients were encouraged to sit up in bed and perform passive functional exercises to strengthen the hip joint, quadriceps, and hamstrings. The patients were allowed touch-toe weight-bearing a maximum of 20 kg for the first 12 weeks with a walker or crutches depending on physical state. After 12 weeks, full weight-bearing gradually progressed according to patient tolerance.

Follow-up

After discharge, the patients were traced using telephone, letter, or e-mail and were asked to return for completing the clinical and radiological postoperative evaluation at 6 weeks, 3 months, 1 year, and annually thereafter. Patients who refused or were unable to return were contacted by two surgeons (S.J.D and J.X.T) to obtain the information in their home.

Data collection

The information included comorbidity, mechanism of injury, fracture type, associated injury, operative time, bleeding amount (including operative blood loss and wound drainage), operative approach, complications, quality of reduction, clinical function, and radiological outcomes. The results from patients who were confirmed to have died from natural causes after 12 months follow-up was included in this study. By contrast, the results from patients who had been lost to follow-up or confirmed to have died from natural causes within 12 months follow-up were excluded. Data from the final follow-up visit were analyzed for this study.

Radiographic and clinical evaluation

Three standard plain preoperative radiographs (anteroposterior pelvis, obturator oblique, and iliac oblique views) were obtained along with computed tomography scans to classify fracture according to Letournel's classification system [12]. Reduction quality was evaluated on the three-standard plain post-operative radiographs and graded as anatomical (0 mm to 1 mm of displacement), imperfect (2 mm to 3 mm displacement), or poor (more than 3 mm displacement) on the basis of the residual displacement as defined by Matta [9].

Clinical function was categorized as excellent (18 points), good (15–17 points), fair (13–14 points), or poor (< 13 points) on the basis of the modified Postel Merle D'Aubigne Score, which includes degree of pain (0–6 points), degree of ambulation (0–6 points), and range of motion (0–6 points) components [9, 13]. Radiological outcome was evaluated on the follow-up postoperative radiographs and was graded as excellent, good, fair, and poor in accordance with Matta criteria [9].

The acetabular fracture types were classified by a senior author (J.Y.S). Reduction quality was evaluated by two surgeons (S.K.Z and Z.S.Z) who did not participate in any of the surgical procedures. Two other surgeons (S.J.D and J.X.T) who were blinded to reduction quality completed the clinical and radiological evaluation. The senior author (J.Y.S) made the final assessment when the results (reduction quality and radiological outcome) were inconsistent. We take the average of the clinical outcomes that were evaluated by the two surgeons.

Statistical analysis

Analysis was performed using STATA version 11.0 (StataCorp LP, College Station TX). Continuous data were expressed as mean ± standard deviation (SD) and were analyzed using t-test or one-way ANOVA. Tukey's test was performed for multiple comparisons. The ordinal data were analyzed with Kruscal–Wallis test. Statistical significance was considered at $p < 0.05$ unless otherwise specified.

Results

Patient characteristics

Of the 62 patients, 7 (11.3%) were lost to follow-up at a mean of 18 months (6–31 months) postoperatively and 2 (3.2%) had died from natural causes within 12 months follow-up, during which all patients had excellent or good clinical function. The nine patients were excluded from this study. The remaining 53 patients (44 males and 9 females) aged 60–90 (mean age: 72.8 ± 6.6 years) were enrolled. The mean follow-up was 52.5 ± 24.1 months (range: 18–110 months). Detailed distribution of patient demographics and characteristics, fracture types, mechanism of injury, and associated injury is shown in Table 1.

Operative variable

Operative approach, operative time, and bleeding amount are shown in Table 2. Anatomical reduction was observed in 28 patients (52.8%), imperfect in 19 (35.8%), and poor in 6 (11.3%). Compared with the old–old patients, the young–old patients were more likely to achieve anatomical reduction (67.9% vs. 36%, $p = 0.024$) (Table 2) but more blood loss (705 mL vs. 591 mL, $p = 0.016$) and longer operative time (145 min vs. 110 min, $p = 0.021$) (Table 2).

Clinical results at the final follow-up

Clinical function was excellent in 19 patients (35.8%), good in 20 (37.7%), fair in 4 (7.5%), and poor in 10 (18.9%). The average clinical score (modified Merle d'Aubigne-Postel score) was 15.6 ± 2.7 points (range: 9–18 points). Two patients in the young–old group (3.8%) underwent THA at 30 and 35 months after their initial injuries. One of the two patients have a femoral head injury and subsequent osteonecrosis of the femoral head (Fig. 1), and the other has a poor reduction and subsequent severely post-traumatic osteoarthritis.

Table 1 Demographics of both groups

Variable	Young-old group ($n = 28$)	Old-old group ($n = 25$)
Mean age (years)	67.8 ± 4.1 (60–74)	78.5 ± 3.5 (75–90)
Sex ratio (male:female)	25: 3	19: 6
Mean BMI (kg/m^2)	22.3 ± 2.8 (17.9–25.5)	22.3 ± 2.1 (21.3–24.8)
Comorbidity (n)		
Hypertension	15	18
Anemia	6	9
Cardiopathy	2	4
Diabetes mellitus	3	2
Pulmonary	1	4
Cerebrovascular accident	1	3
Fracture types		
Associated both column	9	9
T-shaped	6	3
Transverse + posterior wall	5	2
Anterior column	1	4
Posterior wall	3	2
Anterior wall	0	4
Transverse	2	1
Posterior column	1	0
Posterior column + posterior wall	1	0
Mechanism of injury		
Fall at home	2	7
Pedestrian	1	10
Bike accident	2	1
Motorcyclist	4	0
Auto vs. Pedestrian	14	5
Fall from >2 m	5	2
Associated injury		
Splenic rupture	1	0
Sacroiliac joint dislocation	1	0
Thoracic spine and costal fracture	1	0
Head trauma	1	0
Mean follow-up (months)	60.7 ± 26.6 (24–110)	43.3 ± 17.2 (18–84)

Table 2 Operative parameters of both groups ($n = 53$)

Variable	Young-old group (n = 28)	Old-old group (n = 25)	*p*-value
Operative approach			0.022
Kocher-Langenbeck	7	4	
Ilioinguinal	1	8	
Kocher-Langenbeck + Ilioinguinal	20	13	
Mean operative time (min)	145 ± 53	110 ± 54	0.021
Mean bleeding amount (ml)	705 ± 308	591 ± 204	0.012
Quality of reduction			0.024
Anatomic	19	9	
Imperfect	7	12	
Poor	2	4	

Up to 75% of the young–old patients and 72% of the old–old patients can achieve good to excellent clinical function. The clinical scores were comparable in both groups (15.5 ± 3.2 vs. 15.7 ± 2.1, $p = 0.787$); however, comparison of the components of the modified Postel Merle D'Aubigne Score showed that the patients in the young–old group had lower pain scores (4.9 ± 1.2 vs. 5.5 ± 0.7, $p = 0.029$), higher ambulation scores (5.5 ± 1.0 vs. 4.9 ± 0.9, $p = 0.027$), and similar range of motion scores (5.1 ± 1.2 vs. 5.3 ± 0.7, $p = 0.457$) than those in the old-old group (Table 3).

The average clinical scores were significantly higher in the young–old patients with anatomical reduction (16.6 ± 2.4 points; range: 9–18 points) than in those with imperfect reduction (13.3 ± 1.9 points; range: 9–18 points) ($p = 0.015$) and poor reduction (12.0 ± 2.8 points; range: 10–14 points) ($p = 0.005$, Fig. 2).

The average clinical scores in the old–old patients with anatomical, imperfect, and poor reduction were 16.1 ± 2.1 (range: 12–18 points), 15.8 ± 2.1 (range: 12–18 points), and 14.8 ± 2.5 points (range: 12–18 points), respectively. No statistical difference in clinical scores was detected between the different grades in reduction quality ($p > 0.05$, Fig. 2, Fig. 3).

The rate of postoperative complication was slightly higher in the old–old group (44.0%) than in the young–old group (39.3%), but no difference was found between the groups ($p = 0.728$, Table 4). Nine (14.5%) of the 62

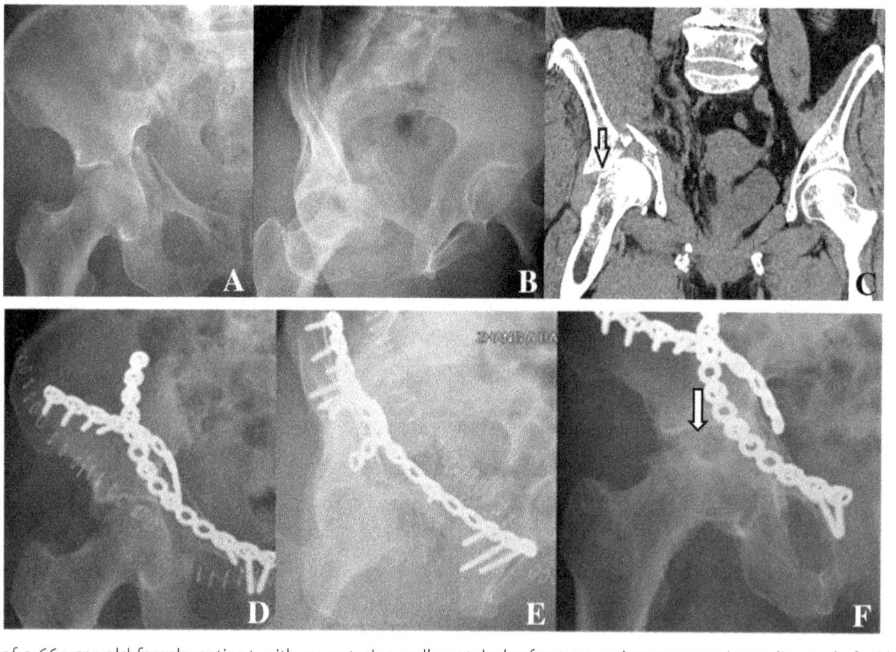

Fig. 1 Radiographs of a 66-year-old female patient with an anterior wall acetabular fracture. **a** Anteroposterior radiograph; **b** Obturator oblique radiograph; **c** CT scan, showing femoral head injury (arrow). **d, e** Immediately after surgery, showing a satisfactory reduction of fracture; **f** The radiograph taken at 30 months postoperatively, showing an osteonecrosis of the femoral head (arrow)

Table 3 Clinical outcomes of both groups at the final follow-up

Variable	Young-old group (n = 28)	Old-old group (n = 25)	p-value
Clinical scores (points)	15.5 ± 3.2	15.7 ± 2.1	0.787
Degree of pain	4.9 ± 1.2	5.5 ± 0.7	0.029
Degree of ambulation	5.5 ± 1.0	4.9 ± 0.9	0.027
Range of motion	5.1 ± 1.2	5.3 ± 0.7	0.457

patients died from natural causes during the follow-up period; of these nine patients, one died at 6 months, one at 9 months, and seven at 18–72 months postoperatively (average: 35 ± 19 months). The average age at the time of surgery of the nine patients was 78.4 ± 6.3 years (range: 68–85 years).

Radiological outcomes at the final follow-up

We found that better clinical function meant fewer patients willing to return for radiological evaluation. For example, only 16 patients have completed radiological evaluation. Of these patients, radiological outcomes were excellent in three patients, good in four patients, fair in three patients, and poor in six patients. The radiological outcomes do not reflect the real situation of all patients because most patients were not assessed. Thus, these outcomes were not included in this analysis.

Discussion

With the increased acetabular fractures in the elderly population, an understanding of how these patients respond to ORIF is important. We compared the postoperative clinical function and complication rates between old–old and young–old patients who underwent ORIF and investigated the influence of patient age on the association of reduction quality and clinical function.

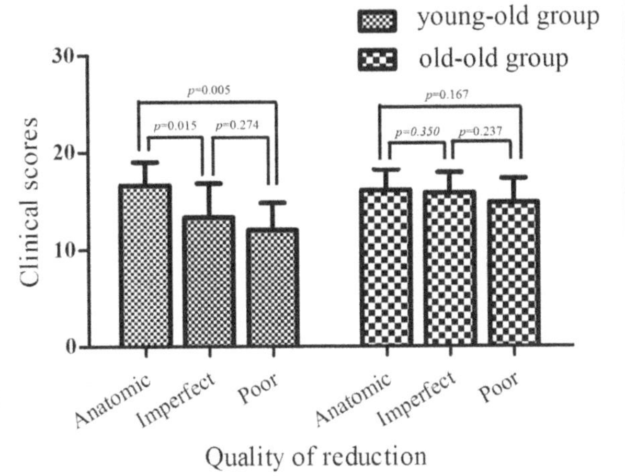

Fig. 2 The relationship between quality of reduction and clinical scores

The clinical scores were similar in both groups (15.5 points vs. 15.7 points, $p = 0.787$). By contrast, previous studies presented an inverse relationship between age and clinical function [4–6, 9]. This discrepancy in results may be attributed to the fact that previous studies [9–11] represent a wide age variety and compare the clinical function between young patients (< 40, 50, and 55 years old) and old patients (> 40, 50, or 55 years old), whereas the present study represents only elderly patients (60–90 years) and a comparator group (young–old patients vs. old–old patients). We also compared the component of clinical score between the two groups and found higher pain scores ($p = 0.029$) and lower ambulation scores ($p = 0.026$) in the old–old patients than in the young–old patients but a comparable range of motion scores ($p = 0.457$). This result may be related to the different pain tolerance levels of patients and the increased pain threshold in the old–old patients.

Although elderly patients often have comorbid medical conditions, few age-related complications were observed and no perioperative death occurred in this study. These findings may be attributed to the rational treatment strategy for elderly patients. This strategy includes optimization of preoperative patient's medical condition to improve surgery tolerance, as well as minimization of operative trauma and time and blood loss to achieve stable internal fixation of fractures rather than to strive for anatomical reduction. When a surgeon strives for an intraoperative anatomical reduction, this procedure often prolonged operative time and increased blood loss that may harm to the older population because older patients, especially those with medical conditions, have weaker blood loss tolerance than young patients. In the present study, the patients in the young–old group showed higher anatomical reduction (67.9% vs.36.0%, $p = 0.024$), blood loss (705 ml vs. 591 ml, $p = 0.016$), and operative time (145 min vs. 110 min, $p = 0.021$) compared with those in the old–old group. This finding may explain the similar complication rate in both groups ($p = 0.728$).

In this study, we found that reduction quality exerted an age-dependent influence on clinical function. The reduction quality in the young–old patients was significantly associated with clinical function ($p = 0.001$), and an anatomical reduction was associated with a good or excellent function. By contrast, no statistical difference

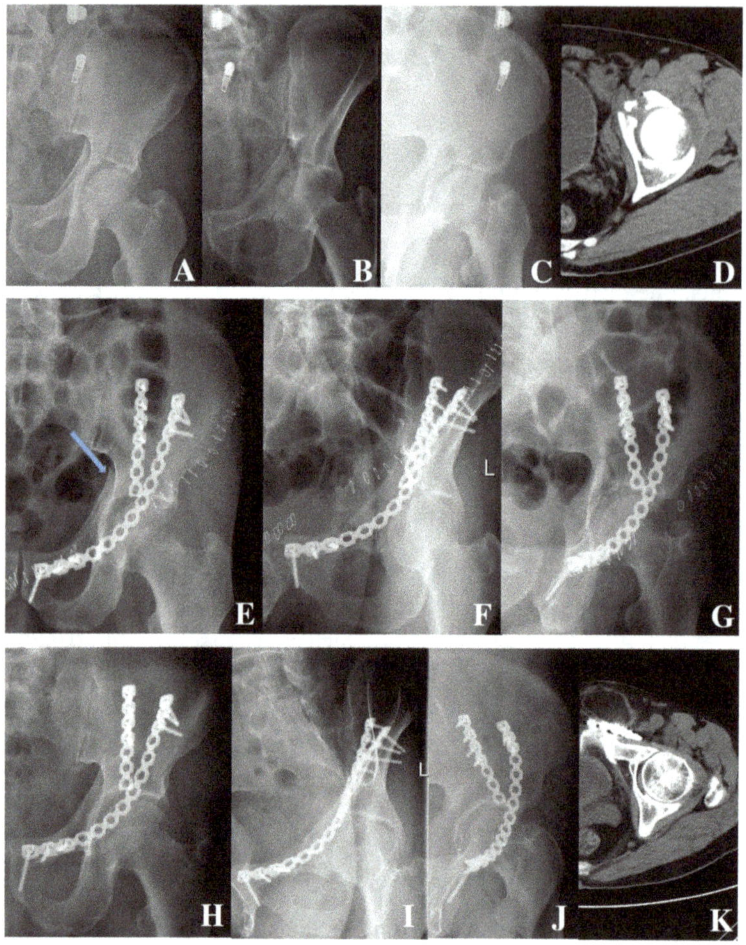

Fig. 3 Radiographs of a 75-year-old male patient with an anterior wall acetabular fracture. **a** Anteroposterior radiograph; **b** Obturator oblique radiograph; **c** Iliac oblique radiograph; **d** CT scan. Radiographs showing imperfect reduction (arrow) of the fracture immediately after the operation. **e** Anteroposterior radiograph; **f** Obturator oblique radiograph; **g** Iliac oblique radiograph. Radiographs showing an excellent radiological outcome at 84 months after the operation and the clinical score was 18 points. **h** Anteroposterior radiograph; **i** Obturator oblique radiograph; **j** iliac oblique radiograph; **k** CT scan

Table 4 Complications and natural death during the follow-up of both groups

Variable	Young-old group (n = 28)	Old-old group (n = 25)	p-value
Complications (n, %)	11 (39.3%)	11 (44.0%)	0.728
Lateral femoral cutaneous nerve palsy	0	2 (8.0%)	
Loss of reduction	0	2 (8.0%)	
Deep venous thrombosis	1 (3.6%)	1 (4.0%)	
Superficial infection	0	1 (4.0%)	
Heterotopic ossification	8 (28.6%)	4 (16.0%)	
Grade I	3	2	
Grade II	3	2	
Grade III	2	0	
Femoral head avascular necrosis	2 (7.1%)	0	
Incisional hernia	0	1 (4.0%)	
Death (n, %)	1 (3.6%)	6 (24.0%)	0.043

was detected among the clinical functions of anatomical, imperfect, and poor reduction in the old–old patients (p = 0.587). We speculated that the old–old patients may have characteristics (e.g., limited life expectancy, low activity level, low functional requirements, and weak muscle strength around the hip) that may reduce the wear and tear of the hip cartilage resulting from non-anatomical reduction and may increase their tolerance to non-anatomical reduction. In addition, the follow-up time of the old–old group was shorter than that of the young–old group (43 ± 17 months vs. 61 ± 27 months) because of the limited life expectancy of the old–old patients (the death rates in the old–old and young–old groups were respectively 24.0% and 3.6%, respectively), and this study included the patients who died. In addition, studies have reported that a precise anatomical reduction highly correlates with the best long-term clinical function rather than the short-term function [9, 14, 15]. Old–old patients with the above-mentioned characteristics may not necessarily need to sacrifice operative time and blood loss to strive for anatomical reduction; a stable fracture reduction that allows early postoperative ambulation may be accepted in old–old patients. In support to our findings, Archdeacon et al. [8] conducted a retrospective study of 26 patients older than 70 years with acetabular fracture and suggested that these patients can tolerate imperfect reduction.

We found that the age-dependent influence on the rate of anatomical reduction was higher in the young–old group than in the old–old group (67.9% vs. 36.0%, p = 0.024) and that the loss of reduction was more likely to occur in the old–old group than in the young–old group (8.0% vs. 0%). This result may be attributed to the fact that old–old patients often have a combination of osteoporosis and comminuted acetabular fractures, which complicate the completion of anatomical reduction and stability [9]. Moreover, accurate reduction was not attempted for some of the old–old patients in this study with the aforementioned characteristics.

Weakness of this study

This study has some limitations. First, the small sample size due to the relatively low incidence of acetabular fractures in elderly patients may compromise the robustness of the results. Second, the mean follow-up times of the young–old and old–old groups were 60.7 and 43.3 months, respectively, which may be too short to draw a definite conclusion on the association between reduction quality and clinical function, particularly in the old–old group. Third, all patients came from a single center, and the results of patients and treatment preferences from this center may not be applicable to other centers. Fourth, the clinical function was evaluated using the modified Postel Merle D'Aubigne Score instead of the patient-centered outcome scores (e.g., EQ5D, SF-12, SMFA, and SF-36). The patient-centered outcome scores for elderly patients may be much helpful. However, the modified Postel Merle D'Aubigne Score is widely applied to assess the clinical function of patients with acetabular fractures, and this scoring system has been routinely used since 1990 [16, 17].

Conclusions

The present findings add evidence to justify performing ORIF in elderly patients with acetabular fractures. Our findings suggest that individuals older than 75 years may achieve similar clinical functions and complications to young–old patients. Moreover, unlike that in the young–old patients, the reduction quality in the old–old patients may be not affecting the clinical function. Therefore, the treatment strategy of acetabular fractures with ORIF may be different according to different age groups. In particular, the goal for young–old patients should be anatomical reduction, whereas that for old–old patients should be to minimize operative time and blood loss, and thus achieve a stable fixation that allows early post-operative ambulation.

Abbreviations

ORIF: Open reduction and internal fixation; THA: Total hip arthroplasty

Acknowledgements

The authors thank Sheng-Jie Dong, and Zhi Yang from the Department of Orthopedic Surgery, Affiliated Hospital of Xuzhou Medical University for the Working Environment for valuable technical assistance and support.

Funding

This work was supported by the Jiangsu Provincial Medical Youth Talent (QNRC2016800), the Science and Technology Planning Project of Xuzhou (KC16SL111), the Foundation of Jiangsu Province commission of Health and Family Planning (H201708l), and the Key Medical Subjects Foundation of Jiangsu Province (BE2015627).

Authors' contributions

ZGC, YXM did the study, analyzed the data, and wrote the manuscript. ZGC, YXM, SYJ, FS, CXY, GKJ was involved in the design, data management, and analysis of the study. SJY, FS, GKJ were involved in the study design, and data analysis. ZGC, YXM, FS, SJY, GKJ contributed to the study design and analysis. All authors read and approved the final manuscript.

Consent for publication

Not applicable.

Competing interests

The authors declare that they have no competing interests.

Author details

[1]Department of Orthopedic Surgery, the Affiliated Hospital of Xuzhou Medical University, No. 99 Huaihai West Road, Xuzhou, Jiangsu 221002,

People's Republic of China. [2]Hyperbaric Oxygen Treatment Center, the Affiliated Hospital of Xuzhou Medical University, No. 99 Huaihai West Road, Xuzhou, Jiangsu 221002, People's Republic of China. [3]Orthopaedic Department, the First Affiliated Hospital of Soochow University, 188 Shizi Street, Suzhou, Jiangsu 215006, People's Republic of China.

References

1. Ferguson TA, Patel R, Bhandari M, Matta JM. Fractures of the acetabulum in patients aged 60 years and older: an epidemiological and radiological study. J Bone Joint Surg Br. 2010;92(2):250–7.
2. Heeg M. Fractures of the acetabulum. Drukkerij van Denderen B.V: Groningen; 1990.
3. Tornetta P 3rd. Displaced acetabular fractures: indications for operative and nonoperative management. J Am Acad Orthop Surg 2001; 9(1):18–28.
4. Tidermark J, Blomfeldt R, Ponzer S, Söderqvist A, Törnkvist H. Primary total hip arthroplasty with a Burch-Schneider antiprotrusion cage and autologous bone grafting for acetabular fractures in elderly patients. J Orthop Trauma. 2003;17(3):193–7.
5. Mouhsine E, Garofalo R, Borens O, Blanc CH, Wettstein M, Leyvraz PF. Cable fixation and early total hip arthroplasty in the treatment of acetabular fractures in elderly patients. J Arthroplast. 2004;19(3):344–8.
6. Herscovici D Jr, Lindvall E, Bolhofner B, Scaduto JM. The combined hip procedure: open reduction internal fixation combined with total hip arthroplasty for the management of acetabular fractures in the elderly. J Orthop Trauma 2010; 24 (5):291–296.
7. Anglen JO, Burd TA, Hendricks KJ, Harrison P. The "Gull sign": a harbinger of failure for internal fixation of geriatric acetabular fractures. J Orthop Trauma. 2003;17(9):625–34.
8. Archdeacon MT, Kazemi N, Collinge C, Budde B, Schnell S. Treatment of protrusio fractures of the acetabulum in patients 70 years and older. J Orthop Trauma. 2013;27(5):256–61.
9. Matta JM. Fractures of the acetabulum: accuracy of reduction and clinical results in patients managed operatively within three weeks after the injury. J Bone Joint Surg Am. 1996;78(11):1632–45.
10. Kreder HJ, Rozen N, Borkhoff CM, Laflamme YG, McKee MD, Schemitsch EH, Stephen DJ. Determinants of functional outcome after simple and complex acetabular factures involving the posterior wall. J Bone Joint Surg Br. 2006; 88(6):776–82.
11. Moed BR, WillsonCarr SE, Watson JT. Results of operative treatment of fractures of the posterior wall of the acetabulum. J Bone Joint Surg Am. 2002;84(5):752–8.
12. Letournel E, Judet R. Fractures of the Acetabulum, 2nd ed. New York: Springer. pp 63–397(1993).
13. D'aubigne RM, Postel M. Functional results of hip arthroplasty with acrylic prosthesis. J Bone Joint Surg Am. 1954;36(3):451–75.
14. Mears DC, Velyvis JH, Chang CP. Displaced acetabular fractures managed operatively: indicators of outcome. Clin Orthop Relat Res. 2003;407:173–86.
15. Marsh JL, Buckwalter J, Gelberman R, Dirschl D, Olson S, Brown T, Llinias A. Articular fractures: does an anatomic reduction really change the result? J Bone Joint Surg Am. 2002;84(7):1259–71.
16. Zha GC, Sun JY, Chen L, Zheng HM, Wang Q, Jin Y. Late reconstruction of posterior acetabular wall fractures using iliac crest. J Trauma Acute Care Surg. 2012;72(5):1386–92.
17. Wei L, Sun JY, Wang Y, Yang X. Surgical treatment and prognosis of acetabular fractures associated with ipsilateral femoral neck fractures. Orthopedics. 2011;34(5):348.

26

The V sign in lateral talar process fractures: an experimental study using a foot and ankle model

Thorsten Jentzsch[1*], Anita Hasler[1], Niklas Renner[1], Manuel Peterhans[2], Reto Sutter[3], Norman Espinosa[4] and Stephan H. Wirth[1]

Abstract

Background: Lateral talar process fractures (LTPF) are often missed on conventional radiographs. A positive V sign is an interruption of the contour of the LTP. It has been suggested, but not proven to be pathognomonic for LTPF. The objective was to study whether the V sign is pathognomonic for LTPF and if it can be properly assessed in different ankle positions and varying fracture types.

Methods: An experimental study was conducted. Two investigators assessed lateral radiographs (n = 108) of a foot and ankle model. The exposure variables were different ankle positions and fracture types. The primary outcome was the correct detection of a V sign. The secondary outcomes were the detection of the V sign depending on ankle position and fracture type as well as the uncertainty.

Results: The interobserver agreement on the V sign and type of fracture were fair ($\kappa = 0.35$, 95% CI 0.18–0.53, $p < 0.001$ and $\kappa = 0.37$, 95% CI 0.26–0.48, $p < 0.001$). The mean sensitivity, specificity, PPV, NPV, and likelihood ratio for the detection of the V sign were 77% (95% CI 67–86%), 59% (95% CI 39–78%), 85% (95% CI 75–92%), 46% (95% CI 29–63%), and 2. The mean uncertainty in the V sign detection was 38%. The V sign identification stratified by ankle position and fracture type showed significant better results with increasing inversion ($p = 0.035$ and $p = 0.011$) and type B fractures ($p = 0.001$ and $p = 0.013$).

Conclusions: The V sign may not be pathognomonic and is not recommended as the only modality for the detection of LTPF. It is better visualized with inversion, but does not depend on plantar flexion or internal rotation. It is also better seen in type B fractures. It is difficult to detect and investigator-dependent. It may be helpful in a clinical setting to point into a direction, but a CT scan may be used if in doubt about a LTPF.

Keywords: Orthopedics and biomechanics, Biomechanics, Imaging, Ankle, Bone, Fracture

Background

Talar fractures constitute less than 1% of all fractures and less than 10% of fractures of the foot [1]. They are usually caused from high-energy trauma. Talar body fractures (61%) are more common than neck and head fractures [2]. Among all body fractures, dome compression and lateral process fractures (24%) are the most common and missed types when using conventional radiography. Lateral talar process fractures (LTPF) are rare, but account for 15% of ankle injuries in snowboarders, who reveal a 17-fold increased risk of sustaining such a fracture [3, 4]. They are caused by forced dorsiflexion, inversion, and potentially external rotation and are commonly missed on anteroposterior and lateral radiographs [5, 6]. In 1965, Hawkins introduced his classification system of these fractures [7]. Type I (42%) fractures are more common than type II (32%) and type III (24%) fractures [8]. Type I and II fractures involve the talofibular and posterior subtalar joint, while type III fractures involve the posterior subtalar joint only. Type I is defined as a simple fracture. Type II constitutes a comminuted fracture of the entire process.

* Correspondence: thorsten.jentzsch@balgrist.ch; thorsten.jentzsch@gmail.com
[1]Department of Orthopaedics, Balgrist University Hospital, University of Zurich, Forchstrasse 340, 8008 Zurich, Switzerland

Type III is an anterior-inferior chip fracture. Type I fractures can be further subdivided according to displacement, with <2 mm in type IA and ≥2 mm in type IIB types. It is vital to diagnose these fractures early to avoid long-term morbidity due to painful arthritis and avascular necrosis.

Usually, the radiographic workup consists of anteroposterior, dorsoplantar, mortise, and lateral views of the foot and ankle. Lateral views of normal ankles demonstrate a V-shaped lateral talar process. Displaced fractures show an interrupted V shape [9]. In other words, radiographic appearance of the lateral talar process resembles an uninterrupted (symmetric) V-shape in healthy individuals, but it appears as an interrupted (asymmetric) V-shape in patients with LTPF. Therefore, it has been suggested, but not proven, that a positive V sign is pathognomonic for displaced LTPF. In theory, the V sign could be important when assessing potential fractures that may occur after ankle sprains [10].

However, the literature on the V sign is sparse and lacks a systematic approach [9, 10]. In clinical emergency practice, standardized weight bearing lateral radiographs are often insufficient for proper ankle assessment. Due to pain and functional deficits, including the inability to bear weight, as well as accompanying ankle injuries and variable imaging techniques, lateral radiographs are highly susceptible to rotational malpositioning. Hypothetically, this could negatively affect the presence of the V sign in normal ankles. In addition, the severity of fractures may influence the prevalence of the V sign as well.

The aim of the study was to investigate the performance of V sign assessment under different ankle positions and varying fracture patterns of the lateral talar process. The null hypothesis was that the V sign is always present in LTPF and that it keeps unchanged when assessed at different positions of the ankle and varying fracture types.

Methods

Study design and setting

An experimental study was conducted at a University Hospital in Switzerland in February 2016 to compare the detection of the V sign in normal and fractured lateral talar processes according to different ankle joint positions and fracture types. A waiver was granted from the local ethics committee (Kantonale Ethikkommission Zürich, BASEC-Nr. Req-2017-00429) and written informed consent was obtained from the patient that is presented as a clinical example.

Model and investigators

Four left, large, high resolution, solid foam, radiopaque distal foot and ankle sawbones (Pacific Research Laboratories, Vashon, WA, USA) were used in this model (Fig. 1). These were evaluated by a fellow and consultant in orthopedic surgery. The gold standard was defined by both investigators, who obtained the x-rays and knew the macroscopic appearance of the model. It reflected the true nature of the model, where the V sign was absent in all intact lateral talar processes (Fig. 1) and present in all LTPF (Fig. 2).

Variables

Exposure variables included varying ankle joint positions during lateral radiographs and different fracture types. First, varying degrees of plantar flexion (0°, 20° and 40°) were examined. Second, varying degrees of inversion (0°, 20° and 40°) were added [11]. Third, varying degrees of internal rotation (0°, 20° and 40°) were added [6]. These angles were chosen according to physiological values for the range of motion of the ankle joint, common relieving postures during ankle pain, and previous reports on mechanisms of injury [6, 11]. There were four different fracture models: no fracture, type A, type B, and type C. This resulted in 27 different radiographs for each group.

The primary outcome variable was the correct detection of a V sign [9]. The secondary outcome variables were the detection of the V sign depending on the ankle position and fracture type according to Hawkins as well as the uncertainty in the evaluation of the V sign [7].

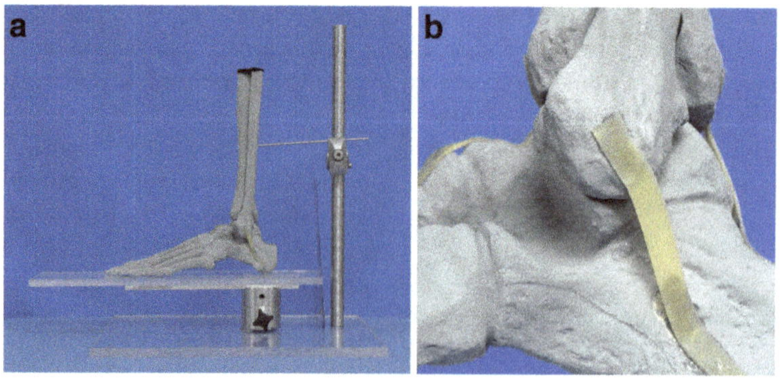

Fig. 1 Photographs of study set up with a mounted distal foot and ankle sawbone model showing an intact lateral talar process. **a** Overview. **b** Hindfoot including lateral talar process

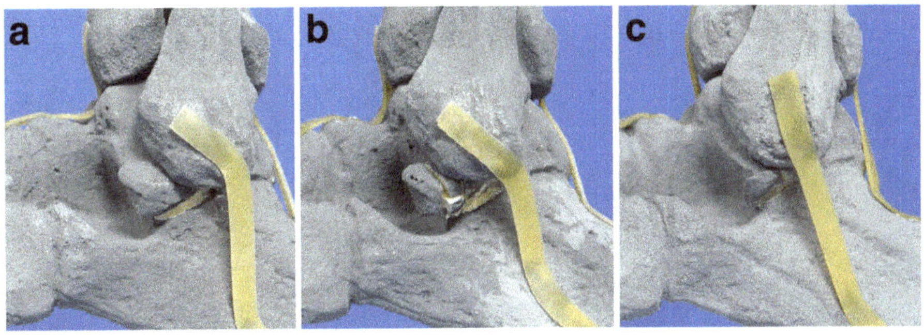

Fig. 2 Photographs of lateral talar process fractures of the distal foot and ankle model. **a** Type A fracture. **b** Type B fracture. **c** Type C fracture

Data sources and measurements

One model was left intact, while the other three models had displaced (5 mm) fractures introduced with increasing severity to resemble different fracture patterns according to the Hawkins classification [7] (Fig. 2). A chisel and hammer were used to create these fractures and double-faced adhesive tape (Beiersdorf AG, Tesa SE, Norderstedt, Germany) was needed to hold these fractures in place. The V sign is illustrated in Fig. 3. Lateral radiographs were acquired for each model and each position by two investigators (Fig. 4). Two other investigators documented their decisions about the V sign in REDCap (version 6.11.5; Vanderbilt University, Nashville, TN, USA).

Radiographic technique

Lateral radiographs were acquired with a fully digital radiographic C-arm system (Ziehm Vision; Ziehm Imaging GmbH, Nurnberg, Germany). The tube voltage was 44 kV, the tube load 1.9 mAs, and the acquisition duration 2 s. Models were placed as close as possible to the image intensifier.

Bias

Choosing different independent investigators for the acquisition and review of radiographs as well as blinding of the latter minimized observer bias. Information bias was addressed by randomizing and numbering the radiographs from 1 to 108 using random number tables (Excel, version 2010; Microsoft Corporation, Redmond, USA). Errors in classifying the radiographs were minimized by training the investigators how to assess the V sign according to the technique published in previous reports [9, 12]. Both investigators received the same instruction prior to the beginning of the study. For this purpose, the investigators received detailed information about the V sign. In addition, examples of radiographs with negative and positive V signs using clinical and model radiographs helped to improve the training sessions.

Calculation of study size

A total of 108 lateral radiographs were obtained. It was assumed that the V sign can be seen in the majority (90%) of radiographs from the fracture group (n = 81), but remains mostly absent (10%) in radiographs of the normal group (n = 27). This would require a minimum of five samples per group and a total number of 10 samples for a power of 80% and a significance level of 5%. The chosen study size surpassed these calculations.

Statistical methods

Data are presented as absolute numbers and their percentages. Groups were compared with the chi-squared test for categorical values. The interobserver measure of agreement was calculated with the kappa (κ) coefficient. Ninety-five percent confidence intervals were calculated with the formula 'estimate ± 1.96 × standard error'. The sensitivity, specificity, negative predictive value (NPV),

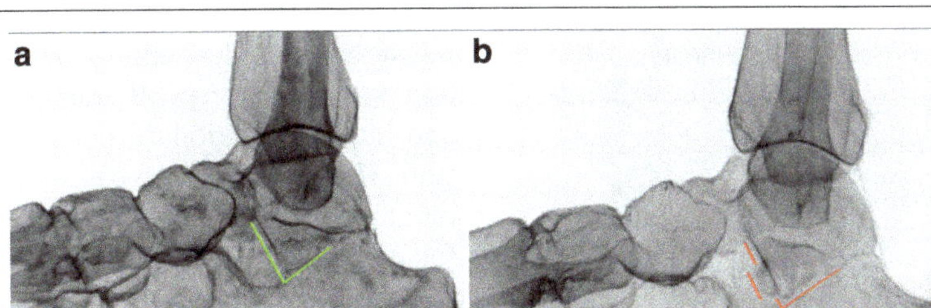

Fig. 3 Illustration of the V sign. **a** Negative (absent) V sign, which is illustrated by the intact (symmetric) V-shape of the lateral talar process depicted in *green*. **b** Positive (present) V sign, which is illustrated by the defective (asymmetric) V-shape of the lateral talar process depicted in *red*

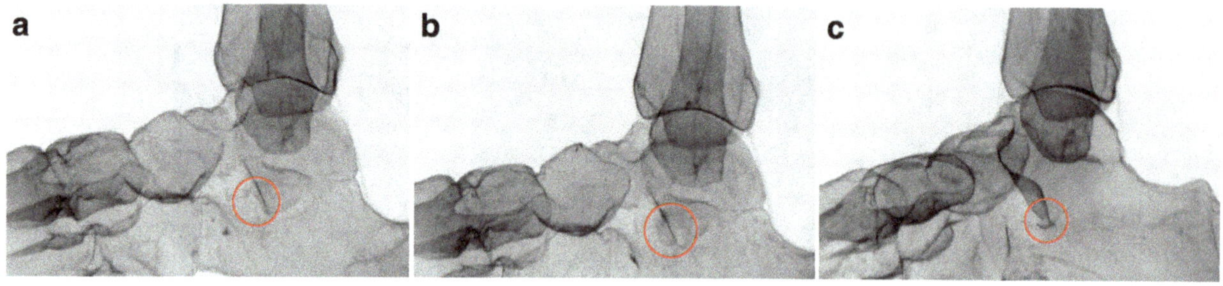

Fig. 4 The V sign on lateral radiographs, as demonstrated in the sawbone models. The *circles* indicate the location of the V sign. **a** Positive V sign; type A fracture. **b** Positive V sign; type B fracture. **c** Positive V sign; type C fracture

positive predictive value (PPV), and likelihood ratio are presented for the V sign. Exact 95% confidence intervals are presented using means of numerators and denominators for both investigators, respectively. New binary variables were created for the correct detection of a V sign for each investigator. There were no missing values. The significance level was set at 5%. Statistical analysis was performed with Stata/IC (version 13.1; StataCorp LP, College Station, TX, USA).

Results

Participants

The interobserver agreement on the V sign and type of fracture were fair (κ = 0.35, 95% CI 0.18–0.53, $p < 0.001$ and κ = 0.37, 95% CI 0.26–0.48, $p < 0.001$, respectively) (Tables 1 and 2). The mean uncertainty of both investigators about the presence of the V sign was 38%. The agreement on the uncertainty of the presence of the V sign and type of fracture were moderate and fair, respectively (κ = 0.51, 95% CI 0.32–0.70, $p < 0.001$ and κ = 0.36, 95% CI 0.18–0.54, $p < 0.001$, respectively).

The mean sensitivity, specificity, PPV, and NPV for the detection of the V sign were 77% (95% CI 67–86%), 59% (95% CI 39–78%), 85% (95% CI 75–92%), and 46% (95% CI 29–63%) (Table 3). The prevalence of a V sign was 75% (81 V signs [and fractures] and 27 absent V signs [no fractures]). The pretest odds, likelihood ratio, and posttest odds were 3, 2, and 6, respectively.

The correct identification of the V sign stratified by ankle position showed significant better results with increasing inversion ($p = 0.035$ and $p = 0.011$ for each investigator, respectively) (Table 4). It was not associated with plantar flexion and internal rotation ($p = 0.31$ and 0.33 for plantar flexion as well as 0.35 and 0.53 for internal rotation for each investigator, respectively). With an inversion of 40°, the V sign was correctly identified in 83 and 89%; without inversion, in 56 and 61%. Furthermore, the correct identification of the V sign stratified by fracture type revealed significant differences between fracture types ($p = 0.001$ and $p = 0.013$ for each investigator, respectively) (Table 5). The V sign was correctly identified most often in fractures types B (89% each), while the V sign was detected least often in cases without a fracture (63 and 56%, for each investigator, respectively).

Table 1 Detection of the V sign by each investigator

V Sign Detection: Investigator 1	V Sign Detection: Investigator 2			Kappa* (95% CI)	*P*-value[†]
	No (n [%])	Yes (n [%])	Total (n [%])		
No	19 (70)	23 (28)	42 (39)	0.35 (0.35–0.42)	<0.001
Yes	8 (30)	58 (72)	66 (61)		
Total	27 (100)	81 (100)	108 (100)		

*Interobserver measure of agreement
[†]Kappa statistic

Discussion

On conventional lateral radiographs, the lateral talar process has an uninterrupted (symmetric) V-shape in healthy individuals, but an interrupted (asymmetric) V-shape in patients with LTPF. In the present study, the interobserver agreement on the V sign and type of a fracture were only fair, demonstrating that the V sign and sole use of lateral radiographs are of limited use in the clinical setting. With a mean uncertainty about the presence of the V sign of 38%, the V sign was difficult to evaluate. While the sensitivity of 77% for the detection of the V sign may be considered somewhat useful, the specificity was too low. A likelihood ratio of 2 indicated that the V sign increased the probability of a LTPF by approximately 15% [13]. The V sign is also more likely to be detected if the ankle assumes an inverted position and in cases of type B fractures, while plantar flexion and internal rotation do not seem to influence its detection. These findings are based on conventional lateral radiographs and no specific radiological view is necessary for better demonstration. If in doubt about the presence or absence of a LTPF, a CT scan may be useful.

In the literature, there are two studies about the V sign. First, in a retrospective cohort study of 23 snowboarders with a mean follow-up of 3.5 years after conservative and

Table 2 Detection of the fracture type by each investigator

Fracture Type Detection: Investigator 1	Fracture Type Detection: Investigator 2					Kappa* (95% CI)	P-value†
	No fracture (n [%])	Type A (n [%])	Type B (n [%])	Type C (n [%])	Total (n [%])		
No fracture	26 (60)	9 (38)	3 (13)	4 (22)	42 (39)	0.37 (0.24–0.50)	<0.001
Type A	7 (16)	12 (50)	6 (26)	2 (11)	27 (25)		
Type B	6 (14)	3 (13)	11 (48)	2 (11)	22 (20)		
Type C	4 (9)	0 (0)	3 (13)	10 (56)	17 (16)		
Total	43 (100)	24 (100)	23 (100)	18 (100)	108 (100)		

*Interobserver measure of agreement
†Kappa statistic

surgical treatment, the American Orthopedic Foot and Ankle Society (AOFAS) hindfoot score was 94 (of 100) points, but subtalar osteoarthritis was found in 45% [9]. It was concluded that the outcome was favorable if the diagnosis was established early and the treatment was adequately tailored to the displacement as well as associated injuries. To establish early diagnosis, a positive pathognomonic V sign was mentioned. Second, a case report described a 31-year old women with a LTPF, originally misdiagnosed as an ankle sprain despite the pathognomonic presence of a V sign [10]. Before using these findings in a clinical setting with confidence, further studies evaluating in vivo findings may be needed.

Conventional radiographic suspicion of LTPF is usually confirmed with computed tomography (CT) to evaluate the extent of the fracture. If CT scans are not available or during intraoperative assessment, the Canale and Harris views may be added to visualize the talar neck and subtalar joint. The mortise view (internal rotation of the ankle by 20°) prevents overlapping of the talus with the fibula for assessment of the lateral talus. Treatment of LTPF usually consists of conservative measures for nondisplaced type III fractures, excision for displaced (>2 mm) fractures with multiple small fragments (type II), and internal fixation for displaced fractures with a large (≥1 cm) fragment (type I) [8, 11, 14, 15].

Selection bias may have been introduced by aberrant fracture patterns resulting in non-differential misclassification of (non-)fracture types potentially under- or overestimating the strength of association. Furthermore, the use of a foot and ankle model may not accurately reflect the setting in humans. However, it is a feasible method

Table 3 Performance of the V sign

	Result (% [95% CI*])
Sensitivity	77 (67–86)
Specificity	59 (39–78)
NPV	85 (75–92)
PPV	46 (29–63)

*Exact 95% confidence intervals are presented using means of numerators and denominators for both investigators, respectively

Table 4 Correctly identified V sign stratified by investigator and ankle position

Correctly Identified V Sign	Ankle position (°)			Total	P-value*
	0 (n [%])	20 (n [%])	40 (n [%])		
	Inversion				
Investigator 1					
No	16 (44)	13 (36)	6 (17)	35 (32)	0.035
Yes	20 (56)	23 (64)	30 (83)	73 (68)	
Total	36 (100)	36 (100)	36 (100)	108 (100)	
Investigator 2					
No	14 (39)	6 (17)	4 (11)	24 (22)	0.011
Yes	22 (61)	30 (83)	32 (89)	84 (78)	
Total	36 (100)	36 (100)	36 (100)	108 (100)	
	Plantar flexion				
Investigator 1					
No	15 (42)	11 (31)	9 (25)	35 (32)	0.31
Yes	21 (58)	25 (69)	27 (75)	73 (68)	
Total	36 (100)	36 (100)	36 (100)	108 (100)	
Investigator 2					
No	10 (28)	9 (25)	5 (14)	24 (22)	0.33
Yes	26 (72)	27 (75)	31 (86)	84 (78)	
Total	36 (100)	36 (100)	36 (100)	108 (100)	
	Internal rotation				
Investigator 1					
No	10 (28)	15 (42)	10 (28)	35 (32)	0.35
Yes	26 (72)	21 (58)	26 (72)	73 (68)	
Total	36 (100)	36 (100)	36 (100)	108 (100)	
Investigator 2					
No	6 (17)	10 (28)	8 (22)	24 (22)	0.53
Yes	30 (83)	26 (72)	28 (78)	84 (78)	
Total	36 (100)	36 (100)	36 (100)	108 (100)	

*Chi-squared test

Table 5 Correctly identified V sign stratified by investigator and fracture type

Correctly Identified V Sign	Fracture Type					*P*-value*
	No Fracture (n [%])	Type A (n [%])	Type B (n [%])	Type C (n [%])	Total (n [%])	
Investigator 1						
No	10 (37)	16 (59)	3 (11)	6 (22)	35 (32)	0.001
Yes	17 (63)	11 (41)	24 (89)	21 (78)	73 (68)	
Total	27 (100)	27 (100)	27 (100)	27 (100)	108 (100)	
Investigator 2						
No	12 (44)	4 (15)	3 (11)	5 (19)	24 (22)	0.013
Yes	15 (56)	23 (85)	24 (89)	22 (81)	84 (78)	
Total	27 (100)	27 (100)	27 (100)	27 (100)	108 (100)	

*Chi-squared test

for standardized evaluation of the ankle joint without causing radiation and potential pain to patients with ankle injuries.

As a clinical example, we briefly report on a 41 year-old male patient with a LTPF after a snowboard accident 1 month ago (Fig. 5). Conventional radiographs were initially obtained at an external institution before he was treated for a low ankle sprain. Due to persisting pain after 1 month, an MRI was obtained and he was referred to our institution for further evaluation. This demonstrated the type I LTPF and adjacent bone marrow edema. Radiographs and computed tomography images were acquired for better assessment of the osseous structures and to confirm the displaced lateral talar process fracture. The fracture was treated with an open reduction and internal fixation with two screws followed by non-weightbearing in a cast for 6 weeks.

In daily practice of every physician that treats traumatic foot and ankle injuries, the first step in the diagnostic cascade after clinical evaluation usually includes the acquisition of a conventional radiograph. The results of this novel experimental study demonstrate that standard lateral x-rays of the foot and ankle are somewhat helpful to avoid missing a commonly missed LTPF and to strengthen the suspicion of a LTPF. If tolerated by patients, the visualization of LTPF may be enhanced by inverting the foot without the need to change flexion or rotation. These findings are particularly interesting to physicians and regions where CT scans or MRIs are not readily available. If the V sign is positive or there is negative V sign but high clinical suspicion of a LTPF, patients may benefit from CT scans or MRIs for better evaluation of the type of fracture and size of fragments in order to plan the best treatment strategy for each patient.

Conclusions

We conclude that the V sign may not be pathognomonic and is not recommended as the only modality for the detection of a LTPF. It is better visualized with inversion of the foot, but does not depend on plantar flexion or internal rotation. It is also better seen in type B fractures. It is difficult to detect and investigator-dependent. It may be helpful in a clinical setting to point into a direction, but a CT scan may be used if in doubt about a LTPF.

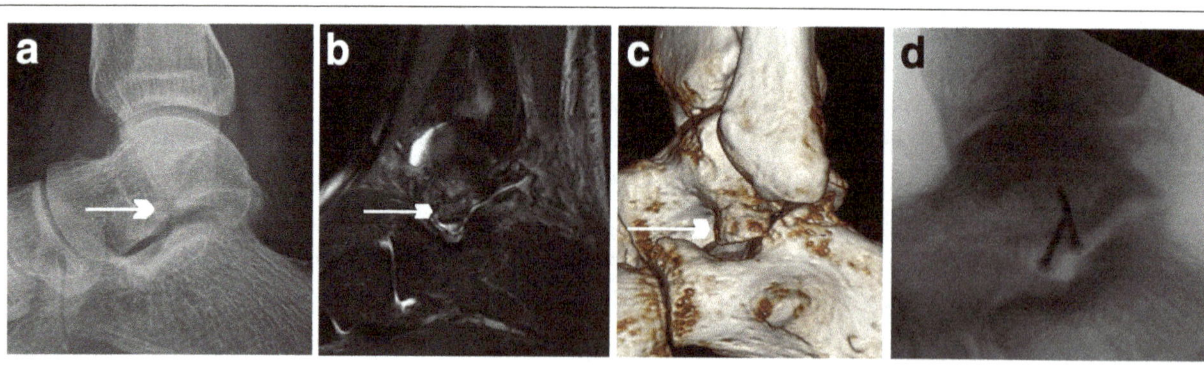

Fig. 5 Clinical example of a patient with a lateral talar process fracture (LTPF). **a** Conventional lateral radiograph. **b** MRI showing a sagittal proton density fat-saturated image, which demonstrates the fracture line (*arrow*). **c** Computed tomography images confirming the displaced lateral talar process fracture (*arrows*). **d** Conventional lateral radiograph after open reduction and internal fixation with two screws

Abbreviations
LTPF: Lateral talar process fractures

Acknowledgements
The authors would like to thank Mr. Elias Bachmann, MSc and Mr. Beda Rutishauser for their valuable help building the mount as well as Mr. Burkhardt Seifert, Prof. Dr. rer. nat., for his support with statistical analysis.

Funding
This work was supported by funding from the Balgrist Foundation. The funders had no role in manuscript preparation.

Authors' contributions
TJ: conception and design, acquisition of data, statistical analysis and interpretation of data, drafting the manuscript; AH and MP: conception and design. NR: acquisition of data; RS: interpretation of data; NE: idea; SW: analysis and interpretation of data, supervision; All: revision of the manuscript, final approval of the version to be published.

Consent for publication
Written informed consent to participate and publish was obtained from the patient illustrated in Fig. 5.

Competing interests
The authors declare that they have no competing interests.

Author details
[1]Department of Orthopaedics, Balgrist University Hospital, University of Zurich, Forchstrasse 340, 8008 Zurich, Switzerland. [2]Department of Orthopaedics, Kantonsspital Aarau, Aarau, Switzerland. [3]Department of Radiology, Balgrist University Hospital, University of Zurich, Zurich, Switzerland. [4]Institute for Foot and Ankle Reconstruction Zurich, Zurich, Switzerland.

References
1. Summers NJ, Murdoch MM. Fractures of the talus: a comprehensive review. Clin Podiatr Med Surg. 2012;29(2):187–203.
2. Dale JD, Ha AS, Chew FS. Update on talar fracture patterns: a large level I trauma center study. AJR Am J Roentgenol. 2013;201(5):1087–92.
3. Kirkpatrick DP, Hunter RE, Janes PC, Mastrangelo J, Nicholas RA. The snowboarder's foot and ankle. Am J Sports Med. 1998;26(2):271–7.
4. Chan GM, Yoshida D. Fracture of the lateral process of the talus associated with snowboarding. Ann Emerg Med. 2003;41(6):854–8.
5. Mukherjee SK, Pringle RM, Baxter AD. Fracture of the lateral process of the talus. A report of thirteen cases. J Bone Joint Surg Br. 1974;56(2):263–73.
6. Boon AJ, Smith J, Zobitz ME, Amrami KM. Snowboarder's talus fracture. Mechanism of injury. Am J Sports Med. 2001;29(3):333–8.
7. Hawkins LG. Fracture of the lateral process of the talus. J Bone Joint Surg Am. 1965;47:1170–5.
8. Perera A, Baker JF, Lui DF, Stephens MM. The management and outcome of lateral process fracture of the talus. Foot Ankle Surg. 2010;16(1):15–20.
9. von Knoch F, Reckord U, von Knoch M, Sommer C. Fracture of the lateral process of the talus in snowboarders. J Bone Joint Surg Br. 2007;89(6):772–7.
10. van Egmond PW, van de Rest H, Nolte PA. Back to the emergency department with a painful ankle. Ned Tijdschr Geneeskd. 2014;158:A7388.
11. Funk JR, Srinivasan SC, Crandall JR. Snowboarder's talus fractures experimentally produced by eversion and dorsiflexion. Am J Sports Med. 2003;31(6):921–8.
12. Melenevsky Y, Mackey RA, Abrahams RB, Thomson NB. Talar Fractures and Dislocations: A Radiologist's Guide to Timely Diagnosis and Classification. Radiographics. 2015;35(3):765–79.
13. McGee S. Simplifying likelihood ratios. J Gen Intern Med. 2002;17(8):646–9.
14. Heckman JD, McLean MR. Fractures of the lateral process of the talus. Clin Orthop Relat Res. 1985;199:108–13.
15. Langer P, Nickisch F, Spenciner D, Fleming B, DiGiovanni CW. In vitro evaluation of the effect lateral process talar excision on ankle and subtalar joint stability. Foot Ankle Int. 2007;28(1):78–83.

27

The risk of violating the posterior malleolar fracture when nailing the ipsilateral concomitant spiral distal tibial fracture

Yu Zhang, Xiaodong Qin, Lijun Song and Xiang Li*

Abstract

Background: For a distal tibial spiral fracture combined with a non-displaced posterior malleolar fragment (PMF), we proposed a hypothesis that the treating surgeon could assess the size of the PMF to determine the need for stabilizing that structure first before rodding the tibia.

Materials and methods: Fifty 3-D models (22 females) of combined distal tibial and posterior malleolar fractures from one trauma center were reconstructed. In each case, a virtual tibial intramedullary nail (vIM nail) with three distal anteroposterior (AP) locking screws (S_{13}, S_{15} and S_{37}, the number indicating the distance from the screw to the nail tip) were inserted into the center of the tibial canal and ended on top of the distal tibial physeal scar. Contact between the screws and the PMF was defined as causing PMF displacement. The relationship between PMF secondary displacement and traumatic anatomic factors (the fragment area and height of the PMF) was explored. Then, the parameters were justified by analyzing intraoperative radiographs of 35 cases treated by nail with single locking screw (S_{15}) design.

Results: In the analog experiment, multiple logistic regression analysis revealed that the height of the PMF could confidently predict the risk of fragment displacement (S_{13}: odds ratio [OR] 1.18, 95% confidence interval [CI] 1.06–1.32; S_{15}: OR 1.15, 95% CI 1.05–1.27). Regarding the height of the PMF, the receiver operating characteristic established a cut-off value of 31.2 mm for preliminary fixation of the fragment with 88.89% sensitivity and 88.89% specificity. In the operation group the nail stopped on the top of distal tibial physeal scar, no PMF secondary displacement occurred when the PMF height was less than 31.2 mm. However, the incidence of secondary displacement was 93.33% when the height of the PMF exceeded 31.2 mm.

Conclusion: When the distal tibial physeal scare was set as the limit of nail insertion depth, the height of the PMF could be used as a reliable reference predicting the risk of PMF secondary displacement caused by distal anteroposterior locking screw.

Keywords: Ankle fracture, Tibial fracture, Morphological measurement, Intramedullary nail

Background

The combination of tibial shaft fracture and posterior malleolar disruption was first reported by Lauge-Hansen in 1946 [1]. Later, other authors recognized that a posterior malleolar fragment (PMF) could predominantly co-occur with a distal tibial spiral fracture [2, 3]. In 1988, Bostman further discussed this special lower limb injury and recommended additional CT scanning of the ankle for distal tibial spiral fractures [4]. Since then, the understanding of this special limb injury has been continuously increasing.

For tibial shaft spiral fractures, either proximal or distal, both a plate and an intramedullary nail can be utilized. However, the existence of the PMF and the "connection line" complicate the fixation selection since they change a tibial shaft fracture from a simple to a more complex intra-articular fracture [5]. Although the multiple distal locking option of the latest nail design greatly improves

* Correspondence: lixiang19801980@163.com
Department of Trauma, the First Affiliated Hospital of Nanjing Medical University and Jiangsu Province Hospital, 300 Guangzhou Road, Nanjing 210029, China

the holding strength of the short distal tibia segment and is compatible with a soft envelope, there is always a major concern about secondary displacement of an initial non-displaced PMF, especially those involving a substantial articular surface area, when inserting an IM nail or distal AP locking screws. The suggestion of indiscriminate PMF fixation with cannulated screws before nailing was made without sufficient supporting evidence and is not an effective solution [6]. This protocol might irritate the adjacent tendon (especially the hallux flexor longus from the posteroanterior screw) and ligaments, cause percutaneous nerve entrapment [7], exaggerate excessive patient radiation exposure and incur extra financial cost. Guo's study also suggested that PMF fixation failed to improve functional outcomes when there was a moderate size PMF combined with a tibial spiral fracture [8]. As the treatment benefit should be balanced against the potential complications and costs, we believe it is wise to tailor the operation protocol for every case.

It could be deduced that when a smaller-sized PMF correlates with a lower risk of nail-induced secondary displacement of the fragment, this indicates that when the PMF size is small enough, the necessity of additional cannulated screw fixation of the fragment can be eliminated if the nail is inserted in the proper position. In this group of patients, a properly inserted IM nail could provide sufficient fixation without disrupting the non-displaced PMF. However, the proper threshold for the fragment size and a reliable anatomic reference for proper nail insertion depth have not been established. This paper investigated the factors influencing the intraoperative secondary displacement of PMFs caused by nail insertion and distal AP screw locking. By conducting radiographic measurements and simulating vIM nail fixation on a reconstructed 3-D model, the core morphological feature of the PMF predicting fragment violation from the nail and AP locking screw tips and its threshold could be determined. Then, an anatomical landmark that serves as a reliable reference for the proper depth of nail insertion could also be established. These results were validated in the same group of patients.

Methods

Patient and fracture evaluation

This is a retrospective study with ethically approved by the institutional review board of our Hospital (No. 2017-SR-121). From June 2011 to February 2017, 765 tibial fracture cases were retrieved from the orthopedic database in a territorial trauma center. The inclusion criteria were a spiral fracture at the distal third of the tibia combined with a posterior malleolar fracture confirmed by thin-slice CT scan (GE Light-Speed CT; Waukesha, WI, USA). Pathological fractures, skeletally immature patients, fractures without CT scan or with PMF contour obscured by an indistinct fracture line and severely comminuted tibial fractures with direct involvement of ankle joints were excluded from the study. Fifty-five patients (22 females) fulfilled the inclusion criteria and were included in the study. All subjects provided informed consent in written to take part in the study. Baseline characteristics of the patients were collected.

Imaging parameters were as follows: 64-detector CT scanner, section thickness, 0.625 mm; tube voltage, 120 kVp; pitch, 1.375; matrix, 512 × 512. Data were saved in DICOM 3.0 format (.dcm) and available in Picture Archiving and Communication System. All the damaged bony structure of the ankle joint was recorded and the PMFs were classified according to Bartoníček's classification scheme [9]. This is a pathoanatomy-oriented classification based on CT examination that takes into account the size, shape and location of the fragment, stability of the tibiotalar joint and integrity of the fibular notch (Fig. 1). The incidence of a "communication line", defined as a fracture line progressing from the spiral tibial fracture to the PMF [5], was also recorded.

3-D reconstruction and implant simulation

3-D models were reconstructed with the program Mimics version 19 (Materialise NV Inc., Leuven, Belgium). The model consisted of two components: the lower leg and the simulated vIM nail. After reconstruction of the leg, the simulated vIM nail was devised step by step with a reproducible method. First, as the ideal position of the tibial nail axis is across the center of the ankle, this point and its sagittal plane projection were established on axial scan according to Cinotti's method [10]. This method is precise [11] and easy to perform by identifying the center of the talar dome originating from the connection of 2 points located in the middle of its anterior and posterior region. The middle points of the talar dome at its anterior and posterior edges were identified with the gauge tool and connected by "line a"; this line is the projection of the center of the ankle in the sagittal plane and represents the central line of the talar dome (Fig. 2a). Second, the geometrical center point of the tibial canal was identified with the area gauge tool of the software. Then, the central sagittal plane of the distal tibia and ankle joint could be determined by connecting "line a" and the aforementioned tibial canal center point. Third, on the central sagittal plane, the tibial canal axis (tCA) was identified using two bisection points of the distal shaft of the tibia described by Yao (Fig. 2b) [12]. The geometrical center point of the tibial canal was also in the tCA which was also the central axis of the vIM nail. On the same plane, the axis of the distal AP locking screws was perpendicular to the tCA (Fig. 2c). Finally, the vIM nail and the distal AP locking screws were reconstructed around their corresponding

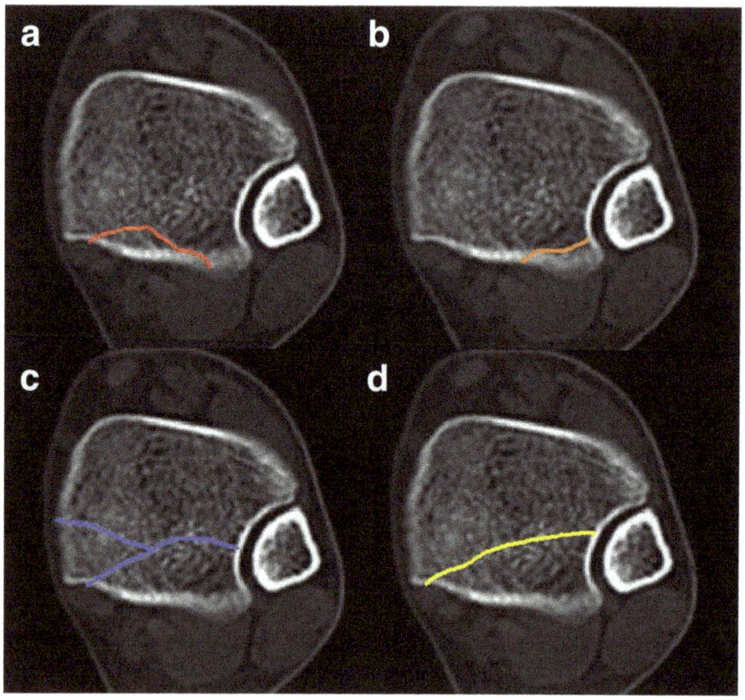

Fig. 1 There are four types of Bartoníček's classification scheme: **a** (type 1): extraincisural fragment with an intact fibular notch; **b** (type 2): posterolateral fragment extending into the fibular notch; **c** (type 3): posteromedial two-part fragment involving the medial malleolus; **d** (type 4): large posterolateral triangular fragment (involving more than one-third of the notch)

axis. In this study, the vIM nail was straight, with a diameter of 10 mm and 5 mm for the AP locking screws.

As a rule, the nail tip was positioned just above the distal tibial physeal scar, which is a discrete anatomic landmark at the distal tibia. Three simulated AP locking screws were set at the distal end of the nail. In the reconstructed tibial nail system, each screw was on the central sagittal plane (CSP) and perpendicular to the vIM nail. The distance from the nail tip to the axis of each of these AP locking screws was 13 mm ($Screw_{13}$, S_{13}), 15 mm ($Screw_{15}$, S_{15}) and 37 mm ($Screw_{37}$, S_{37}) to mimic the designs of two widely available tibial nails (TRIGEN META-NAIL Tibial Nail, Smith & Nephew Inc., Massachusetts, USA, and ETN, Depuy Synthes Inc., Zuchwil, Switzerland).

Radiographic measurements

With the gauge tool Mimics, measurements were conducted separately by two orthopedic surgeons and agreement was reached by consensus. The research method developed by Yao and Haraguchi et al. [12, 13] was applied in the current study. The measured parameters included the height of the PMF (HP), the fragment area ratio (FAR), the minimal distance from nail tip to the PMF (DNP) and the distance from the distal AP locking screw to the PMF (DSP).

The height of the PMF (HP)

After identification of the tCA, another line (tCA') was drawn in parallel through the apex of the PMF (Fig. 2c). The HP was defined as the greatest distance from the apex of the fragment to the point where the tCA' crossed the articular surface of the ankle.

The FAR

At the level of the tibial plafond, the posterior fragment area (s) and the remaining cross-sectional area of the tibia (S) were measured. The ratio of the fragment area to the total cross-sectional area of the tibial plafond was calculated using ($FAR = s / [s + S]$).

The distance from the distal AP locking screws to the PMF (DSP)

The distance from the distal edge of each locking screw to the PMF was measured (Fig. 2c). If the locking screw completely or partially penetrated the PMF, the measured distance was defined as negative and the condition as PMF violation. When the locking screw avoided the PMF, the distance was defined as positive and the condition was defined as fragment spared.

The distance from the nail tip to the PMF (DNP)

On the axial plane, the minimal distance from tip of the nail to the PMF was measured (Fig. 2d). When there

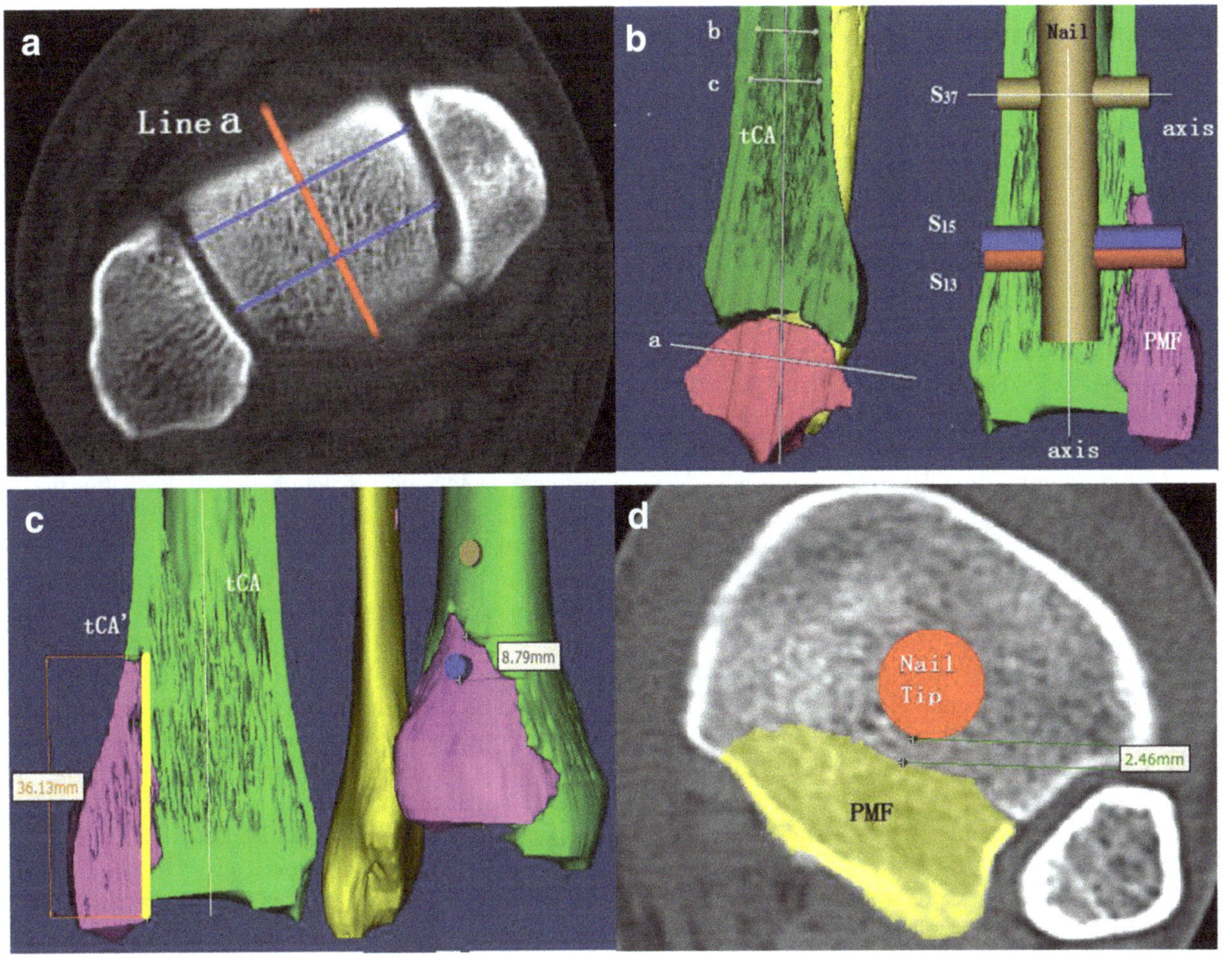

Fig. 2 a "Line a" is the projection line of the centers of the talar dome. **b** After the central sagittal plane (CSP) is determined, on this plane the tIN and three AP locking screws (S13, S15 and S37) are simulated. The relationship between AP locking screws and the PMF is demonstrated. **c** Measurements on reconstructed 3D model: the fragment height (FH) and the minimal distance from distal AP locking screw tip to the PMF (DSF). **d** Measurements on axial scan: minimal distance from the nail tip to the PMF (DNF)

was no violation from the nail tip to the PMF, the distance was defined as positive. When the nail tip violated the PMF, the measurement was defined as negative.

Interobserver reliability

Two senior orthopedic trauma surgeons analyzed all the CT scans in separate sessions and were blinded to each other's measurements. The interobserver reliability and 95% CI were excellent for all variables: 0.967 (95% CI, 0.957 to 0.975) for the HP, 0.974 (95% CI, 0.965 to 0.983) for the FAR, 0.967 (95% CI, 0.954 to 0.976) for the DNP, 0.971 (95% CI, 0.962 to 0.983) for the DSP and 0.957 (95% CI, 0.945 to 0.983) for the incidence of secondary fracture line.

Surgical technique

The patient was supine and fitted with an inflated tourniquet. The subpatellar approach was preferred, and the tibial canal was opened. The fracture was closely reduced by longitudinal manual distraction and maintained with reduction forceps. With the help of the reducer and the Poller screw technique, the guide wire was inserted precisely in the center of the ankle joint in the anteroposterior and lateral view. After gauging and reaming, the tibial nail was inserted with the tip located just above the top of the distal physeal scar in every case, and a lateral radiograph was taken to detect any displacement of the PMF. With a SURESHOT Targeting System (Smith & Nephew Inc., Massachusetts, USA), the most distal AP locking screw was inserted first. The drilling process was monitored under lateral radiography, and any noticeable displacement of the PMF terminated drilling. The PMF was percutaneously reduced with forceps and stabilized with one or two posteroanterior cannulated screws. After confirmation of the PMF reduction, the locking process continued.

Statistical analysis

The summary measurements were presented as the mean and standard deviation, proportions or as median with Q25 and Q75. Comparisons between the types of posterior malleolar fractures in the incidence of PMF violation were conducted with *t* tests for continuous variables and chi square tests for categorical variables. Two-tailed p values of < 0.05 were considered significant.

Variables with p values of < 0.2 were manually entered into the multiple logistic regression analysis to model the sparing of the PMF. A variable remained in the model when its p value was < 0.05 or when it had a significant impact on the − 2 log likelihood value. The logistic regression model results were presented as ORs with 95% CIs.

Receiver operating characteristic analyses were performed for continuous variables to test for diagnostic accuracy and determine optimal thresholds. Variables with an area under the ROC curve of > 0.80 were considered adequate for investigation [14]. A sensitivity of > 90% was used as the criterion for an optimal threshold.

Results

Fifty-five patients were included in this study with mean age of 45.18 years (range, 24 to 81 years), and 33 of them were male (60%). The measured FAR and HP of the PMF are listed in Table 1. The DNP was 4.29 mm [range, 1.5–8.54 mm] and all the measurements were positive, which indicated no PMF penetration from the vIM nail tip. Among the three AP locking screws, the S_{13} entailed the highest probability of PMF violation, followed by the S_{15} and S_{37}.

Table 1 Patient demographics and fracture characteristics

Clinical characteristics	n
FAR *(%)*[a]	19.06 ± 8.6
HP *(mm)*	33.38 ± 10.06
Incidence of displaced PMF *(%)*	25.45
Incidence of a "connection line" *(%)*	78.18
Mean displacement of the PMF *(mm)*[b]	1.50 (1.03–1.83)
Incidence of PMF violation *(%)*	
S_{13}	50.91
S_{15}	43.64
S_{37}	1.82
Distance from the nail tip to the PMF *(mm)*	4.29 (1.5–8.54)
Distance from distal AP locking screws to the violated PMF *(mm)*	
S_{13}	−7.41 (−13.07 to −5.17)
S_{15}	−6.34 (−10.53 to − 5.73)
S_{37}	− 1.18

Posterior malleolar fragment (PMF), height of posterior malleolar fragment (HP), fragment area ratio (FAR), anteroposterior (AP)
[a]The values are given as the mean and the standard deviation. [b]The values are given as the median with Q25 and Q75

According to Bartoníček's classification, no case fit the description of type 1, and the entire 55 cases could be divided into types 2 to 4. Among those three types, there were significant differences in the incidence of the secondary fracture line ($p = 0.004$), FAR ($p < 0.001$), HP ($p = 0.0013$) and the risk of PMF violation ($p = 0.004$ for the S_{13}, and $p = 0.015$ for the S_{15}) (Table 2).

Univariate analysis revealed that for the S_{13}, the difference between the spared and violated PMF was significant in FAR ($p = 0.004$), HP ($p < 0.001$) and Bartoníček's classification distribution ($p = 0.004$). There were also significant differences between the two groups in FAR ($p = 0.003$), HP ($p < 0.001$) and Bartoníček's classification distribution ($p = 0.015$) for the S_{15} (Table 3). Multiple logistic regression analysis showed the HP as an independent factor for predicting spared PMF for the S_{13} (OR 1.18, 95% CI 1.06–1.32, $p = 0.002$) and the S_{15} (OR 1.15, 95% CI 1.05–1.27, $p = 0.005$).

For the S_{13} and the S_{15}, the only continuous radiographic variable with an adequate AUC value in the ROC was the HP (0.909 for S_{13} and 0.882 for S_{15}). For the S_{13}, the HP cutoff value of 31.2 mm was 88.89% sensitive and 88.89% specific for spared PMF, corresponding to a positive and negative predictive value of 85.71% and 88.89%, respectively. An HP cutoff value of 31.2 mm was 88.89% sensitive and 88.89% specific for spared PMF, corresponding to a positive and negative predictive value of 85.71% and 88.89%, respectively. For the S15, this cutoff was 80.65% sensitive and 87.50% specific for PMF violation, corresponding to a positive and negative predictive value of 89.29% and 77.78%, respectively.

From the same group, tibial IM nails (TRIGEN META-NAIL Tibial Nail, Smith & Nephew Inc., Massachusetts, USA) were applied to 35 cases with no significant initial displacement of the PMF. The HP in 18 patients was less than 31.2 mm. Of the 18 cases, 6 patients experienced distal migration of the nail and physeal scar penetration during nail insertion. Five of 6 had PMF secondary displacement caused by S_{15} screws (Fig. 3). The remaining 12 cases whose IM nails were properly positioned had no secondary displacement. Among the 17 cases with PMF height exceeding 31.2 mm, 3 cases had distal physeal scar penetration. Fourteen cases had secondary displacement of PMF caused by an S_{15} screw, including three physeal scar penetrating cases.

Discussion

After Lauge-Hansen's discussion [1], Weber's series including 14 similar cases evoked interest in this topic [3]. Then, other authors conducted further studies investigating the injury mechanism, radiographic features, and associated injuries resulting from the treatment protocol [15–17]. The greatest improvement was made in summarizing the radiographic characteristics of this specific

Table 2 Comparison of demographic and fracture morphology between three types of Bartoníček's classification

	Bartoníček's classification			Coefficient value	*p-value*
	Type 2	Type 3	Type 4		
No. of patients	9	7	39		
Age *(yr)*	49.33 ± 14.54	43.00 ± 21.51	44.61 ± 12.07	F = 0.522	0.596
Sex[a]				$\chi^2 = 4.105$	0.128
Female	7	2	24		
Male	2	5	15		
Secondary fracture line				$\chi^2 = 10.878$	0.004
Negative	4	4	4		
Positive	5	3	35		
FAR *(%)*	0.05 (0.04–0.09)	0.16 (0.14–0.30)	0.24 (0.19–0.26)	H = 20.585	< 0.001
HP *(mm)*	26.37 (21.51–28.18)	30.98 (26.30–39.40)	33.77 (29.99–39.76)	H = 13.258	0.0013
Incidence of PMF violation					
S_{13}				$\chi^2 = 11.205$	0.004
PMF spared	9	3	15		
PMF disrupted	0	4	24		
S_{15}				$\chi^2 = 8.414$	0.015
PMF spared	9	3	19		
PMF disrupted	0	4	20		

Height of posterior malleolar fragment (HP), fragment area ratio (FAR), posterior malleolar fragment (PMF)
[a]The values are given as the number of patients

lower injury. When plain radiography was the primary tool for fracture assessment, Werken stated that a concomitant posterior malleolar fragment was actually an isolated fracture [2]. However, Hou's study revealed that the incidence of a "connection line" in concomitant tibial shaft fracture and ipsilateral ankle injury was as high as 92.71% [5]. In agreement with that conclusion, our study verified the high occurrence of this distinct radiographic sign (78.18%). When evaluated by CT scan only, our results confirmed that the "connection line" was a reliable indicator of concomitant posterior malleolar fracture and distal tibial spiral fracture.

The optimal treatment has been a topic of debate in recent years. One source of disagreement is the optimal implantation selection. Intramedullary nails and minimal invasive plating techniques can both be utilized to fix a tibial fracture. Generally, IM nails with locking screws can provide sufficient fixation stability with minimal soft tissue dissection [18, 19]. Furthermore, the fixation stability of distal tibial shaft fractures has been substantially improved by multiple-level/multiple-direction locking options and the Poller screw technique [20, 21]. Recently, most authors have preferred the IM nail rather than plating to treat this injury [2, 5, 6, 16, 22–24].

Another subject of interest has been how to treat PMF. It is clear that a considerably displaced PMF requires reduction and fixation to reconstruct the tibial plafond articular surface to congruency [25]. However,

Table 3 Univariate analysis results for factors related to posterior malleolar fragment violation of S_{13} and S_{15}

Clinical features	S_{13}		*p-value*	S_{15}		*p-value*
	PMF spared	PMF disrupted		PMF spared	PMF disrupted	
FAR *(%)*[a]	0.14 (0.07–0.24)	0.24 (0.19–0.26)	0.004	0.14 (0.08–0.24)	0.24 (0.19–0.27)	0.003
HP *(mm)*	27.23 (23.6–0.71)	37.22 (33.12–41.03)	< 0.001	28.16 (24.69–30.98)	37.22 (33.17–41.24)	< 0.001
Bartoníček's classification[b]			0.004			0.015
Type 2	9	0		9	9	
Type 3	3	4		3	4	
Type 4	15	24		19	20	

Posterior malleolar fragment (PMF), height of posterior malleolar fragment (HP), fragment area ratio (FAR)
[a]The values are given as the median with Q25 and Q75. [b]The values are given as the number of patients

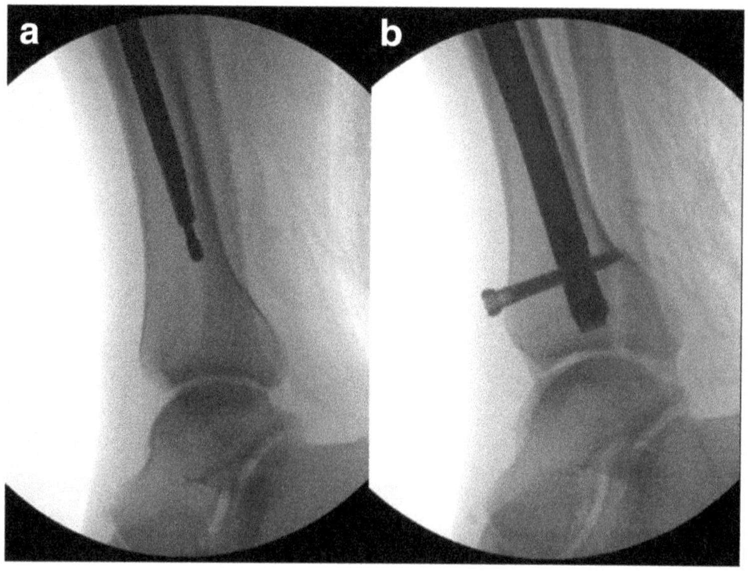

Fig. 3 a Demonstrating a non-displaced PMF before intramedullary nail insertion. **b** The penetration of distal tibial physeal scar from nail tip resulted in a secondary displacement of the PMF from distal AP locking screw

the present study revealed that in most cases, the PMF was non-displaced (74.55%), and the mean FAR was 19.06 ± 8.6%, much smaller than the proposed critical size for a posterior malleolar fracture fragment, which is one-quarter to one-third of the articular surface [26]. From the standpoint of rehabilitation, the fixed PMF might provide the theoretical benefit of allowing early active/passive ankle flexion exercise and even early partial weight bearing. However, biomechanical study has revealed that in normal ankles, the contact stresses are centrally located in plantar flexion and move to an anterior location as the ankle moves toward dorsiflexion. Therefore, a large area of the cartilage at the periphery of the joint is not loaded during the motion cycle. Under physiological conditions, the posterior articular surface of the ankle bears little load during the range of motion [25]. Thus, when a non-displaced PMF is left unfixed, the non-weight-bearing exercise of ROM would be unlikely to cause secondary displacement.

To gain a better holding strength on the distal tibial segment, deeper insertion of the IM nail was advocated. However, when nailing a tibial shaft fracture concurrent with ipsilateral posterior malleolar fracture, the PMF is within the pathway of the nail and distal AP screws. An increased depth of the nail would exaggerate the proximity between the nail/screw and the PMF. As a result, the reaming of the canal or the drilling of the AP locking screw might cause secondary displacement of the PMF. Therefore, the only indication for PMF fixation might be the necessity of eliminating the risk of secondary displacement of this intra-articular fracture during tibial nailing.

To quantify the actual risk of secondary displacement of the PMF during nail insertion and screw locking, we devised a simulated operation, and the results were confirmed by actual operations. In this study, the distal tibial physeal scar was used as the reference for nail insertion depth to gain the best holding strength because this structure is consistent in almost every case [8, 27]. It is also a durable bone plate that can withstand further advancement of the nail and provide obvious biomechanical benefits to fixation stability.

After the standardization of the IM nail insertion depth, a vIM nail with multiple AP locking screw options was simulated. The DNP measurement revealed that setting the advancement limit of the nail tip provided a safe space between the nail and the PMF (4.29 mm [1.5–8.54]). Therefore, the nail itself would not greatly exacerbate the posterior malleolar fracture displacement when the nail tip depth was properly determined. Subsequent study revealed that secondary displacement was almost caused by distal AP locking screws S_{13} and S_{15}. Further comparison between the violated and spared PMF groups revealed that the FAR and HP were significantly different (Table 3). This result confirmed that the morphological features of the PMF would significantly influence the risk of PMF violation.

As a morphological classification, Bartoníček's classification highly correlated with the risk of PMF violation during nailing. For S_{13} and S_{15}, there were significant differences among the three types in the rate of PMF violation ($p = 0.004$ and $p = 0.015$), and the highest group was type 4 (61.54% and 48.72%), followed by type 3. This result suggested that the surgeon should be alerted to the risk of PMF secondary displacement when the cross-section area and height of the PMF are large. To further quantify the risk factors, univariate analysis and multiple logistic regression analysis identified HP as the single significant factor relating to the violation of PMF by S_{13} and S_{15}. ROC analysis revealed that HP < 31.2 mm could be a reliable independent protective factor for PMF violation. According to the study design, this parameter was established using the distal tibial physeal scar as the consistent nail depth limitation. When the nail stopped proximally to this reference, the risk of PMF violation was reduced accordingly, while the mean distance measured from S_{13} and S_{15} to the edge of the violated PMF was − 7.4 mm (from − 2.32 to − 24.52) and − 6.34 mm (from − 2.08 to − 22), respectively. It can be postulated that withdrawal of the inserted vIM nail by 1.5 cm could significantly reduce the risk of PMF violation for both S_{13} (from 50.91% to 9.09%) and S_{15} (from 43.64% to 5.45%). The threshold of the HP is a very precise number and we believe it is unnecessary to normalize this figure according to patient's height or body build. The risk of PMF secondary displacement is mainly determined by the fragment's own anatomic features. Furthermore, there is no evidence that height or body build could significantly alter the position of the distal tibial physeal scar. Although the length of the tibial nail is significantly influenced by the height variance among patients, the distal locking screw arrangement in a tibial nail of any size is standardized.

The results of this simulation study were subsequently validated in the actual patients. Of the 55 patients, 35 patients had non-displaced PMF; therefore, their intraoperative and postoperative radiography were investigated. When the height of the PMF was less than 31.2 mm, avoiding distal tibial physeal scar penetration by the nail tip could act as a protective factor of the PMF from distal AP locking screw violation (S_{13} and S_{15}). However, this effect was not significant when the HF exceeded 31.2 mm. For those cases, to eliminate the risk of PMF secondary displacement, advanced PMF fixation by a cannulated screw before nail insertion is suggested.

We acknowledge the inherent limitations of the current study. Foremost, we used a relatively small sample size; however, we believe the use of non-paired objects of study provided sufficient sample heterogeneity. Furthermore, the relatively narrow ranges of our confidence intervals suggest that the sample size was sufficient for the observed variability. Second, the simulated nail fixation process was devised under idealized conditions that might not fully reflect reality; thus, the conclusion of this study could not cover all the fractures, especially when a PMF is more complex, such as with large size, substantial displacement or incarcerated fragments. However, this result was justified by our retrospective analysis of the authentic operation radiographic data. Our study provided concrete support for Guo's suggestion [8] that the traditional indication can be used to guide the treatment of a PMF. Third, our vIM nail does not cover all types of authentic tibial nails. Actually, it is impractical to make the virtual model represent all nail designs. To the best of our knowledge, the two prototypes are among the most widely used tibial intramedullary nails and both are characterized by an extremely distally located locking screw design. Therefore, we believe this virtual model has certain representativeness.

Conclusion

In this paper, the potency of Bartoníček's classification in directing the treatment of a PMF combined with a distal tibial spiral fracture was confirmed. We further found three key factors underpinning the risk of PMF secondary displacement: (1) the height of the PMF, (2) the space relationship between the nail tip and the distal tibial physeal scar and (3) the position of the distal anteroposterior locking screw in the tibial intramedullary nail. Among all the factors, the HP and the physeal scar were consistent variants and out of the surgeon's control. Identification of them could help the treating surgeon eliminate the risk of PMF secondary displacement by using a simple mathematical calculation. Other than preliminary PMF fixation, the surgeon could either draw the tibial nail (with a distal locking screw arrangement similar to the vIM nail) back a little to maintain a safe distance between the nail tip and the physeal scar, or change to another tibial nail with a more proximal tibial anteroposterior locking screw design.

Abbreviations

AP: anteroposterior; CI: confidence interval; DNP: distance from the nail tip to the PMF; DSP: distance from the distal AP locking screw to the PMF; FAR: fragment area ratio; HP: height of the PMF; OR: odds ratio; PMF: posterior malleolar fragment; S_{13}: $Screw_{13}$; S_{15}: $Screw_{15}$; S_{37}: $Screw_{37}$; tCA: tibial canal axis; vIM: nailvirtual tibial intramedullary nail

Acknowledgements

We gratefully acknowledge the support of all the doctors in our department.

Funding

No funding was obtained for this study.

Authors' contributions

LX and ZY performed the study. QXD and SLJ participated in the operation and data collection/interpretation for the study. ZY performed the statistical analysis. QXD conceived of the study and participated in its design. LX was responsible for coordination, data collection/interpretation and proofreading the final manuscript. All authors read and approved the final manuscript.

Consent for publication

Not applicable.

Competing interests

The authors declare that they have no competing interests.

References

1. Lauge-Hansen. Injuries caused by abnormal movements of the foot. Oxford: Nord. Med; 1946.
2. Van der Werken C, Zeegers EV. Fracture of the lower leg with involvement of the posterior malleolus; a neglected combination? Injury. 1988;19:241–3.
3. Weber, BG: Die Verletzungen des oberen Sprunggelenkes. 1sted. Bern: Hans Huber; 1966.
4. Böstman OM. Displaced malleolar fractures associated with spiral fractures of the tibial shaft. Clin Orthop Relat Res. 1988;(228):202–7.
5. Hou Z, Zhang L, Zhang Q, Yao S, Pan J, Irgit K, Zhang Y. The "communication line" suggests occult posterior malleolar fracture associated with a spiral tibial shaft fracture. Eur J Radiol. 2012;81:594–7. https://doi.org/10.1016/j.ejrad.2011.01.039.
6. Kempegowda H, Maniar HH, Richard R, Tawari A, Jove G, Suk M, Beebe MJ, Han C, Tornetta P 3rd, Kubiak EN, Horwitz DS. Posterior malleolar fractures associated with Tibial shaft fractures and sequence of fixation. J Orthop Trauma. 2016;30:568–71. https://doi.org/10.1097/BOT.0000000000000629.
7. Patel A, Charles L, Ritchie J. A complication of posterior malleolar fracture fixation. J Foot Ankle Surg. 2016;55:383–6. https://doi.org/10.1053/j.jfas.2014.12.040.
8. Guo J, Liu L, Yang Z, Hou Z, Chen W, Zhang Y. The treatment options for posterior malleolar fractures in tibial spiral fractures. Int Orthop. 2017;10 https://doi.org/10.1007/s00264-016-3388-8.
9. Bartoníček J, Rammelt S, Kostlivý´ K, Vaněček V, Klika D, Trešl I. Anatomy and classification of the posterior tibial fragment in ankle fractures. Arch Orthop Trauma Surg. 2015;135:506–16. https://doi.org/10.1007/s00402-015-2171-4.
10. Cinotti G, Sessa P, Rocca AD, Ripani FR, Giannicola G. Effects of tibial torsion on distal alignment of extramedullary instrumentation in total knee arthroplasty. Acta Orthop. 2013;84:275–9. https://doi.org/10.3109/17453674.2013.792032.
11. Cinotti G, Sessa P, D'Arino A, Ripani FR, Giannicola G. Improving tibial component alignment in total knee arthroplasty. Knee Surg Sports Traumatol Arthrosc. 2015;23(12):3563–70. https://doi.org/10.1007/s00167-014-3236-6.
12. Yao L, Zhang W, Yang G, Zhu Y, Zhai Q, Luo C. Morphologic characteristics of the posterior malleolus fragment: a 3-D computer tomography based study. Arch Orthop Trauma Surg. 2014;134:389–94. https://doi.org/10.1007/s00402-013-1844-0.
13. Haraguchi N, Haruyama H, Toga H, Kato F. Pathoanatomy of posterior malleolar fractures of the ankle. J Bone Joint Surg Am. 2006;88:1085–92. https://doi.org/10.2106/JBJS.E.00856.
14. Bradley AP. The use of the area under the ROC curve in the evaluation of machine learning algorithms. Pattern Recogn. 1997;30:1145–59.
15. Robinson CM, McLauchlan GJ, McLean IP, Court-Brown CM. Distal metaphyseal fractures of the tibia with minimal involvement of the ankle. Classification and treatment by locked intramedullary nailing. J Bone Joint Surg Br. 1995;77:781–7.
16. Purnell GJ, Glass ER, Altman DT, Sciulli RL, Muffly MT, Altman GT. Results of a computed tomography protocol evaluating distal third tibial shaft fractures to assess noncontiguous malleolar fractures. J Trauma. 2011;71:163–8. https://doi.org/10.1097/TA.0b013e3181edb88f.
17. Schottel PC, Berkes MB, Little MT, Lazaro LE, Nguyen JT, Helfet DL, Lorich DG. Predictive radiographic markers for concomitant ipsilateral ankle injuries in tibial shaft fractures. J Orthop Trauma. 2014;28:103–7. https://doi.org/10.1097/BOT.0b013e31829e71ef.
18. Vallier HA, Cureton BA, Patterson BM. Randomized, prospective comparison of plate versus intramedullary nail fixation for distal tibia shaft fractures. J Orthop Trauma. 2011;25(12):736–41. https://doi.org/10.1097/BOT.0b013e318213f709.
19. Yavuz U, Sökücü S, Demir B, Yıldırım T, Ozcan C, Kabukçuoğlu YS. Comparison of intramedullary nail and plate fixation in distal tibia diaphyseal fractures close to the mortise. Ulus Travma Acil Cerrahi Derg. 2014;20(3):189–93. https://doi.org/10.5505/tjtes.2014.92972.
20. Krettek C, Miclau T, Schandelmaier P, Stephan C, Möhlmann U, Tscherne H. The mechanical effect of blocking screws ("Poller screws") in stabilizing tibia fractures with short proximal or distal fragments after insertion of small-diameter intramedullary nails. J Orthop Trauma. 1999;13:550–3.
21. Vallier HA. Current evidence: plate versus intramedullary nail for fixation of distal tibia fractures in 2016. J Orthop Trauma. 2016;30(Suppl 4):S2–6. https://doi.org/10.1097/BOT.0000000000000692.
22. Kukkonen J, Heikkilä JT, Kyyrönen T, Mattila K, Gullichsen E. Posterior malleolar fracture is often associated with spiral tibial diaphyseal fracture: a retrospective study. J Trauma. 2006;60:1058–60. https://doi.org/10.1097/01.ta.0000196700.74272.10.
23. Boraiah S, Gardner MJ, Helfet DL, Lorich DG. High association of posterior malleolus fractures with distal tibial spiral fractures. Clin Orthop Relat Res. 2008;466:1692–8. https://doi.org/10.1007/s11999-008-0224-5.
24. Tsai CE, Su YP, Feng CK, Chen CM, Chiu FY, Liu CL. Concomitant tibial shaft and posterior malleolar fractures can be readily diagnosed from plain radiographs: a retrospective study. J Chin Med Assoc. 2014;77:95–100. https://doi.org/10.1016/j.jcma.2013.10.002.
25. Fitzpatrick DC, Otto JK, McKinley TO, Marsh JL, Brown TD. Kinematic and contact stress analysis of posterior malleolus fractures of the ankle. J Orthop Trauma. 2004;18:271–8.
26. Jaskulka RA, Ittner G, Schedl R. Fractures of the posterior tibial margin: their role in the prognosis of malleolar fractures. J Trauma. 1989;29:1565–70.
27. Grenier S, Benoit B, Rouleau DM, Leduc S, Laflamme GY, Liew A. APTF: anteroposterior tibiofibular ratio, a new reliable measure to assess syndesmotic reduction. J Orthop Trauma. 2013;27:207–11. https://doi.org/10.1097/BOT.0b013e31826623cc.

Anterior inferior plating versus superior plating for clavicle fracture

Jie Ai[1,2,3], Shun-Li Kan[2], Hai-Liang Li[2], Hong Xu[2], Yang Liu[2], Guang-Zhi Ning[2*] and Shi-Qing Feng[2*]

Abstract

Background: The position of plate fixation for clavicle fracture remains controversial. Our objective was to perform a comprehensive review of the literature and quantify the surgical parameters and clinical indexes between the anterior inferior plating and superior plating for clavicle fracture.

Methods: PubMed, EMBASE, and the Cochrane Library were searched for randomized and non-randomized studies that compared the anterior inferior plating with the superior plating for clavicle fracture. The relative risk or standardized mean difference with 95% confidence interval was calculated using either a fixed- or random-effects model.

Results: Four randomized controlled trials and eight observational studies were identified to compare the surgical parameters and clinical indexes. For the surgical parameters, the anterior inferior plating group was better than the superior plating group in operation time and blood loss ($P < 0.05$). Furthermore, in terms of clinical indexes, the anterior inferior plating was superior to the superior plating in reducing the union time, and the two kinds of plate fixation methods were comparable in constant score, and the rate of infection, nonunion, and complications ($P > 0.05$).

Conclusions: Based on the current evidence, the anterior inferior plating may reduce the blood loss, the operation and union time, but no differences were observed in constant score, and the rate of infection, nonunion, and complications between the two groups. Given that some of the studies have low quality, more randomized controlled trails with high quality should be conduct to further verify the findings.

Keywords: Anterior inferior plating, Superior plating, Clavicle fracture, Meta-analysis

Background

Clavicle fracture was one of the most common fractures, the overall incidence of it was 64 per 100,000 per year according to previous studies [1, 2]. Many different techniques were developed to treat it. The therapeutic methods for clavicle fracture have been well studied and the differences between non-operative management and operative management have been compared in many studies [3–5]. Furthermore, more and more evidences based on randomized controlled trials with high quality confirmed that non-operative intervention may increase the initial fracture displacement, the incidence of nonunion and the time to return to sports [6–8]. Hence, there was a growing appreciation that operative treatment could be more helpful than non-operative intervention for patients with clavicle fracture.

In addition, various methods can be used for clavicle fracture, and the plate and screw constructs were two most common methods [3]. Furthermore, the anterior inferior plating and superior plating were two techniques which were used in plate fixation and some studies have been performed to compare the two different methods for clavicle fracture. Nevertheless, the positions of plate remained controversial. Zlowodzki and colleagues presented that superior plating was associated with more symptoms [5]. In addition, evidences indicated that the anterior inferior plating may reduce the risk of damaging the underlying neurovascular bundle and implant prominence [9–13]. However, Robertson and colleagues demonstrated that compared with the anterior inferior plating, the superior plating was preferred because of an advantage in fracture fixation, which could be seen in routine activity [13]. Furthermore, a previous studies reported that the superior plating had greater biomechanical stability [14].

* Correspondence: ninggz_tmu@foxmail.com; sqfeng@tmu.edu.cn
[2]Department of Orthopaedics, Tianjin Medical University General Hospital, 154 Anshan Road, Heping District, Tianjin 300052, China
Full list of author information is available at the end of the article

Because of these contradictory results, we conducted this meta-analysis to provide an overview and quantitative estimate of the two different plating technologies for clavicle fracture based on the current evidences.

Methods

The present meta-analysis was performed according to the recommendations of the Cochrane Handbook for Systematic Reviews of Interventions and was reported in compliance with the PRISMA (Preferred Reporting Items for Systematic Reviews and Meta-Analyses statement) guidelines [15, 16].

Search strategy and study selection

PubMed, EMBASE, the Cochrane Library, Sciencedirect, CNKI and WanFang were searched by two researchers independently from inception to June 21, 2016. We combined MeSH terms with text words in the electronic search to identify the relevant literature. The search terms regarding to "clavicle fracture" were combined with terms related to "anterior inferior plating" and "superior plating". In addition, we also manually examined the systematic reviews, meta-analyses, and the included articles for further studies. There was no language restriction. Based on the titles and abstracts, two investigators picked out the potential eligible studies. And then the full text of the remaining studies were reviewed for eligibility. Any disagreement was resolved by discussion or consulting a third reviewer.

Eligibility criteria

(1) Participants: Patients who had clavicle fracture and underwent anterior inferior plating or superior plating were considered eligible for the inclusion criteria.
(2) Intervention and comparison: The group in which patients underwent anterior inferior plating for clavicle fracture was regarded as intervention group, and the control group enrolled patients with clavicle fracture who underwent superior plating. Patients who had clavicle fracture but didn't receive anterior inferior plating or superior plating were excluded.
(3) Outcomes: Blood loss and operation time were selected as surgical parameters, and we also extracted the union time, constant score, and the incidences of infection, nonunion and complications as clinical indexes.
(4) Study design: Randomized controlled trials, cohort studies, and case-control studies that compared anterior inferior plating with superior plating in patients with clavicle fracture were considered qualified.

Data extraction and outcome measures

Two reviewers independently extracted data from the eligible articles using a standard data extraction form. If any disagreements appeared, another reviewer was consulted. The following information was extracted from each included article:

Characteristics of each study: type of research, author name, year of publication, total number of patients, number of patients in intervention group and control group, duration of follow-up, and number of clavicle fracture of different sides.

Characteristics of patients: mean age and sex distribution.

Interventions: in intervention group, patients with clavicle fracture were treated by anterior inferior plating, and in control group, superior plating was chose.

Outcomes: surgical parameters (blood loss and operation time); clinical indexes (union time, constant score, infection, nonunion, and complications). We will choose the longest follow-up time as the measurement time point for all of the outcomes.

Assessment of methodological quality

We evaluated the risk of bias of randomized controlled trails based on the Cochrane Handbook. The items which we assessed were showed as following: random sequence generation, allocation concealment, blinding of participants and personnel, blinding of outcome assessors, incomplete outcome data, selective outcome reporting and other bias (baseline balance and fund). According to evaluation, all of the randomized controlled trails were determined as low risk of bias, high risk of bias, or unclear risk of bias.

The Newcastle-Ottawa Scale (NOS) [17], which included three domains with eight items, was used to assess the methodological quality of cohort studies. Furthermore, a semi quantitative principle of star system with a maximum score of nine stars was used to evaluate the quality of articles. Four of nine stars represented the appropriate selection of exposure and non-exposure cohort participants, two of nine stars represented the comparability of cohort, and the assessment of outcomes and follow-up were represented by three stars. Five or more stars out of a total of nine stars was regarded as good quality.

Statistical analysis

We used a descriptive analysis to describe the characteristics of studies included. Review Manager, version 5.3 was used to analysis the data. For dichotomous outcomes, we calculated relative risk (RR) with 95% confidence interval (CI), and for continuous outcomes, standardized mean difference (SMD) and 95% CI were calculated. We used I^2 to estimate the heterogeneity among different studies [18]. If I^2 was greater than 50%, significant heterogeneity was considered. When I^2 exceeded 50%, a random-effects model was used. Otherwise, a fixed-effects model was used. Furthermore, we also conducted meta-regression analyses using Stata, version 12.0 (Stata Corp, College Station, TX) to explore the effect of mean age and duration of follow-up on different outcomes. The Egger's linear regression test and funnel plots were used to examine the possibility of publication bias if more than ten studies were included [19]. P value of less than 0.05 denoted statistically significant difference.

Results

Study search

Eight hundred ninety-three potentially relevant records were identified. One hundred sixty-eight records were ruled out due to duplicates. After screening the titles and abstracts, 34 records potentially fit our eligibility criteria. Then with full text screened, 12 studies were included [13, 20–30] in the final analysis. And the flowchart of literature selection are shown in Fig. 1.

Study characteristics

Of the 12 articles included in our quantitative analysis, eight studies were retrospective studies [13, 21–24, 26, 29, 30], and the other four articles were randomized controlled trails [20, 25, 27, 28]. Only one study was multicenter study [13], and the rest of them were single-center study. Three studies included clavicle fracture of the aged [22, 25, 27], and midshaft clavicle fracture was studied in four studies [21, 23, 24, 26]. In addition, of the 12 articles, only one study reported the patient-reported symptoms and subjective outcome scores [26]. Finally, 954 patients (anterior inferior plating = 456, superior plating = 498) were included in our quantitative analysis. None of the studies received industry found. The information of study characteristics are presented in Table 1.

Methodological quality of the included studies

Risk of bias of randomized controlled trials

There were four studies [20, 25, 27, 28] which were reported as randomized controlled trails. Only one study was regarded as low risk of bias [20], and other studies were considered to be at unclear risk of bias for the reasons of lacking enough information of random sequence generation, allocation concealment, blinding of the participants, and blinding of outcome assessment. In addition, only one study described the random sequence generation and allocation concealment detailedly [20]. Besides, none of the studies received foundation from any industries or other non-profit organizations. The outcomes of risk of bias of are presented in Fig. 2.

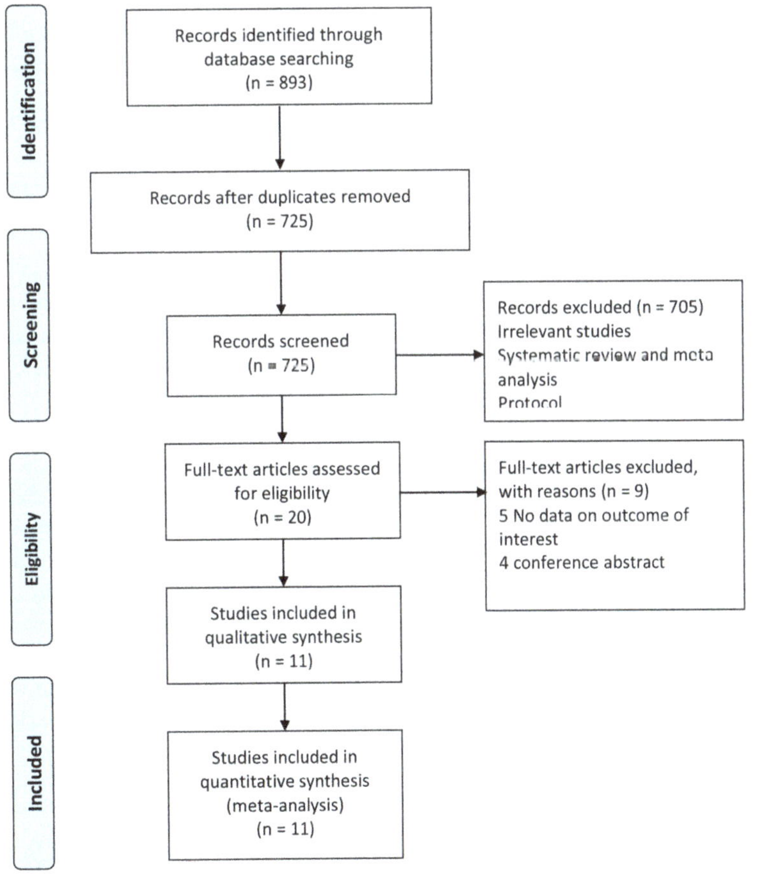

Fig. 1 The flow diagram of study selection

Table 1 Baseline characteristics of studies included in the meta-analysis

Source	Total no. of patients	Intervention	No. of patients	Follow-up, mo	Mean age, y	Fracture side			Gender	
						Left	Right	Bilateral	Male(%)	Female(%)
Cao 2015 [21]	42	Anterior inferior plating	23	-	46.4 ± 5.20	15	8	-	19	4
		Superior plating	19	-	48.5 ± 9.30	16	3	-	14	5
Qiu 2011 [28]	200	Anterior inferior plating	100	12	29	90	90	20	100	100
		Superior plating	100	12						
Deng 2008 [29]	67	Anterior inferior plating	29	6	28	54	50	-	59	50
		Superior plating	38	6						
Formaini 2013 [26]	105	Anterior inferior plating	43	2.00 ± 1.57	36.9 ± 13.2	21	22	-	27(63)	16(37)
		Superior plating	62	3.34 ± 2.01	36.1 ± 14.3	28	34	-	46(74)	16(26)
Hulsmans 2016 [13]	99	Anterior inferior plating	39	27 ± 19	38.6 ± 14.6	20	19	-	36(92)	3(8)
		Superior plating	60	21 ± 11	40.3 ± 11.5	29	31	-	55(92)	5(8)
Li 2013 [25]	66	Anterior inferior plating	33	6	68 ± 1.2	19	47	-	42	24
		Superior plating	33	6						
Qiu 2014 [22]	78	Anterior inferior plating	39	6.0	-	27	51	-	23	16
		Superior plating	39	6.0	-				24	15
Sohn 2015 [20]	37	Anterior inferior plating	18	16.7 ± 3.56	50.4 ± 17.36	7	11	-	18	1
		Superior plating	19	20.2 ± 9.85	46.7 ± 13.46	7	11	-	18	1
Xiao 2013 [23]	74	Anterior inferior plating	37	18	42.25 ± 2.92	17	20	-	19	18
		Superior plating	37	18	43.23 ± 3.16	18	19	-	20	17
Zhang 2012 [27]	92	Anterior inferior plating	46	6.0	67.9 ± 7.8	27	65	-	56	36
		Superior plating	46	6.0						
Zhao 2013 [24]	88	Anterior inferior plating	37	19.3	40.7	-	-	-	21	17
		Superior plating	51	19.3	42.5	-	-	-	38	13
Zheng 2006 [30]	25	Anterior inferior plating	13	16	36.5	-	-	-	16	9
		Superior plating	12	16						

Methodological quality of cohort studies

There were eight studies which were reported as cohort study [20–24, 26, 29, 30]. All of them were considered as good quality. Five studies reported the ascertainment of exposure [13, 21–23, 26], and all of the eight studies laid down the period of follow-up appropriately before assessment. Furthermore, only two studies fully considered the comparability between different groups [13, 26]. The detailed information about risk of bias of these cohort studies are showed in Table 2.

Surgical parameters

Operation time

There were seven studies ($n = 475$) provided available data for operation time [20–23, 25–27]. Of them, four studies were cohort studies [21, 22, 25, 27] and three studies were reported as randomized controlled trials [20, 23, 26]. The result of our meta-analysis showed that the operation time of anterior inferior plating was shorter than superior plating (SMD = −0.58, 95% CI −0.97 to −0.19, $P = 0.004$; $I^2 = 77\%$; Fig. 3a). In addition, meta-regression analysis was preformed to explore whether mean age had an effect on the operation time. The result showed that the mean age did not have an effect on it ($P = 0.48$, see Additional file 1: Figure S1).

Blood loss

Six studies reported the estimated blood loss during the operation [21–23, 25–27]. Among the six studies, four of them were retrospective studies [21–23, 26]. Most of them did not report the detailed information regarding fracture pattern, and only one study [26] reported the OTA classification. The result showed that blood loss in the experiment group was less than that in the control group (SMD = −0.78, 95% CI −1.15 to −0.40, $P < 0.0001$; $I^2 = 73\%$; Fig. 3b). Furthermore, the meta-regression analysis showed that no effect of mean age on blood loss ($P = 0.22$, see Additional file 1: Figure S2).

Clinical indexes

Union time

Seven studies with 521 patients reported the union time [20, 22–27]. Three of them [20, 25, 27] were randomized controlled trials, but only one study [20] reported the

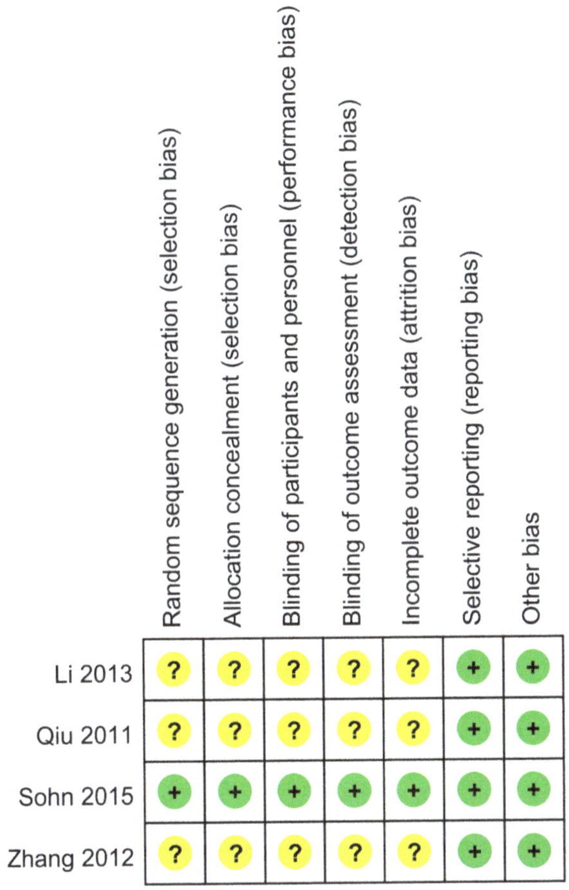

Fig. 2 Risk of bias assessment of randomized controlled trials

detailed information of time schedule for follow up and demonstrated that there was no difference in union time between the two groups ($P > 0.05$). However, in the other two randomized controlled studies, the results indicated that the anterior inferior plating had a significant advantage in union time over the superior plating ($P < 0.05$). Moreover, the other four studies were retrospective ones and showed that the anterior inferior plating was superior to the superior plating, but only one study showed statistically significant differences between the two groups.

Constant score

Three studies with 199 patients [20, 23, 24] contributed to the analysis of constant score, and the constant score in the anterior inferior plating group was similar to that in the superior plating group (SMD = 0.49, 95% CI −0.34 to 1.31, $P = 0.25$; $I^2 = 87\%$; Fig. 4a).

Infection

There were four studies [13, 20, 22, 26] reporting the outcome of infection, and no significant difference were observed between two groups (RR = 0.89, 95% CI 0.29 to 2.66, $P = 0.83$; $I^2 = 21\%$; Fig. 4b).

Nonunion

The data regarding nonunion were available in four studies with 424 patients [13, 20, 24, 28]. No significant difference was found between the two groups (RR = 0.39, 95% CI 0.15 to 1.05, $P = 0.06$; $I^2 = 0\%$; Fig. 4c).

Complications

Eight studies with 675 patients reported complications [13, 20, 23, 24, 26, 28–30], such as infection, implant breakage, nonunion, screw pullout, irritation, and fracture deformity. Compared with the superior plating, the anterior inferior plating was not associated with a significant reduction in complications (RR = 0.52, 95% CI 0.25 to 1.06, $P = 0.07$; $I^2 = 82\%$; Fig. 4d). Furthermore, meta-regression analyses demonstrated that no relationship was observed between duration of follow-up and complications ($P = 0.16$, see Additional file 1: Figure S3), but the mean age affected the rate of complications ($P = 0.02$, see Additional file 1: Figure S4), i.e., trials with higher age presented higher rate of complications.

Table 2 Methodological quality of cohort studies

Study	Selection				Comparability	Outcome			Score
	Representativeness of exposed cohort	Selection of non-exposed group	Ascertainment of exposure	Outcome of interest	Comparability of cohorts	Assessment of outcome	Length of follow-up	Adequacy of Follow-up	
Cao 2015 [21]	1	1	1	1	1	1	1	1	8
Deng 2008 [29]	1	1	0	0	1	1	1	1	6
Formaini 2013 [26]	1	1	1	1	2	1	1	1	9
Hulsmans 2016 [13]	1	1	1	1	2	1	1	1	9
Qiu 2014 [22]	1	1	1	1	1	1	1	1	8
Xiao 2013 [23]	1	1	1	1	1	1	1	1	8
Zhao 2013 [24]	1	1	0	0	1	1	1	1	6
Zheng 2006 [30]	0	1	0	0	1	1	1	1	5

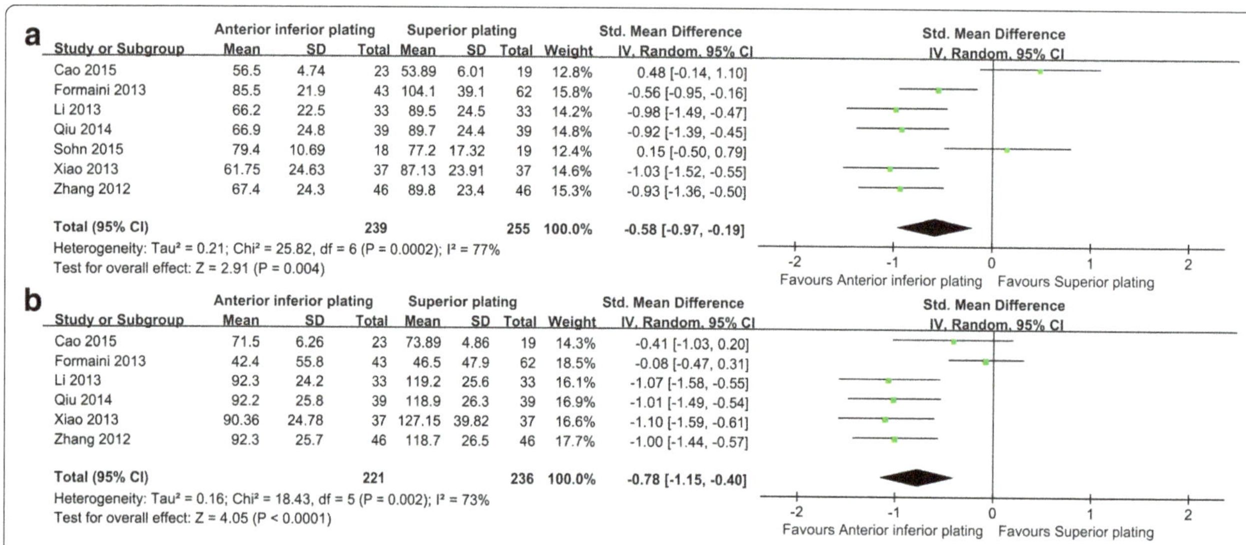

Fig. 3 Comparison of operation time (**a**) and blood loss (**b**) in patients undergoing anterior inferior plating versus superior plating for clavicle fracture

Discussion

Plate fixation has been regarded as an effective treatment for clavicle fracture, which may result in a high rate of union and low rates of associated complications [31–33]. Anterior inferior plating and superior plating are two different plate fixation procedures [34]. As both of them have their certain advantages and disadvantages, which approach is more effective and safety is still in dispute. So we performed this meta-analysis to compare the effectiveness and safety between anterior inferior plating and superior plating for patients with clavicle fracture, and to our knowledge, this study was the first meta-analysis to fill this gap.

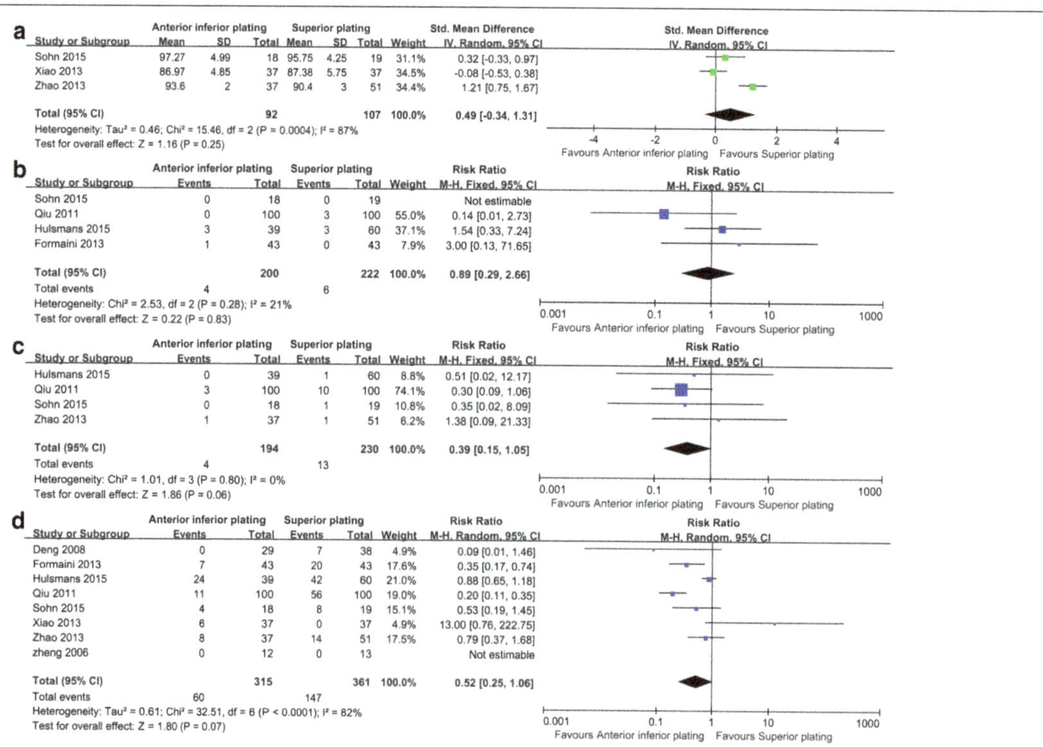

Fig. 4 Comparison of constant score (**a**), infection (**b**), nonunion (**c**), and complications (**d**) in patients undergoing anterior inferior plating versus superior plating for clavicle fracture

In this meta-analysis, we pooled the most recent evidence from both randomized and nonrandomized controlled trials, and provided the most reliable evidence. For surgical parameters, the results regarding operation time and blood loss demonstrated that the anterior inferior plating was better than the superior plating, which were consistent with Michael's study [5]. This outcome may be explained by the following reasons. First, patients was supine during operation. When surgeon aligned the plate with the clavicle in an anteroinferior-to-posterior direction, the diameter of anterior inferior clavicle aspect was broader than the superior clavicle aspect, which may help surgeon operate smoothly and save much operation time. Second, in terms of plate bending, the anterior inferior plating could be more easily bent along the shape of the contralateral clavicle than the superior plating [20, 23]. However, four [21–23, 26] of those studies which reported the result of blood loss were retrospective review of the patients, and the method for calculating blood loss was based on the documentation recorded in the operation room, but not the reduced Hg after operation. And the other two randomized controlled studies [25, 27] also did not describe how they calculate the blood loss. Furthermore, all of them did not report the detailed information of fracture pattern which may also influence the blood loss. So this result may be biased.

For the clinical index of union time, there were seven studies reported this outcome [20, 22–27]. Four of them were retrospective studies [22–24, 26], and the other three studies [20, 25, 27] were randomized controlled trials. However, most of them did not report the detailed time schedule for follow up to evaluate the union time. Considering that different surgeons had different time schedule to evaluate the bone healing time, we could not merge the data to calculate the pooled effects. And all results showed that the anterior inferior plating had an advantage over the superior plating in reducing union time. The possible benefit of the anterior inferior plating is less skin irritation and less vascular compromise during the surgery. Furthermore, the placement of screws was away from the infraclavicular neurovascular structure [20], which may explain why the anterior inferior plating contributed to the union of clavicle fracture.

Besides, based on the pooled estimates, we found that the anterior inferior plating was similar with the superior plating in the rate of nonunion and complications. This was different from previous studies [35, 36]. In biomechanical studies, the superior plating presented superiority over the anterior inferior plating in fracture rigidity and the bending load to failure; however, the anterior inferior plating was superior in stability regarding bending rigidity [37, 38]. Both of them have their own advantages, so no differences were observed in nonunion and complications between two groups.

The strengths of this meta-analysis are presented as following. First, to the best of our knowledge, this is the first meta-analysis providing comprehensive insights into the comparison of the effectiveness and safety between the anterior inferior plating and the superior plating for clavicle fracture, which would provide a more reliable evidence for clinical practice. Second, we used strict retrieval conditions to identify the possible articles. Both randomized and non-randomized studies were included to provide sufficient sample size so that the inference is more reliable. Third, we also conducted meta-regression analyses to explore whether mean age and duration of follow-up were independent predictive factors for union time, operation time, blood loss, infection, nonunion and complications.

In addition, there were also several limitations which must be declared in this study. First, only 973 patients were included in this study. The number of patients was relatively small, which would limit the statistical power. Second, only four randomized controlled trials were included, and three of them were regarded as unclear risk of bias, which may influence the outcomes. Third, given that only five studies provided data for the number of each fracture side and the reasons of clavicle fracture, we could not conduct subgroup analyses to explore whether the fracture side or the reasons of clavicle fracture may influence the effect of surgery.

Conclusions

Based on the current evidence, the anterior inferior plating may reduce the blood loss, the operation and union time, but no differences were observed in constant score, and the rate of infection, nonunion, and complications between the two groups. Given that some of the studies have low quality, more randomized controlled trails with high quality should be conduct to further verify the findings.

Additional file

Additional file 1: Figure S1. Meta-regression analysis of influence of mean age on operation time. The circles represent each study. The size of the circle represents the power of the study. The solid line indicates the weighted regression line. **Figure S2.** Meta-regression analysis of influence of mean age on blood loss. The circles represent each study. The size of the circle represents the power of the study. The solid line indicates the weighted regression line. **Figure S3.** Meta-regression analysis of influence of mean age on union time. The circles represent each study. The size of the circle represents the power of the study. The solid line indicates the weighted regression line. **Figure S4.** Meta-regression analysis of influence of duration of follow-up on complications. The circles represent each study. The size of the circle represents the power of the study. The solid line indicates the weighted regression line. **Figure S5.** Meta-regression analysis of influence of mean age on complications. The circles represent each study. The size of the circle represents the power of the study. The solid line indicates the weighted regression line. (DOCX 257 kb)

Abbreviations

CI: Confidence interval; NOS: Newcastle-Ottawa Scale; PRISMA: Preferred Reporting Items for Systematic Reviews and Meta-Analyses statement; RR: Risk ratio; SMD: Standardized mean difference

Funding

This work was supported by State Key Program of National Natural Science Foundation of China (81330042), Special Program for Sino-Russian Joint Research Sponsored by the Ministry of Science and Technology, China (2014DFR31210), International Cooperation Program of National Natural Science Foundation of China (81620108018) and Key Program Sponsored by the Tianjin Science and Technology Committee, China (13RCGFSY19000, 14ZCZDSY00044). The funders had no role in study design, data collection and analysis, decision to publish, or preparation of the manuscript.

Authors' contributions

SQF, GZN, JA and SLK conceived, designed and coordinated the experiments and drafted the manuscript. JA, SLK and HLL contributed to data acquisition. JA, HLL, HX and YL analyzed and interpreted the data. JA, HX and YL revised the manuscript. All authors read and approved the final manuscript.

Competing interests

The authors declare that they have no competing interests.

Consent for publication

Not applicable.

Author details

[1]Tianjin Medical University, 22 Qixiangtai Road, Heping District, Tianjin 300070, China. [2]Department of Orthopaedics, Tianjin Medical University General Hospital, 154 Anshan Road, Heping District, Tianjin 300052, China. [3]Department of Orthopaedics, Yuci People's Hospital, 262 Jingwei Road, Jinzhong, Shanxi Province 030600, China.

References

1. Postacchini F, Gumina S, De Santis P, Albo F. Epidemiology of clavicle fractures. J Shoulder Elbow Surg. 2002;11(5):452–6.
2. Nordqvist A, Petersson C. The incidence of fractures of the clavicle. Clin Orthop Relat Res. 1994;300:127–32.
3. McKee RC, Whelan DB, Schemitsch EH, McKee MD. Operative versus nonoperative care of displaced midshaft clavicular fractures: a meta-analysis of randomized clinical trials. J Bone Joint Surg Am. 2012;94(8):675–84.
4. Robinson CM, Goudie EB, Murray IR, Jenkins PJ, Ahktar MA, Read EO, Foster CJ, Clark K, Brooksbank AJ, Arthur A, et al. Open reduction and plate fixation versus nonoperative treatment for displaced midshaft clavicular fractures: a multicenter, randomized, controlled trial. J Bone Joint Surg Am. 2013;95(17): 1576–84.
5. Zlowodzki M, Zelle BA, Cole PA, Jeray K, McKee MD. Treatment of acute midshaft clavicle fractures: systematic review of 2144 fractures: on behalf of the Evidence-Based Orthopaedic Trauma Working Group. J Orthop Trauma. 2005;19(7):504–7.
6. Robinson CM, Court-Brown CM, McQueen MM, Wakefield AE. Estimating the risk of nonunion following nonoperative treatment of a clavicular fracture. J Bone Joint Surg Am. 2004;86-A(7):1359–65.
7. Hill JM, McGuire MH, Crosby LA. Closed treatment of displaced middle-third fractures of the clavicle gives poor results. J Bone Joint Surg. 1997;79(4):537–9.
8. Robertson GA, Wood AM. Return to sport following clavicle fractures: a systematic review. Br Med Bull. 2016;119:111–28.
9. Collinge C, Devinney S, Herscovici D, DiPasquale T, Sanders R. Anterior-inferior plate fixation of middle-third fractures and nonunions of the clavicle. J Orthop Trauma. 2006;20(10):680–6.
10. Kloen P, Sorkin AT, Rubel IF, Helfet DL. Anteroinferior plating of midshaft clavicular nonunions. J Orthop Trauma. 2002;16(6):425–30.
11. Shen WJ, Liu TJ, Shen YS. Plate fixation of fresh displaced midshaft clavicle fractures. Injury. 1999;30(7):497–500.
12. Sinha A, Edwin J, Sreeharsha B, Bhalaik V, Brownson P. A radiological study to define safe zones for drilling during plating of clavicle fractures. J Bone Joint Surg. 2011;93(9):1247–52.
13. Hulsmans MH, van Heijl M, Houwert RM, Timmers TK, van Olden G, Verleisdonk EJ. Anteroinferior versus superior plating of clavicular fractures. J Shoulder Elbow Surg. 2016;25(3):448–54.
14. Celestre P, Roberston C, Mahar A, Oka R, Meunier M, Schwartz A. Biomechanical evaluation of clavicle fracture plating techniques: does a locking plate provide improved stability? J Orthop Trauma. 2008;22(4):241–7.
15. Higgins JP, Green S. Cochrane handbook for systematic reviews of interventions version 5.1.0. The Cochrane Collaboration. 2011. Available from: http://www.handbook.cochrane.org.
16. Liberati A, Altman DG, Tetzlaff J, Mulrow C, Gotzsche PC, Ioannidis JP, Clarke M, Devereaux PJ, Kleijnen J, Moher D. The PRISMA statement for reporting systematic reviews and meta-analyses of studies that evaluate health care interventions: explanation and elaboration. J Clin Epidemiol. 2009;62(10):e1–34.
17. Wells GA, Shea B, O'Connell D, Peterson J, Welch V, Losos M, Tugwell P. The Newcastle-Ottawa Scale (NOS) for assessing the quality of nonrandomized studies in meta-analysis. 2011. Available from: www.ohri.ca/programs/clinical_epidemiology/oxford.asp.
18. Higgins JP, Thompson SG, Deeks JJ, Altman DG. Measuring inconsistency in meta-analyses. BMJ (Clinical research ed). 2003;327(7414):557–60.
19. Egger M, Davey Smith G, Schneider M, Minder C. Bias in meta-analysis detected by a simple, graphical test. BMJ (Clinical research ed). 1997;315(7109):629–34.
20. Sohn HS, Shon MS, Lee KH, Song SJ. Clinical comparison of two different plating methods in minimally invasive plate osteosynthesis for clavicular midshaft fractures: A randomized controlled trial. Injury. 2015;46(11):2230–8.
21. Cao JS, Wang X, Chen BL, Li J. A comparative study of internal fixation with praevia versus superior reconstruction plate for treatment of middle clavicular fractures in adults. J Tradit Chin Orthop Traumatol. 2015;01:27.
22. Qiu WH, Luo CQ, He XZ. The clinical effect of old person with clavicle fracture treated with anterior plate. Chin J Mod Drug Appl. 2014;13:68–9.
23. Xiao ZL, Qi LH. The curative effect comparison between anterior and upper reconstruction plate internal fixation for middle clavicular fractures. Chin J Mod Med. 2013;15(4):68–70.
24. Zhao YP, Tang PF, Guo XD, Zhang LH, Chen H, Wang Y. Clinical analysis of the reconstruction plate for complicated midshaft clavicle fracture: anterior versus superior. Prog Mod Biomed. 2013;13(21):4053–72.
25. Li WF. The clinical effect of 33 old patients with clavicle fracture treated with anterior plating. Nei Mongol J Tradit Chin Med. 2013;29:73.
26. Formaini N, Taylor BC, Backes J, Bramwell TJ. Superior versus anteroinferior plating of clavicle fractures. Orthopedics. 2013;36(7):e898–904.
27. Zhang D, Xu Y. The clinical effect of old patients with clavicle fracture treated with anterior plating. Chin J Prim Med Pharm. 2012;24:19.
28. Qiu CT, Chen LQ. The effect of anterior plating of clavicular fractures. Chin Mod Doct. 2011;09:49.
29. Deng D, Cao CF, Ji B, Jiang YX, Zhou JJ, Shi JX, Cheng XY, Shi WJ, Zhao Y, Wang Z. Retrospective study of fore-lying reconstruction plate in treating fracture of collar bone. Chin J Tradit Med Traum Orthop. 2008;16(10):3–4.
30. Zheng JH, Zeng G, Luo XJ, Gao J, Guo YZ. The clinical effect of anterior versus superior plating of clavicular fractures. Anatomy Clinics. 2006;04:11.
31. Drosdowech DS, Manwell SE, Ferreira LM, Goel DP, Faber KJ, Johnson JA. Biomechanical analysis of fixation of middle third fractures of the clavicle. J Orthop Trauma. 2011;25(1):39–43.
32. Wilson DJ, Scully WF, Min KS, Harmon TA, Eichinger JK, Arrington ED. Biomechanical analysis of intramedullary vs. superior plate fixation of transverse midshaft clavicle fractures. J Shoulder Elbow Surg. 2016;25(6):949–53.
33. Society. COT. Nonoperative treatment compared with plate fixation of displaced midshaft clavicular fractures. A multicenter, randomized clinical trial. J Bone Joint Surg Am. 2007;89(1):1–10.

Permissions

All chapters in this book were first published in MD, by BioMed Central; hereby published with permission under the Creative Commons Attribution License or equivalent. Every chapter published in this book has been scrutinized by our experts. Their significance has been extensively debated. The topics covered herein carry significant findings which will fuel the growth of the discipline. They may even be implemented as practical applications or may be referred to as a beginning point for another development.

The contributors of this book come from diverse backgrounds, making this book a truly international effort. This book will bring forth new frontiers with its revolutionizing research information and detailed analysis of the nascent developments around the world.

We would like to thank all the contributing authors for lending their expertise to make the book truly unique. They have played a crucial role in the development of this book. Without their invaluable contributions this book wouldn't have been possible. They have made vital efforts to compile up to date information on the varied aspects of this subject to make this book a valuable addition to the collection of many professionals and students.

This book was conceptualized with the vision of imparting up-to-date information and advanced data in this field. To ensure the same, a matchless editorial board was set up. Every individual on the board went through rigorous rounds of assessment to prove their worth. After which they invested a large part of their time researching and compiling the most relevant data for our readers.

The editorial board has been involved in producing this book since its inception. They have spent rigorous hours researching and exploring the diverse topics which have resulted in the successful publishing of this book. They have passed on their knowledge of decades through this book. To expedite this challenging task, the publisher supported the team at every step. A small team of assistant editors was also appointed to further simplify the editing procedure and attain best results for the readers.

Apart from the editorial board, the designing team has also invested a significant amount of their time in understanding the subject and creating the most relevant covers. They scrutinized every image to scout for the most suitable representation of the subject and create an appropriate cover for the book.

The publishing team has been an ardent support to the editorial, designing and production team. Their endless efforts to recruit the best for this project, has resulted in the accomplishment of this book. They are a veteran in the field of academics and their pool of knowledge is as vast as their experience in printing. Their expertise and guidance has proved useful at every step. Their uncompromising quality standards have made this book an exceptional effort. Their encouragement from time to time has been an inspiration for everyone.

The publisher and the editorial board hope that this book will prove to be a valuable piece of knowledge for researchers, students, practitioners and scholars across the globe.

List of Contributors

Brita Stanghelle
Faculty of Health Sciences, Department of Physiotherapy, Oslo and Akershus University College of Applied Sciences, St. Olavs plass, 0130 Oslo, Norway

Hege Bentzen
Department of Physiotherapy, Oslo and Akershus University College of Applied Sciences, Oslo, Norway

Lora Giangregorio
Department of Kinesiology, University of Waterloo, Waterloo, Canada

Are Hugo Pripp
Faculty of Health Sciences, Oslo and Akershus University College of Applied Sciences, Oslo, Norway

Astrid Bergland
Faculty of Health Sciences, Leader of the research group Age, Health and Welfare and the PhD-program in Health Sciences, Oslo and Akershus University College of Applied Sciences, Oslo, Norway

Yu Zhang, Xiaodong Qin, Lijun Song and Xiang Li
Department of Trauma, the First Affiliated Hospital of Nanjing Medical University and Jiangsu Province Hospital, 300 Guangzhou Road, Nanjing 210029, China

Thorsten Jentzsch, Anita Hasler, Niklas Renner and Stephan H. Wirth
Department of Orthopaedics, Balgrist University Hospital, University of Zurich, Forchstrasse 340, 8008 Zurich, Switzerland

Manuel Peterhans
Department of Orthopaedics, Kantonsspital Aarau, Aarau, Switzerland

Reto Sutter
Department of Radiology, Balgrist University Hospital, University of Zurich, Zurich, Switzerland

Norman Espinosa
Institute for Foot and Ankle Reconstruction Zurich, Zurich, Switzerland

Xue-Mei Yang
Hyperbaric Oxygen Treatment Center, the Affiliated Hospital of Xuzhou Medical University, No. 99 Huaihai West Road, Xuzhou, Jiangsu 221002, People's Republic of China

Jun-Ying Sun
Orthopaedic Department, the First Affiliated Hospital of Soochow University, 188 Shizi Street, Suzhou, Jiangsu 215006, People's Republic of China

Chang Ho Shin, Doo Jae Lee, In Ho Choi, Tae-Joon Cho and Won Joon Yoo
Department of Orthopaedic Surgery, Seoul National University College of Medicine, 101 Daehak-ro Jongno-gu, Seoul, 03080, Republic of Korea

Daniel Jerrhag, Magnus K. Karlsson and Bjorn E. Rosengren
Clinical and Molecular Osteoporosis Research Unit, Departments of Clinical Sciences and Orthopedics Malmö, Skåne University Hospital, Lund University, SE 20502 Malmo, Sweden

Martin Englund
Department of Clinical Sciences Lund, Orthopedics, Clinical Epidemiology Unit, Lund University, Faculty of Medicine, Lund, Sweden
Clinical Epidemiology Research and Training Unit, Boston University School of Medicine, Boston, MA, USA

Aldo Okamura and Gabriel Maciel de Mendonça
Hospital Municipal do Campo Limpo Dr. Fernando Mauro Pires da Rocha, Estrada de Itapecerica, 1661 - Campo Limpo, São Paulo, SP 05835-005, Brazil

Jorge Raduan Neto, Vinicius Ynoe de Moraes, Flavio Faloppa and João Carlos Belloti
Hand, Arm and Shoulder Surgery Unit, Department of Orthopedics and Traumatology, Universidade Federal de São Paulo, UNIFESP/EPM, Rua Borges Lagoa, 778 Vila Clementino, São Paulo, SP, Brazil

Moritz Crönlein, Marc Beirer, Dominik Pförringer, Chlodwig Kirchhoff, Peter Biberthaler and Karl F. Braun
Department of Trauma Surgery, Klinikum rechts der Isar, Technical University of Munich, Ismaninger Strasse 22, 81675 Munich, Germany

Martin Lucke
Department of Trauma Surgery, Chirurgisches Klinikum München Süd, Am Isarkanal 30, 81379 Munich, Germany

Sebastian Siebenlist
Department of Trauma Surgery, Klinikum rechts der Isar, Technical University of Munich, Ismaninger Strasse 22, 81675 Munich, Germany
Department of Orthopaedic Sports Medicine, Klinikum rechts der Isar, Technical University of Munich, Ismaninger Strasse 22, 81675 Munich, Germany

Guo-Chun Zha, Shuo Feng, Xiang-Yang Chen and Kai-Jin Guo
Department of Orthopedic Surgery, the Affiliated Hospital of Xuzhou Medical University, No. 99 Huaihai West Road, Xuzhou, Jiangsu 221002, People's Republic of China

Johnny Paulsson, Josefine Corin Stig and Ola Olsson
Department of Orthopedics, Helsingborg Hospital, S-251 87 Helsingborg, Sweden

Jonathan D. Adachi
McMaster University, 501-25 Charlton Ave E., Hamilton, ON L8N 1Y2, Canada

Henry G. Bone
Michigan Bone and Mineral Clinic, 22201 Moross Rd, Detroit, MI 48236, USA

Nadia S. Daizadeh, Paula Dakin, Andrea Wang, Celia J. F. Lin and Rachel B. Wagman
Amgen Inc., One Amgen Ctr Dr., Thousand Oaks, CA 91320, USA

Socrates Papapoulos
Leiden University Medical Center, Albinusdreef 2, 2333, ZA, Leiden, Netherlands

Peyman Hadji
Krankenhaus Nordwest, Steinbacher Hohl 2-26, 60488 Frankfurt am Main, Germany

Chris Recknor
United Osteoporosis Centers, 2350 Limestone Pkwy, Gainesville, GA 30501, USA

Michael A. Bolognese
Bethesda Health Research Center, 10215 Fernwood Rd Ste 40, Bethesda, MD 20817, USA

Serge Ferrari
Geneva University Hospital, Rue Gabrielle-Perret-Gentil 4, 1205 Genève, Switzerland

Tengbo Yu, Hao Tao, Chengdong Zhang and Guangjie Zhou
Department of Orthopaedic Surgery, Affiliated Hospital of Qingdao University, Qingdao, Shandong 266000, People's Republic of China

Fenglei Xu
Department of Radiology, Affiliated Hospital of Qingdao University, Qingdao, Shandong 266000, People's Republic of China

Yanling Hu
Department of Orthopaedic Surgery, Affiliated Hospital of Qingdao University, Qingdao, Shandong 266000, People's Republic of China
Department of Orthopaedic Surgery, Affiliated Hospital of Qingdao University, 59 Haier Road, Qingdao City 266003, Shandong Province, China

Joep Kitzen, Martijn G. M. Schotanus and Pieter B. J. Tilman
Department of Orthopaedic Surgery, Zuyderland Medical Centre, Postbus 5500, 6130 MB Sittard-Geleen, the Netherlands

Herbert S. W. Plasschaert
Department of Pathology, Zuyderland Medical Centre, Sittard-Geleen, the Netherlands

Frans-Jan H. Hulsmans
Department of Radiology, Zuyderland Medical Centre, Sittard-Geleen, the Netherlands

David Wennergren, Stina Stjernström, Michael Möller, Mikael Sundfeldt and Carl Ekholm
Department of Orthopaedics, Sahlgrenska University Hospital, SE-413 45 Gothenburg, Mölndal, Sweden

Teemu P. Hevonkorpi and Antti P. Launonen
Department of Orthopedics and Trauma Surgery, Tampere University Hospital, Tampere, Finland

Tuomas T. Huttunen
Department of Anesthesia, Tampere University Hospital, Tampere, Finland

Pekka Kannus
School of Medicine, University of Tampere, Tampere, Finland
Injury & Osteoporosis Research Center, UKK Institute for Health Promotion Research, Tampere, Finland

Seppo Niemi
Injury & Osteoporosis Research Center, UKK Institute for Health Promotion Research, Tampere, Finland

Ville M. Mattila
Department of Orthopedics and Trauma Surgery, Tampere University Hospital, Tampere, Finland
School of Medicine, University of Tampere, Tampere, Finland
Department of Clinical Science, Intervention and Technology, Karolinska Institutet, Division of Orthopedics and Biotechnology, Karolinska Institutet and Department of Orthopedics at Karolinska University Hospital, Karolinska Institutet, Solna and Huddinge, Sweden

Brady J. Hurtgen, Beth E. P. Henderson, Catherine L. Ward, Stephen M. Goldman, Koyal Garg, Sarah M. Greising, Joseph C. Wenke and Benjamin T. Corona
Extremity Trauma and Regenerative Medicine Task Area, US Army Institute of Surgical Research, 3698 Chambers Pass, BHT1, Fort Sam Houston, TX 78234, USA

Todd O. McKinley
Department of Orthopaedic Surgery, Indiana University School of Medicine, Indianapolis, IN, USA

Wei Xu, Chao Chen, Yifan Li, Xiaodong Zhu and Zhikun Li
Department of Orthopedics, Tongren Hospital, Shanghai Jiao Tong University School of Medicine, 1111 XianXia Road, Shanghai 200336, People's Republic of China

Yunhan Ji
Medical Services Section, Tongren Hospital, Shanghai Jiao Tong University School of Medicine, 1111 XianXia Road, Shanghai 200336, People's Republic of China

Silian Wang
Department of Radiology, Tongren Hospital, Shanghai Jiao Tong University School of Medicine, 1111 XianXia Road, Shanghai 200336, People's Republic of China

You-Shui Gao, Yan-Jie Guo, Xin-Gang Yu, Yang Chen, Chen Chen and Nan-Ji Lu
Department of Orthopaedic Surgery, Shanghai Jiao Tong University Affiliated Sixth People's Hospital, Shanghai 200233, China

Bowen Su and Roger Newson
Department of Primary Care & Public Health, School of Public Health, Imperial College London, W6 8RP, London, UK

Harry Soljak
Department of Anaesthetics, St Peter's Hospital, Chertsey KT16 0PZ, UK

Michael Soljak
Department of Primary Care & Public Health, School of Public Health, Imperial College London, W6 8RP, London, UK
Centre for Population Health Sciences (CePHaS), Lee Kong Chian School of Medicine, Nanyang Technological University, Singapore 308232, Singapore

Alvin Chao-Yu Chen, Chun-Jui Weng, Ying-Chao Chou and Chun-Ying Cheng
Department of Orthopaedic Surgery, Bone and Joint Research Center, Chang Gung Memorial Hospital-Linkou & University College of Medicine, 5th, Fu-Shin St., Kweishan District, Taoyuan 333, Taiwan, Republic of China

Leif Mattisson
Department of Clinical Science and Education, Södersjukhuset, Karolinska Institutet. Department of Orthopaedics, Stockholm South General Hospital, 11883 Stockholm, Sweden

Alicja Bojan
Department of Orthopaedics, Sahlgrenska University Hospital Gothenburg/Mölndal, 431 80 Mölndal, Sweden

R. Kellersmann
Department of Vascular Surgery, Klinikum Fulda, Fulda, Germany

Anders Enocson
Department of Clinical Science and Education, Södersjukhuset, Karolinska Institutet. Department of Orthopaedics, Stockholm South General Hospital, 11883 Stockholm, Sweden
Department of Molecular Medicine and Surgery, Karolinska University Hospital, Karolinska Institutet, 17176 Stockholm, Sweden

Tien-Yu Yang, Tsan-Wen Huang and Po-Yao Chuang
Chang Gung University College of Medicine, Taoyuan, Taiwan
Department of Orthopaedic Surgery, Chang Gung Memorial Hospital, Chiayi, Taiwan

Kuo-Chin Huang
Chang Gung University College of Medicine, Taoyuan, Taiwan
Department of Orthopaedic Surgery, Chang Gung Memorial Hospital, Chiayi, Taiwan
Putz City, Taiwan

F. Gilbert
Department of Orthopaedic Trauma, Hand, Plastic and Reconstructive Surgery, University Hospital Würzburg, Würzburg, Germany
Department of Trauma Hand Plastic and Reconstructive Surgery, University Munich Germany, Julius-Maximilians-University of Würzburg Oberdürrbacherstr, 6 D-, 97080 Würzburg, Germany

C. Schneemann, R. Wildenauer and U. Lorenz
Department for General Visceral, Vascular & Paediatric Surgery, University Hospital Würzburg, Würzburg, Germany

C. J. Scholz
Core Unit Systems Medicine IZKF, University Hospital Würzburg, Würzburg, Germany

R. Kickuth
Department of Diagnostic and Interventional Radiology, University Hospital Würzburg, Würzburg, Germany

R. H. Meffert
Department of Orthopaedic Trauma, Hand, Plastic and Reconstructive Surgery, University Hospital Würzburg, Würzburg, Germany

A. Busch
Department for General Visceral, Vascular & Paediatric Surgery, University Hospital Würzburg, Würzburg, Germany
Department for Vascular and Endovascular Surgery Klinikum rechts der Isar, Technical University Munich, Munich, Germany

Cecilie Mullerup Kiel and Michael Rindom Krogsgaard
Section for Sports Traumatology M51, Bispebjerg-Frederiksberg Hospital (Part of IOC Research Center Copenhagen), University of Copenhagen, Bispebjerg Bakke 23, DK-2400 Copenhagen, NV, Denmark
Danish Patient Compensation Association, Kalvebod Brygge 45, 1560 Copenhagen, NV, Denmark

Kim Lyngby Mikkelsen
Danish Patient Compensation Association, Kalvebod Brygge 45, 1560 Copenhagen, NV, Denmark

Hengrui Chang, Zhanle Zheng, Yiyang Yu, Jiasheng Shao and Yingze Zhang
Department of Orthopaedic Surgery, the Third Hospital of Hebei Medical University, NO.139 Ziqiang Road, Shijiazhuang, Hebei 050051, People's Republic of China
Key laboratory of biomechanics of Hebei Province, Shijiazhuang, Hebei 050051, People's Republic of China

Cheng-Tzu Wang, Chiang-Sang Chen, Wen-Chih Chen, Jwo-Luen Pao and Chih-Hung Chang
Department of Orthopaedic Surgery, Far Eastern Memorial Hospital, No. 21, Sec. 2, Nanya S. Rd., Banciao Dist, New Taipei City 220, Taiwan

Jia-Wan Chen
Department of Mechanical Engineering, Oriental Institute of Technology, New Taipei City, Taiwan

Karl Wu and Tsung-Yu Lan
Department of Orthopaedic Surgery, Far Eastern Memorial Hospital, No. 21, Sec. 2, Nanya S. Rd., Banciao Dist, New Taipei City 220, Taiwan
Department of Mechanical Engineering, Oriental Institute of Technology, New Taipei City, Taiwan

Joseph J. Knapik, Marilyn A. Sharp and Scott J. Montain
US Army Research Institute of Environmental Medicine, 10 General Greene Ave, Natick, MA 01760, USA

Ji-Qi Wang, Bing-Jie Jiang, Wei-Jun Guo and You-Ming Zhao
Department of Orthopaedics, The Second Affiliated Hospital and Yuying Children's Hospital of Wenzhou Medical University, 109# Xue Yuan Xi Road, Wenzhou, Zhejiang 325000, China

Jie Ai
Tianjin Medical University, 22 Qixiangtai Road, Heping District, Tianjin 300070, China
Department of Orthopaedics, Tianjin Medical University General Hospital, 154 Anshan Road, Heping District, Tianjin 300052, China
Department of Orthopaedics, Yuci People's Hospital, 262 Jingwei Road, Jinzhong, Shanxi Province 030600, China

Shun-Li Kan, Hai-Liang Li, Hong Xu, Yang Liu, Guang-Zhi Ning and Shi-Qing Feng
Department of Orthopaedics, Tianjin Medical University General Hospital, 154 Anshan Road, Heping District, Tianjin 300052, China

Index

www.ingramcontent.com/pod-product-compliance
Lightning Source LLC
LaVergne TN
LVHW080712210926
848485LV00003B/456